Statistics for the
Health Sciences

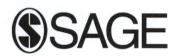

Statistics for the Health Sciences

A Non-Mathematical Introduction

Christine Dancey | John Reidy | Richard Rowe

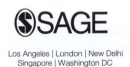

Los Angeles | London | New Delhi
Singapore | Washington DC

SAGE Publications Ltd
1 Oliver's Yard
55 City Road
London EC1Y 1SP

SAGE Publications Inc.
2455 Teller Road
Thousand Oaks, California 91320

SAGE Publications India Pvt Ltd
B 1/I 1 Mohan Cooperative Industrial Area
Mathura Road
New Delhi 110 044

SAGE Publications Asia-Pacific Pte Ltd
33 Pekin Street #02-01
Far East Square
Singapore 048763

Library of Congress Control Number: 2012930387

British Library Cataloguing in Publication data

A catalogue record for this book is available from the British Library

ISBN 978-1-84920-335-7
ISBN 978-1-84920-336-4 (pbk)

Typeset by Cenveo Publisher Services
Printed and bound in Great Britain by Ashford Colour Press Ltd
Printed on paper from sustainable resources

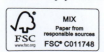

Christine would like to dedicate this book to Professor M. Rachel Mulvey, in celebration of all the shades of grey.
'Le cœur a ses raisons que la raison ne connaît point.'

(Blaise Pascal, 1623–1662)

John would like to dedicate this book to Lisa, Issy and Ollie … thank you for all your love and support … tomato!

Richard would like to dedicate this book to his wonderful family: Richard (senior), Catherine, Becky, Emily and Lucy.

Contents

About the Authors

Professor Christine Dancey has been working in the School of Psychology at UEL since 1990, teaching research methods and statistics and health psychology. Christine is a chartered health psychologist and chartered scientist, and she leads the Chronic Illness Research at UEL. She has conducted research into a wide range of physical illnesses including Mal de Débarquement Syndrome, Chronic Fatigue Syndrome/Myalgic Encephalopathy (CFS/ME), Inflammatory Bowel Disease and Irritable Bowel Syndrome, and has publications and books in this area. In the area of statistics, together with John Reidy, Christine has written *Statistics Without Maths for Psychology*, now in its fifth edition.

Dr John Reidy is a Principal Lecturer at Sheffield Hallam University and has worked at the University for over 12 years. John teaches research methods to students at all levels from first years to masters and PhD students. John is an active health researcher and has a particular interest in the anxiety experienced by people related to behaviours such as blood donation and attending dental appointments.

Richard Rowe is a Senior Lecturer at the University of Sheffield. Richard has taught research methods to students of psychology at all levels and also taught postgraduate courses for students across the Social Science Faculty. Richard's research interests focus on the development of antisocial behaviour.

Preface

In 1999 we (John and Christine) wrote *Statistics Without Maths for Psychology*, we wrote it for our psychology students, most of whom disliked mathematics, and could not understand why they had to learn mathematical formulae and hand-work calculations when their computer software performed the calculations for them. Many did not believe that working through calculations gave them a conceptual understanding of the statistical tests – and neither did we. We wanted students to have a conceptual understanding of statistics, and for them to feel confident in carrying out the analysis using computer software, and to be able to understand how to interpret the statistics.

Statistics Without Maths for Psychology (the fifth edition was published in 2011) was very successful, so much so that students from different subject areas, both undergraduate and postgraduate, in the UK and internationally, found the book really helpful in their studies. Among the reasons for the success of the book are the accessible style and the fact that the statistical concepts are explained clearly to students without the inclusion of statistical formulae. For psychologists, the British Psychological Association stipulates which quantitative methods in psychology should be covered in undergraduate programmes, and so the tests we covered reflected that. All the examples we used were taken from journals relating to psychology. This meant that for students of other disciplines the benefits of the book were limited, and yet there was a need for such a book specifically tailored for such students. John and Christine asked Richard to join them in writing such a book. Richard was already a fan of the approach taken in *Statistics Without Maths for Psychology*, and had been recommending it as core reading for his undergraduate research methods courses.

This book is an introductory textbook intended for undergraduate students of all health sciences and allied subjects. Unlike in psychology and the social sciences, students in the healthcare sciences have more of a need to understand reported statistics in scientific articles rather than in primary data analysis. The majority of students perceive themselves as weak at mathematics and it is with this in mind that *Statistics for the Health Sciences: A Non-mathematical Introduction* was written. With clear explanations of statistical concepts along with the absence of formulae, this book will be particularly well suited to students who study a wide range of subjects which relate to the health sciences and allied professions. In the UK alone there are in the region of 70,000 nursing students in training in addition to the students of allied disciplines such as physiotherapy. This book will help such students understand the rationale and concepts underlying the use of statistical analyses as well as explain how these analyses are applied in health science research. Although we are psychologists, all of us have taught basic, intermediate and advanced statistics to large groups of students in our respective universities. We have talked to staff and students in departments of health and allied professions, and we have a good understanding of the type of quantitative statistics that students in the health sciences need to know. All the examples within the text are taken from journals relating to subjects within health sciences. Some of the research we discuss is taken from our own work, much of which is related to health. Christine, for instance, leads the Chronic Illness Research Team at the University of East London. John has published research addressing general anxiety as well as anxiety related to donating blood and attending dental appointments. Richard has published many papers addressing child psychopathology.

We have tried to simplify complex concepts in this book, and in simplifying there is a trade-off with accuracy. We have tried to be as accurate as possible, while giving the simplest explanations. As an introductory text, this book cannot tell you everything you need to know. This means that in some places we refer you to other, more advanced books. Also, we know that not everyone uses SPSS. However, this is the most commonly employed statistical package in the health sciences, which is why the text is tied so closely to SPSS. Students not using this package should be able to understand our examples anyway. For those of you who use R or SAS, we refer you to our companion website.

We hope that you enjoy our explanations and the examples we give, and that this enables you to understand the statistical explanations given in the journals you read.

Christine P. Dancey
John G. Reidy
Richard Rowe

Acknowledgements

We would like to thank the following:

Michael Carmichael, Rachel Eley, Sophie Hine, and Alana Clogan of SAGE.

Also thanks go to Aparna Shankar of Cenveo Publisher Services.

To L.C. Mok and I.F.-K. Lee for allowing us to use their scattergrams, and D. Hanna, M. Davies and M. Dempster for allowing us to use their dataset.

And finally, to our reviewers: Professor Duncan Cramer and Dr Dennis Howitt at Loughborough University and Dr. Merryl Harvey of Department of Child Health at Birmingham City University. We greatly appreciate their sincere and honest criticisms which has led to important improvements to the final version of the book.

Companion Website

Be sure to visit the companion website (www.sagepub.co.uk/dancey) to find a range of teaching and learning material for both lecturers and students.

For lecturers:

- **Full PowerPoint Slides**: Slides are provided for each chapter and can be edited as required for use in lectures and seminars
- **Multiple Choice Questions**: Test students' knowledge with a downloadable MCQ Testbank organised by chapter

For students:

- **Multiple Choice Questions**: Check your understanding of each chapter or test yourself before exams
- **SPSS Exercises**: Additional SPSS exercises are available for each chapter for you to practice what you've learned. Bonus documents are also included, which illustrate sampling error and sample size, as well as guidance on generating random number sequences in SPSS
- **Guidance for Using R and SAS**: Extra guidance for conducting statistical analyses using R and SAS is provided, organised by chapter

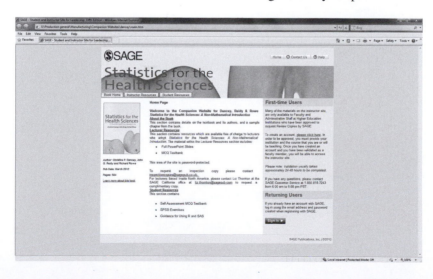

An Introduction to the Research Process

1

Overview

In this chapter we will introduce you to concepts that are important for understanding the research process, including:

- Research hypotheses
- Hypothesis testing
- Evidence-based practice
- Typical research designs

We do not assume any prior knowledge of statistics or of conducting research. All that you need to understand the concepts in this chapter is your brain.

Brains at the ready here we go …. Today there was a report on the radio suggesting that eating more blueberries will reduce the chances of getting cancer. This is not an uncommon type of report in the media these days. How do we know whether to believe all of the reports relating to health that the media present to us? Well, the best thing to do is to read the original research reports and make up our own minds about the adequacy of the research itself, as well as the validity of the conclusions that authors have drawn from their research.

This is how science works. Of course if you wish to work as a health professional there is an even greater need for you to be able to evaluate research evidence. This book will provide you with all of the tools necessary to be able to critically evaluate the research of other health professionals. Not only that, you will gain a working knowledge of how to conduct your own research and how to run some quite sophisticated statistical analyses on your data.

'But I don't want to be a researcher … I have no need to know about statistical analyses' we hear you say. This is a comment we often hear and in many ways it is a valid point. Many students who are training for careers in the health sciences will not be conducting their own research. However, they will need to have an understanding of how research is conducted and how to evaluate that work in order to make appropriate decisions about various forms of treatment. We would hope that the most appropriate form of treatment for any ailment would be chosen on the basis of research evidence. This in essence is what is meant by *evidence-based practice* and you will come across this term quite a bit in this book. An additional benefit of reading and working through this book is that you will then be able to evaluate the many claims about health that are thrown at us by the media, and you will be making people like Ben Goldacre[1] very happy indeed.

So why would you want to learn about statistics? Well, there are many reasons that we can think of:

1) It is a very interesting subject ☺
2) You will learn crucial skills underpinning evidence-based practice
3) You will be able to understand much of the jargon printed in published research
4) You will be able to evaluate the quality of published (and unpublished – where you find it) research
5) You will be able to design and conduct your own research
6) You will be able to draw valid conclusions from any research that you care to conduct
7) You will be able to impress your friends at parties

We think that statistics is a very interesting topic if only because it leads you to appreciate that many of the phenomena that we may observe in our lives are simply down to chance factors. This is the theme of an interesting book by Mlodinow (2008), and it is a book that is worth reading as it shows the pervasive influence of chance in all our lives. Because of this pervasive influence of chance we need to be able to somehow measure it, so that we can discount it as a reason for our research findings. For example, suppose that you attended Pilates classes and you noticed that not a single member of your group had a cold or flu during one particular winter. You might reasonably conclude that Pilates has some kind of protective effect against common viruses. How, though, do you know that all the people in your class that year were not simply lucky enough to avoid these common viruses for the whole winter? How do you know how common such an occurrence is in everyday life? For example, perhaps in the pub next door one of the regular drinkers had also noticed that none of her drinking companions had contracted a cold or flu that winter. We thus need to take account of all sorts of factors when drawing conclusions from our observations. This is exactly the same for research as it is for anecdotal evidence such as that described in the above examples. One of the key issues that you will discover from working through this book is the importance of taking account of chance findings and assessing the probability that observed research results occurred due to chance.

THE RESEARCH PROCESS

What is research? Well, let us start answering this question by posing another. Why do we want to conduct research? The reason we as researchers want to conduct research is because we wish to answer interesting (well interesting to us anyway) questions about the world. For example, *Is smoking related to cancer? Does eating blueberries protect us from developing cancer? Do simple cognitive strategies increase the likelihood of people eating blueberries? Do sugar pills (placebos) make people feel better?* These are all research questions and we as researchers would design and carry out research in order to find evidence to help us answer such questions.

Deriving Research Hypotheses

In Figure 1.1 you can see one possible conceptualisation of the research process. Usually a researcher has some experience of the research in a particular field, whether it be research into the effectiveness of an intervention for the common cold or the possible causes of in-growing toenails. It is likely that researchers will have taken the time to read the previously published research in a particular area. To do this they will have searched for papers published in peer-reviewed journals using a variety of databases such as *Pubmed* in order to identify the most relevant and important research in the area. Knowledge of previous research has a number of benefits for researchers planning to conduct their own research. First of all they can see how others have tackled similar research questions. This saves them having to re-invent the wheel every time they have an interesting question to answer. Second, when researchers publish their work they often flag up future avenues of research and this can then

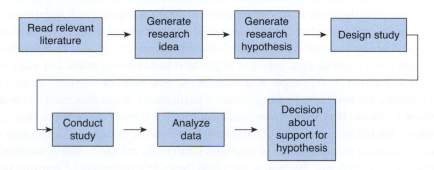

Figure 1.1 Schematic representation of the research process

guide the would-be researcher in their choice of research questions. Third, knowledge of previous research lets the researchers know whether or not they might be heading up a blind alley, or whether other researchers have already answered their research question, which may save them a lot of time and effort in running a study that is unlikely to demonstrate anything useful or interesting. It cannot be stressed enough that before conducting your own research you should make sure that you know what others have done before you. To paraphrase a great scientist (Isaac Newton): make sure you stand on the shoulders of giants, that way you can see a whole lot more before you set off on your research journey.

One of the biggest benefits of knowing the previous research in the area is that it allows you to ask the most important and relevant questions yourself. For example, suppose we want to try to encourage people to give up smoking. Knowledge of the factors that best predict quitting would be essential for us to design an effective health intervention. We might look at the effectiveness of patches, of psychological interventions such as hypnosis, or health promotion activities such as advertising on TV. We would want to look at the published evidence of the effectiveness of all these previously used interventions before designing our own intervention. In addition to this we would want to draw on any research expertise that we had in order for us to accurately measure the effectiveness of our own intervention. Only through a well-designed study could we tell whether our intervention has led to an increase in people quitting smoking.

Activity 1.1

Take a good look at Figure 1.1 and see if you can think of any problems with the way it suggests that research is conducted (the answer can be found at the end of the book).

The Research Question

Once you are familiar with a topic that interests you, and you have a thorough grounding in what has been researched before and what theories have been proposed to account for the findings of that published research, you are ready to start asking research questions.

Research questions can be framed in a number of ways. A useful way of categorising these is that some questions you ask will focus on differences between groups of individuals and other questions will focus on how concepts might be related to each other. For example, you might ask the question: Is treatment X useful for the treatment of tinnitus? In this sort of research question we would be looking to see if participants given treatment X have fewer symptoms of tinnitus. Alternatively, we could ask whether the degree of stress that a person experiences is related to the severity of symptoms of psoriasis. In this sort of question we are interested in whether the symptoms of psoriasis seem to be related to the amount of stress that a person is experiencing. We will come on to these different ways of framing research questions later in this chapter when we discuss typical research designs in more detail.

You need to understand that the way we frame our research question has a dramatic effect on our research design, and indeed the type of statistical analysis that we can conduct on the research data that we end up collecting. For example, if we were interested in the relationship between stress and symptoms of psoriasis we need to measure participants' stress (say in the form of a questionnaire) and also get an independent assessment of the severity of their symptoms of psoriasis. We can then run some statistical analyses to see how closely these two factors might be related to one another. Similarly, if we were interested in whether a new treatment for tinnitus was effective we would want to give the treatment to one group of participants and compare this group with another group who don't get the treatment. We would then run statistical analyses which can tell us if there are any differences in the severity of tinnitus across these two groups of participants. You will find in this book that we have different statistical techniques for these sorts of research situations.

Students often ask us what statistical test is best for a particular research topic, and our initial answer will invariably be to ask the student to think about their research question. But more specifically we would ask the students to think about something called a research hypothesis. We discuss this a little further in the following section.

The Research Hypothesis

Once you have suitable research questions you can then start to formulate testable hypotheses. There is a subtle difference here between research question and research hypothesis. A research question may be a little vague in nature, for example: Is there a link between personality and ability to quit smoking? A research hypothesis should really be much more precise. Thus we would need to identify which aspect of personality we think might be related to ability to quit smoking, e.g. whether there is a relationship between neuroticism and ability to quit smoking or whether participants who are high in extroversion and low in neuroticism will find it easier to quit smoking than those high in neuroticism and low in extroversion. It is extremely important to be as precise as possible with research hypotheses in quantitative research, as the sort of research hypothesis that you have will determine the research designs you use and the statistical techniques that will be appropriate to analyse your data. You should always remember that in order to analyse your data you have to test a hypothesis. We will cover hypothesis testing in more detail in Chapter 4, but when you precisely set out your hypotheses it helps you make decisions about how to design your research and to choose appropriate statistical techniques to test those hypotheses.

CONCEPTS AND VARIABLES

When we try to understand the world around us we often conceptualise the phenomena of interest. For example, we might have a *concept* of 'health' or perhaps 'illness' or 'treatment'. These are all concepts that a health scientist/practitioner might be interested in. Concepts can be thought of as the focus of our research. We might want to know how one concept relates to another concept, e.g. how a particular treatment relates to a particular illness. Concepts can be abstract, e.g. the concept of 'health', or they can be more concrete, e.g. 'heart-rate'. When we conduct research we have to *operationalise* these concepts into something that we can observe and measure. These measured concepts are called *variables*. Thus variables can be thought of as concepts that have been measured in some way. They are called variables simply because they vary, i.e. take on different values, from one person or situation or time to another. We might operationalise the concept of 'health' by asking people to give a rating for how healthy they feel on a scale of 1 to 7, or we might operationalise the concept of 'heart-rate' by using a heart-rate monitor. In the remainder of this book we will be focussing on variables, but it is important to appreciate this relationship between concepts and variables.

When we conduct research we are interested in variables. We are interested in variables because we want to try to find out how they might vary and why they might vary. Thus, we are not really interested in blood pressure for the sake of it, but rather we want to understand what causes blood pressure to be too high or too low and perhaps how we can prevent this from happening. In order to try to identify why variables vary as they do, we often need to look at other variables to see how they might vary in relation to our target variable. For example, we might look at salt intake to see how that is related to blood pressure. If we find that high salt intake tends to be associated with high blood pressure then we might suggest that lowering salt intake might lower blood pressure.

You should be able to see from the foregoing discussion that in science we are interested in variables and more specifically we are interested in the relationships between variables. More often than not we are trying to identify causal relationships between variables. We have to be very careful when thinking about which variable causes changes in another variable. For example, if we simply measured salt intake and found that it seems to be related to blood pressure we could not conclude that high salt intake causes high blood pressure. It might be that high blood pressure causes high salt intake. It might be, for example, that when we have high blood pressure we crave salty foods more and this leads to an increase in salt intake. We could look to see the direction of the causal link between these two variables by setting up an *experiment* (we take a closer look at experiments later in the chapter). We could deliberately alter the amount of salt that people have in their diets and see if this leads to a change in blood pressure. Alternatively, we could try to manipulate a person's blood pressure to see if it leads to an increase in salt intake. In this way we can establish the causal relationship between these two variables.

Sometimes it is not possible to look at variables by conducting experiments because we are not able to manipulate the variables that we are interested in. For example, we cannot manipulate a person's age, they are the age they are and we cannot change that. Also, it is often unethical to manipulate variables, for example we would not want to burn someone to see what effect this has on their

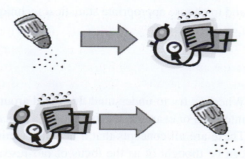

heart-rate. Often our ethical guidelines mean that we just would not want to manipulate the variable that we are interested in. For example, we would not want to manipulate a person's blood pressure because of the potential harm it might cause them. In such situations we would simply measure naturally occurring levels of such variables and see how they might be related to other variables of interest. In such studies we are simply observing and measuring variables and then establishing how they might be related to each other. These are often called *correlational* studies.

When you focus on variables, you will begin to see that not all variables have the same characteristics. For example, the sex of a person is a variable (that is, it varies from one person to the next). This is classed as a *categorical variable* as the values that it can take are simply categories, in this case the categories are *male* and *female*. Other examples of categorical variables are illness diagnosis, thus a person could have muscular dystrophy or not have muscular dystrophy. Or you might classify participants in your study as having generalised anxiety disorder, social phobia or panic disorder. In these cases the diagnosis is the variable. The category that people are placed in varies as function of the symptoms they may or may not have. Another type of variable might be the actual number of symptoms a person has. For example, if we look at the criteria for a diagnosis of chronic fatigue syndrome (CFS) there are quite a large number of symptoms[2] including:

- Severe fatigue
- Muscular pain, joint pain and severe headaches
- Poor short-term memory and concentration
- Difficulty organising your thoughts and finding the right words
- Painful lymph nodes (small glands of the immune system)
- Stomach pain and other problems similar to irritable bowel syndrome, such as bloating, constipation, diarrhoea and nausea
- Sore throat
- Sleeping problems, such as insomnia and disturbed sleep
- Sensitivity or intolerance to light, loud noise, alcohol and certain foods
- Psychological difficulties, such as depression, irritability and panic attacks
- Less common symptoms, such as dizziness, excess sweating, balance problems and difficulty controlling body temperature

People who have CFS will vary in the number of these symptoms that they have at any particular time, and thus the number of symptoms of CFS could be a variable of interest in our research. It is clear that this variable is different from the categorical variables described earlier as we are counting the number of symptoms rather than classifying things or people. We might suggest that such a variable is called *discrete* as we are counting whole numbers of symptoms here and thus the values that the variable can take are only in terms of discrete whole numbers of symptoms.

A final form of variable is a variable that we might call *continuous*. Such a variable can take on any value on the scale that we are measuring. A good example might be reaction times.

Let us suppose that we are wishing to test the effects of a new hay fever treatment. We are concerned that it might have the effect of slowing a person's responses. We would want to obtain a measure of patients' responses when they have taken the medication and also when they are medication free. In such a study we might ask the participants to press a response button as fast as they can when they see a certain target picture appear on the computer screen. We would then record how long it took the participants to respond in this task before and after taking the new medication. We would get the computer to measure the time between the target being presented and the instant that the participant responds. Usually in such tasks we measure reaction times in milliseconds. But response times might be measured even more precisely than this if we had suitable equipment. Response times in this study would be classed as a continuous variable.

It is important to note here that there is a difference between the underlying concept and the way we measure it. It might be that the underlying concept can be considered to vary on a continuous scale (e.g. time) but we choose to measure it on an interval scale (e.g. in days or seconds) or on a categorical scale (BC and AD). Just because we have measured a variable in a particular way does not mean that the concept varies on the same scale of measurement.

LEVELS OF MEASUREMENT

The sorts of statistical tests that we conduct on our research data depend very much on the sort of variables we are measuring. Usually, in order to determine which tests might be most appropriate we look at the *level of measurement* that we have.[3] Level of measurement relates to how we have measured the variables that we are interested in. For example, if we are interested in response times we might classify participants as being 'like lightning' if their response to a question was faster than one second or as being 'slow coaches' if their response was slower than one second. Alternatively, we could ask a judge in a study to give a rating on a five-point scale of how fast they thought participants had responded (where 1 indicates extremely slow and 5 indicates super quick). Alternatively, we could simply use a stopwatch to measure response times. The point that we are making here is that when we conduct research we will need to make decisions about how we measure the concepts that we are interested in (remember this is called operationalisation). These decisions that we make can have a big impact on the types of statistical tools that we are able to use to analyse our data and this is largely because we have different tools for different levels of measurement.

The lowest level of measurement is called a *nominal* scale. Such measurements are typically frequency counts of participants in a category. For example, if we were interested in sex differences in the diagnosis of autism we would count up the number of males and females with the diagnoses and compare them, perhaps using a test like chi-square (see Chapter 9). The crucial characteristic of nominal level data is not only are they classed as categories but there is also no order to the categories, you couldn't say that one category is higher or lower than another (such variables are thus categorical). Thus, we wouldn't be able

to say that being female is better or worse, higher or lower, than being male. We are simply counting how many cases there are in each category. Another good example of a nominal level variable is religion. Here we can't say that being a Christian or Muslim is higher or lower on the scale than say being a Jew or a Hindu. They are simply different categories.

The second level of measurement is the *ordinal scale*. Here we have some sort of order to the different categories on our scale. A good example is the rating scales that are often used to get participants' opinions about things. So we might be interested in how good patients rate their accident and emergency (A & E) department to be on a five-point scale where 1 equals *an absolute shambles* and 5 equals *absolutely fabulous*. Take a look at the rating scale below. How good do you think your A & E department is?

An absolute shambles	Not very good	Neither good or bad	Quite good	Absolutely fabulous
1	2	3	4	5

Using this scale we can see that someone rating the A & E department as a 5 considers this better than someone giving a rating of 3 or 4. Also someone giving a rating of 1 thinks the department is worse than someone giving a rating of 2 or 3. Thus there is some order of magnitude to the data from the lowest rating to highest. The important point to note about such a scale though is that we do not have equal intervals between adjacent points on the scale. Thus we couldn't necessarily say with confidence that the difference between a 1 and 2 on the scale is the same as the difference between 3 and 4 on the scale. That is, the difference between *An absolute shambles* and *Not very good* is not necessarily the same as that between *Neither good or bad* and *Quite good*. Thus, although there is an ordering of the categories on the scale we do not have equal intervals between the adjacent scores. This means that many of the statistical tests that are discussed in this book are not appropriate for such data. We would usually, when dealing with data from ordinal scales, use what we call *non-parametric* tests (see Chapter 4, for example), although as we suggested earlier there is still some debate concerning this.

The next level of measurements is those that involve *interval* scales. In these sorts of measurement scales the difference between adjacent points on the scale are equal. That is, there are equal intervals along the scale. Perhaps the best example of an interval scale is one of the scales that we use to measure temperature, e.g. the Fahrenheit scale. Measuring temperature on such a scale we know that the difference between 0° and 1° Fahrenheit is exactly the same as the difference between 11° and 12°, which is the same as that between 99° and 100°. Once we start using scales that are interval level we have much greater choice in terms of the statistical tools available to us for data analysis. Provided we meet certain assumptions we are able to use both parametric and non-parametric statistical tests (see Chapter 4). One of the problems with interval level scales like temperature is that they do not have a fixed zero. Realistically speaking we don't have an absolute point where we have zero temperature (e.g. zero Fahrenheit and Centigrade do not equate to zero temperature), the zero points on

the scales that we use to measure temperature today in many ways are arbitrary zero points (Centigrade reflecting the freezing point for water and Farhenheit being even more arbitrary). Why is not having a fixed zero important? The answer to this is that if we do not have a fixed zero then we cannot calculate ratios using the measurement scale. Thus we would not be able to say that 10° is twice as hot as 5°, or that 50° is half as warm as 100°. When you have a fixed zero on the scale you can calculate such ratios. An example of a scale that has a fixed zero is number of symptoms of an illness. When someone has a score of zero on this scale they have absolutely no symptoms. With such a scale we can say that someone who has eight symptoms has twice as many symptoms as someone who has four symptoms and four times as many symptoms as someone who has only two symptoms. Thus, when we have such scales they allow us to calculate such ratios. Not surprisingly such scales are called *ratio* level measurements.

We can view the different levels of measurement in order of level as follows:

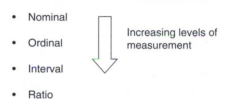

- Nominal
- Ordinal
- Interval
- Ratio

Increasing levels of measurement

Activity 1.2

Have a go at categorising the following variables in terms of their level of measurement:

- Types of jobs undertaken by staff in an intensive care ward
- Ratings for job satisfaction of A & E staff
- Number of visits to a family doctor after a hospital stay for heart transplant patients
- Length of time to regain consciousness after a general anaesthetic
- Number of fillings given to primary school children
- Temperatures of children after being given 5 ml of ibuprofen
- Ethnicity of patients

HYPOTHESIS TESTING

Once we have set out our research hypothesis we can then proceed to design research which tests this hypothesis. When we have a clear hypothesis this will have a big influence on how we design our study and which statistical tests we should use to analyse our data. Let us look at a general research question, say: Is high salt intake linked to high blood pressure? We might frame our hypothesis in two ways. We might say that people who have a high salt intake will have higher blood pressure than those who have a low salt intake. Here we are

interested in differences between groups of people – those who have high salt intake compared to those who have low salt intake. If we set the study up in this way we would use a statistical technique which tests for differences between groups of people (e.g. the t-test or the Mann–Whitney test, see Chapter 7). We might frame the research hypothesis in a slightly different way. We might simply state that we think there will be a relationship between salt intake and blood pressure such that increasing salt intake is associated with increases in blood pressure. In this sort of study we would use statistical techniques which measure relationships among variables (e.g. Pearson's Product-Moment Correlation coefficient, see Chapter 10). In these two examples we are designing studies and running statistical analyses to test hypotheses. The statistical analyses help us decide whether or not we have support for our hypotheses.

EVIDENCE-BASED PRACTICE

What is evidence-based practice? Well, we guess we have to go right back to ask the question: What is the purpose of scientific research? One answer to this question is that we use scientific research to understand our world better. If we understand our world then we can behave more appropriately in response to our new understanding. For example, if we found out that improving sanitation leads to much lower levels of infections then we would want to ensure that we had the highest levels of sanitation possible. If we find that using the MMR vaccine leads to increased incidence of autism we would want look for other ways of inoculating against measles, mumps and rubella. The changes that we make in response to research evidence constitute evidence-based practice (EBP). Thus, given that there appears to be no link between the MMR vaccine and autism we should look to using this route to inoculation rather than separate inoculations for these three diseases, as the latter is associated with much higher risks of infection and long-term harm to children. These are both examples of EBP. Essentially, the ethos of EBP is that we look at the available research evidence and we base our plans, behaviours and practice on such evidence.

There is one important requirement for engaging with EBP, and that is that you need to understand what constitutes evidence. Generally, evidence comes out of conducting scientific research and testing research hypotheses. Thus improving your knowledge of research will enhance your ability to engage with EBP.

RESEARCH DESIGNS

In this section we wish to introduce you to some of the main ways in which researchers design and conduct their research. We will cover experimental and correlational designs as well as single-case designs. In our research we might be interested in differences between conditions, e.g. the difference in blood pressure between a no-salt and low-salt group of high blood pressure patients. Alternatively, we might want to focus on relationships between variables, e.g. the relationship between anxiety/stress and waiting times in an A & E centre. Let us first look at differences between groups.

Looking for Differences

Quite often in health research we are interested in differences between the means of different groups. For example, we might be interested in the difference between a new treatment group and a standard treatment group in recovery from septicaemia. We might compare the length of time it takes participants to recover from the illness in these two groups. Another example of looking at differences would be to compare the same group of patients under two separate conditions. For example, we might want to see if we can improve brain injured patients' ability to navigate a hospital by training them using a virtual reality (VR) tool. In this sort of study we might assess navigation ability before and after training with the new VR tool. If we had undertaken the type of research in the first example above we would have used what we call a *between-groups* or *between-participants* design. If we had conducted that research in the second example then we would have used a *within-groups* or *within-participants* design.

Between-Groups Designs

The key feature of a between-groups design is that you have different participants in each condition that you are comparing. By 'condition' we mean the conditions under which people participate in the research. In a between-groups design these conditions will be different for each group of participants in the study. The beauty of this sort of study from the perspective of statistical analyses is that each group is usually independent, that is a person in one group cannot influence the results of a person in another group. The observations on the variables that we are interested in are completely independent from each other. Most of the statistical tests we use assume that the scores from participants are independent of each other. When we have two separate groups of participants like this it is sometimes called an *independent groups* design to emphasise the fact that the data from each group are independent of each other.

Randomised Control Trials

A classic example of a between-groups design is the *randomised control trial*. Let us look at the first example given above, the difference in septicaemia recovery times between a new treatment and a placebo treatment group. In such a study we would randomly allocate participants to each of these two groups. We would then give patients treatment (either the new treatment or the placebo treatment) and compare the groups in terms of recovery times. There are some important features of this sort of design that make it the gold standard for research in the health sciences (we discuss these in much more detail in Chapter 14). First of all we need to randomly allocate patients to the various conditions in such a design.

Using such a process, when we came across a patient who was willing to take part in the study we would use random number tables or toss a coin to decide whether they got the new or the standard treatment. Such research designs are often also called *experimental designs*. In an experimental design the researcher manipulates one variable called the *independent variable* to see if there is an effect on another variable called the *dependent variable*. In the example given earlier in this paragraph the treatment group is the variable being manipulated: we have decided to give one group of patients a new treatment and another group of patients a placebo treatment. We have manipulated what sort of treatment each group of participants receives and this is therefore the independent variable. Also in this example we want to see if there is a difference between the new treatment and placebo treatments in the recovery times from septicaemia. Recovery time is thus the dependent variable in this study. Students learning about experimental designs often have difficulty working out which variables in a study are the independent and dependent variables, and so it is worth making the effort now to understand these.

In an experimental design it is important that the participants are randomly allocated to the various conditions of the independent variable. The reason for such random allocation of participants is that it reduces the risk of there being systematic differences between your two treatment groups, which may end up compromising the conclusions that you can draw from your study. For example, suppose we allocated the first patients to volunteer for the study to the new treatment condition and then all other participants to the standard treatment condition. It could be that the first volunteers were the more-urgent cases and thus we would expect longer recovery times than for the less-urgent cases. If we used such a process of non-random method of participant allocation and we found a difference between our conditions in terms of recovery times we would not know if it was a result of the treatment or the severity of the illness. We would have introduced a *confounding variable* into the study.

Confounding variables are variables that are not central to your study but which may be responsible for the effect that you are interested in. Whenever you let confounding variables into your study designs then you have less ability to draw firm conclusions about the differences between your treatment conditions. Random allocation helps us guard against potential confounding variables, and if we do not randomly allocate participants to conditions we have to be acutely aware of the increased problem of potential confounds.

You might ask why wouldn't every researcher use random allocation of participants to conditions when it is such a good safeguard against such confounds. Well, it is quite often the case that we want to compare groups of people who cannot be randomly allocated to conditions. For example, we might want to find out whether there is a difference in the number of back injuries suffered by male and female nurses. Here we are interested in the difference between male and female nurses. We cannot randomly allocate participants to our target groups as they are already either male or female. We thus have to be aware that there are more potential confounds with this sort of study. When you investigate differences between intact groups such as males and females, or those diagnosed with a disease compared to those without a diagnoses you are said to be undertaking *quasi-experimental* research.

This is not quite an experimental design as you have not been able to randomly allocate your participants to the conditions that you are interested in.

Activity 1.3

Try to identify the independent and dependent variables in the following example studies:

1. Examining the difference between paracetamol and aspirin in the relief of pain experienced by migraine sufferers
2. Examining the effects of consultants providing full information about a surgical procedure to patients (rather than minimal information) prior to surgery on time to be discharged post surgery
3. Examining the difference between wards with matrons and those without on in-patient satisfaction
4. Examining the uptake of chlamydia screening from family doctor surgeries with and without chlamydia health promotion leaflets

---

Within-Groups Designs

Sometimes in research we might not be necessarily interested in comparing across different groups but rather in comparing one group of people across a number of different tasks or comparing the same group of people on a number of different occasions. For example, we might want to know whether patients with Alzheimer's disease have bigger decrements in memory when in new situations as compared with at home, or we might be interested in comparing the short-term memory capacity of Alzheimer's patients from one year to the next. Such designs are called *within-groups* or *within-participants* designs. One of the problems with between-groups designs is that you have different groups of people in each of your conditions. This means that by chance your groups might be different on some important variable that undermines your ability to draw causal inferences about how your variables are related to each other. Remember, we suggested that random allocation of participants to conditions is the best way of limited the impact of this sort of problem. Another way of limiting this is through the use of within-groups designs. In such designs you have the same group of people being measured on multiple occasions or under multiple conditions. This means that you don't get the differences across groups as a result of individual differences, as each participant is effectively compared against her- or himself, they act as their own control. Another positive feature of using within-groups designs is that because you only need one group of participants you need to recruit fewer of them to take part in your study. Imagine you had a study where you wanted to see if a new treatment for migraine was more effective than ibuprofen. You could recruit 40 migraine sufferers and randomly allocate them to either the new treatment or the ibuprofen group and then compare them to see which participants experienced the most pain relief. Alternatively, you could recruit one group of 20 participants, and the first time they had a migraine they would take one of the treatments and the second time they would take the other treatment, and on each occasion you would

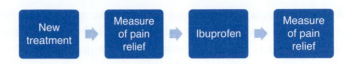

Figure 1.2   Order of events for the within-groups pain relief study

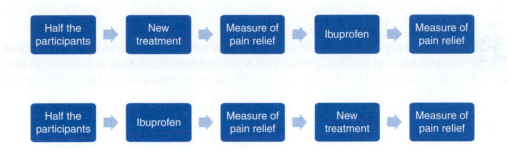

Figure 1.3   An illustration of the order of conditions in a counterbalanced study

record how much pain relief they experienced. You can see here that you only need half the number of people for the within-groups design as you would for the equivalent between-groups design.

One of the problems with this arrangement of conditions is that all the participants have received the treatments in the same order. Because of this we do not know whether there might be some bias in the way they report their experiences of pain relief. Or perhaps some participants drop out of the study and so do not complete the second stage of the study. If this is the case then the lost participants would all be from the ibuprofen condition and this would lead to a less-sensitive study. One way around such problems in within-groups design is to use *counterbalancing*. In a counterbalanced study half the participants would receive the treatments in the order indicated in Figure 1.2, and the other half of participants would receive the ibuprofen followed by the new treatment as in Figure 1.3.

In the counterbalanced study, if there is bias in the study it is spread equally across both the new treatment and the ibuprofen conditions. If participants drop out from the study it is quite likely that they will do so from both of the pain relief conditions.

Correlational Designs

Quite often in research we are not interested in looking at differences among groups but rather in how one variable might change as another variable changes. For example, it seems to be the case that as we increase the wealth in a society the weight of the citizens becomes greater. Thus, in most western societies we are currently experiencing a dramatic increase in rates of people who are overweight. Another example could be that as the number of cigarettes smoked by a person increases their life expectancy decreases. What we are dealing with here are *relationships* among variables. We want to know how one variable varies in relation to another variable. In such research designs we simply take measures of the variables that we are interested in and then look to see how they vary in relation to each other. Such designs are called *correlational designs*. We can use statistical techniques such as Pearson's Product-Moment Correlation coefficient or Spearman's rho to give us a measure of how strongly any two variables are related to (or correlated with) each other. We cover these sorts of designs and analyses in Chapter 10. A useful way of representing the relationship between two variables is to plot a scattergram (see Chapter 10 for more on these) we have presented two examples of these in Figure 1.4 (these graphs were generated using hypothetical data).

In Figure 1.4(a) you should be able to see that as annual income increases (as you move to the right along the *x*-axis) there is a trend for the percentage of people classified as overweight to increase too. The dots on the graphs cluster around an imaginary line running

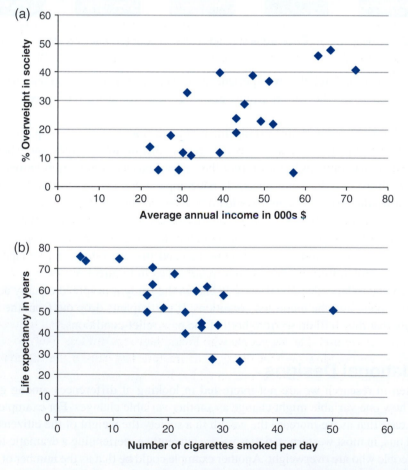

Figure 1.4 Scattergrams showing: (a) the relationship between annual income and percentage of people overweight, and (b) between number of cigarettes smoked per day and life expectancy

from the bottom left-hand corner to the top right-hand corner of the graph. We call such a pattern of findings a positive relationship. In a positive relationship between two variables as one variable increases so does the other. In Figure 1.4(b) however, you should be able to see that as the number of cigarettes smoked per day increases, life expectancy seems to decrease. The dots on the graph seem to cluster around an imaginary line that runs from the top left-hand corner to the bottom right-hand corner of the graph. We call such a pattern of results a negative relationship between the variables. In such relationships as one variable increases the other decreases.

Activity 1.4

See if you can describe a study which uses an experimental design looking at the link between childhood exercise levels and symptoms of Attention Deficit Hyperactivity Disorder (ADHD) (if you are unsure of this please have another look at the section on 'Randomised Control Trials' above). When you have done that see if you can design a study which uses a quasi-experimental design (please bear in mind what the difference is between experimental and quasi-experimental designs). Finally, do the same again but use a correlational design (remember when we are doing correlational research we simply measure the variables of interest and then see how they are related to each other).

Causation

Quite often in research we want to know what causes a variable of interest to change. For example, we might want to find out what has caused an increase in asthma over the past decade or whether an increase in the dosage of a drug causes a decrease in the symptoms of a particular disease. If we are interested in such causal relationships we often run experimental studies. In an experimental study we manipulate one variable called the *independent variable* (IV) and see what effect this manipulation has on another variable called the *dependent variable* (DV). In such a study we can see what causal effect a change in the IV has on the DV. Thus we might manipulate the dosage of a drug to see what effect it has on the symptoms of a disease. When we deviate from such experimental designs we are less able to draw causal conclusions. For example, suppose we were interested in the difference between people who fracture their arms and those who fracture their legs in the uptake of physiotherapy. If we find that the people who break their legs are less likely to turn up for physiotherapy we couldn't say that the type of fracture has caused the difference in the uptake of physiotherapy. It could be for example, that certain types of people (e.g. males) are more likely to have leg fractures and it is their sex that is responsible for them not taking up physiotherapy opportunities. When we have quasi-experimental designs like this, more possibilities for confounding variables creep in.

If we look at correlational designs it is also very difficult to determine the causal direction of the relationship between variables. Suppose we find that there is a positive correlation between alcohol consumption and blood pressure, which of these variables has caused a change in the other? It could be that consuming higher levels of alcohol causes an increase in blood pressure, or it is perhaps equally plausible that those with high blood pressure self-medicate by drinking more. The causal direction of the relationship between these two variables is unclear. We return to this issue again in Chapters 5 and 10.

Summary

We have now introduced you to many of the basic concepts of research design. Armed with knowledge of these concepts, the statistical techniques that we cover in the rest of the book should make a little more sense. In addition, the research that you read about in journals may make more sense. Furthermore, you will be able to scrutinise the claims people make about the causal relationships among the variables that they have investigated.

MULTIPLE CHOICE QUESTIONS

1. What is the difference between a research question and a research hypothesis?
   a) Usually research questions are more precise than hypotheses
   b) Usually research questions are more vague than research hypotheses
   c) Usually research questions are exactly the same as research hypotheses
   d) None of the above

2. What are the benefits of knowing about the previous research in a particular field of interest?
   a) We can see how others have tackled similar research problems
   b) We can see what other researchers have suggested needs following up in future research
   c) It saves us undertaking research that may be pointless
   d) All of the above

3. According to the description of the research process in this chapter how do we decide whether there is support for a particular research hypothesis?
   a) We rely on previous research to test a new research hypothesis
   b) We need to interview other researchers to see if they agree with our hypothesis
   c) We design a study and then collect and analyse our data in such a way as to test our hypothesis
   d) We see if the research hypothesis makes logical sense

4. Which of the following constitute the main focus of interest for us when conducting quantitative research?
   a) Participants' demographic details
   b) The questionnaires that we use
   c) Publishing our research
   d) Variables

5. Which of the following could be considered as a ratio level variable?
   a) Occupation of participants
   b) Time taken to complete a programme of physiotherapy
   c) Ratings on a five-point scale for satisfaction with out-patient services
   d) None of the above

6. Why is it that temperature scales cannot be classed as ratio level variables?
   a) They are too complicated
   b) They contain arbitrary intervals between adjacent values on the scales
   c) There are too many scales for consistent measurements
   d) They do not have a fixed/absolute zero

7. In the scheme outlined in this chapter which of the following represents the correct ordering of the levels of measurements?
   a) Nominal, ordinal, interval, ratio
   b) Ordinal, ratio, interval, nominal
   c) Ratio, ordinal, interval, nominal
   d) Interval, nominal, ordinal, ratio

8. What is the defining characteristic of interval level data?
   a) You can put the categories you have in order of magnitude
   b) You have a fixed zero
   c) You have categories which cannot be ordered in a meaningful way
   d) You have equal intervals between adjacent points on the scale

9. Correlational designs tell us about:
   a) Differences between conditions
   b) The causal relationships between variables
   c) The relationships between variables
   d) None of the above

10. What is a quasi-experiment?
   a) A study where you simply measure the relationship between two variables
   b) A study where you are interested in the difference between intact groups
   c) A study where you randomly allocate participants to your experimental conditions
   d) A study looking at the reflexes of the hunchback of Notre Dame

11. In an RCT study how should you allocate your participants to experimental conditions?
   a) Randomly
   b) By matching participants in each condition on the bases of demographic variables such as age
   c) Put all those to volunteer first in one condition and then the remainder in the other condition
   d) All of the above are appropriate ways of allocating participants to conditions

12. Why are confounding variables such a problem in research?
   a) They are difficult for participants to give responses to
   b) They make questionnaires too long for participants to complete
   c) They lead to high attrition rates for studies
   d) They make it difficult to draw conclusions about the relationships between the main variables in the study

13. In which of the following designs are you least likely to have a problem with confounding variables?
    a) Experimental designs
    b) Quasi-experimental designs
    c) Correlational designs
    d) Both a) and c) above

14. Which of the following designs are best for establishing causal links between variables?
    a) Experimental designs
    b) Quasi-experimental designs
    c) Correlational designs
    d) Both a) and c) above

15. Take a look at the following scattergram. What can you conclude about the relationship between the two variables?

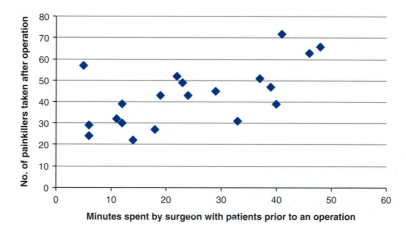

a) That there is a negative relationship between minutes spent with patients and painkillers taken
b) That there is no relationship between the two variables
c) That there is a positive relationship between minutes spent with patients and painkillers taken
d) No conclusions can be drawn from this scattergram

Notes

1 Ben Goldacre writes a column for *The Guardian* called 'Bad Science' in which he critically appraises many of the claims made about health in the media … it really is a good read, as is his book of the same name.
2 Taken from the NHS Chronic Fatigue web pages (http://www.nhs.uk/Conditions/Chronic-fatigue-syndrome/Pages/Symptoms.aspx).
3 There is though some debate about the importance of levels of measurement in the choice of statistical tests. However, we feel that it is instructive to discuss these here as they provide a useful framework for understanding the different types of variables that we deal with in health science research.

Computer–Assisted Analysis

2

Overview

In this chapter we will introduce you to three widely used statistical software packages, namely SPSS, R and SAS®. For each of these packages we will:

- Provide an overview of the interfaces
- Describe how data is set up
- Provide examples of how data might be analysed
- Provide links for the companion website where appropriate

Of the many statistical packages on the market why have we chosen these three? We have chosen SPSS as it is one of the most widely used statistical packages and it uses a Windows-based menu system. This makes it relatively easy for a newcomer to statistics to run analyses with some simple point and click instructions. We have included instructions for SAS on the companion website as this is a very popular statistical package in the health sciences. However, it is a little more complicated as analyses are set up and run using mini-programs. This may sound daunting at this stage but is fairly straightforward. We also felt that it would be useful to include some instructions relating to R as this is a relatively new system which is free to all users, provides excellent graphical outputs and is growing in popularity. This package is

(Continued)

(Continued)

command-line driven, which means you have to learn the commands to run each particular analysis.

In this chapter we will provide introductions to each of these software packages and then in the rest of the book we will provide guidance on running the analyses with SPSS only. We provide the extra instructions relating to SAS and R on the companion website.

OVERVIEW OF THE THREE STATISTICAL PACKAGES

SPSS, SAS and R are very different in the way they expect you to interact with them. SPSS likes you to show it what to do by pointing and clicking at menus and dialogue boxes. SAS likes you to give it lists of things to do in the form of a program, whereas R prefers more direct commands or orders as you go along. However, what you always need to remember with any of these software packages is that you are in charge … you are telling them what to do and they won't do anything that you don't tell them to do. But as with most computer programs you generally have to tell them exactly what to do (you can't be vague about it … stats packages don't like us to be vague … they like to know exactly what we want from them). What this means is that we have to be clear what we want and be sure to tell the software this.

We like to think of SPSS as being like a robot that you have to control using a remote control handset, whereas SAS is a bit like those people at IKEA who generate the instructions for building flat pack furniture (and initially SAS can seem that complicated), and R is much more like your mother-in-law barking individual orders at you (Figure 2.1). With practice these software packages become quite simple to use and, as with any skill, the more you practise the easier it becomes. This is why we provide you with plenty of practice exercises in each chapter.

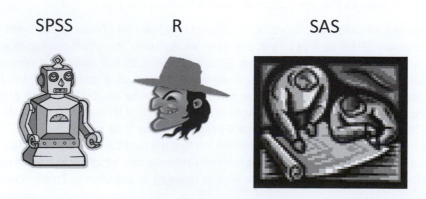

SPSS   R   SAS

Figure 2.1   A comparison of the three statistical packages

To illustrate again the differences between the packages, below we outline how to run a simple analysis on some data. Don't worry about trying to understand what we are asking the software to do at this stage, simply focus on the differences in the way that we tell the software what to do.

If we wanted to generate scattergrams which graphically illustrate the relationship between two variables (see Chapters 1 and 10) in SPSS we would select the *Graphs*, then *Legacy Dialogs* followed by *Scatter/Dot* menu items and this would bring up a dialogue box (Screenshot 2.1).

We would then click on the *Simple Scatter* option and obtain another dialogue box (Screenshot 2.2).

We would move the two variables across to the relevant boxes, click on *OK* and this would then give us the scattergram (Screenshot 2.3).

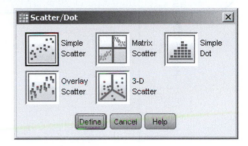

Screenshot 2.1

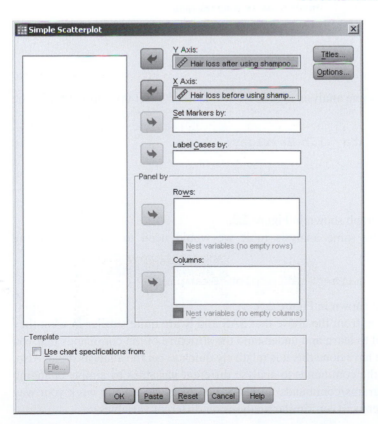

Screenshot 2.2

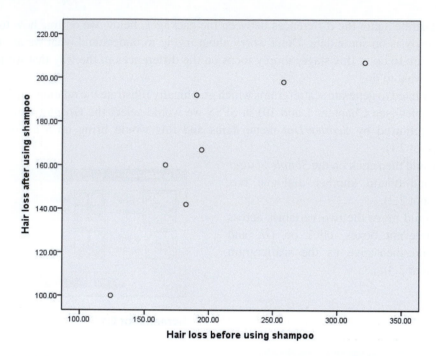

Screenshot 2.3

If we wanted to run the same analysis in SAS we would need to set up a program like the one below:

```
data working; set Data _ lib.Hairloss;
Proc gplot;
plot After*Before;
run;
```

This would give us the graph shown in Figure 2.2.

In terms of running the same analysis in R we would need to use the following commands:

```
plot(Before, After, main="Scatterplot Example")
```

This will give the output shown in Figure 2.3.

You should be able to see from the above that SAS and R are quite similar in what they expect from you. You need to learn and understand the structure of the commands that you are typing in, but once you have done this it is relatively quick to get the analysis done. Also, it is quite easy to modify the commands to analyse different variables by simply changing variable names in the programs/commands. In SPSS, however, you have to work your way by clicking through the menus to run similar analyses on different variables.[1]

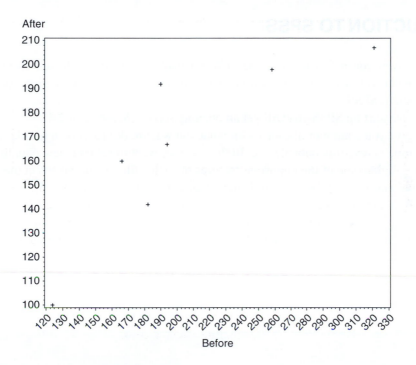

Figure 2.2   Scatterplot generated by SAS

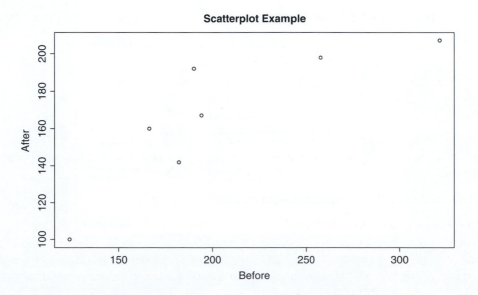

Figure 2.3   Scatterplot generated by R

INTRODUCTION TO SPSS

We have given you a feel for how the different packages want you to tell them what to do (remember you are doing the telling here). In this section we will give you a basic introduction to SPSS.

When you start up SPSS you will get an opening screen (Screenshot 2.4).

It will give you a number of choices for what you want to do: running a tutorial; entering data; opening an existing data file, etc. In this case we want to set up a new data file so that we can highlight some of the important features of such a file to you. So select the 'Type in data option' and you will be presented with a blank data file (Screenshot 2.5).

You will notice that the data file consists of a large number of blank 'cells'. These blank cells will contain the data when we have typed it in. At the bottom left-hand corner of the screen you will notice two 'tabs' labelled *Data View* and *Variable View*. As a default SPSS shows us the *Data View*. In this view you are presented with the actual data that you type in.

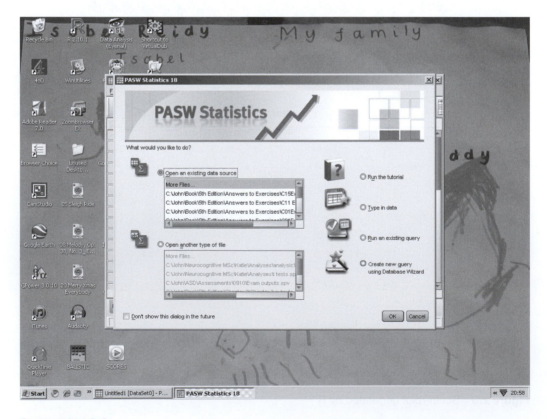

Screenshot 2.4

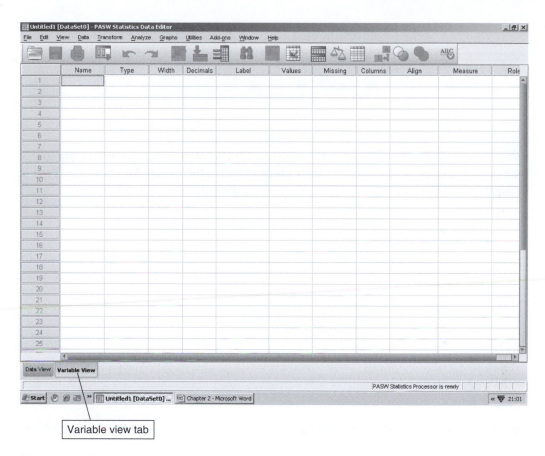

Variable view tab

Screenshot 2.5

In the *Variable View* part of the screen you will be presented with the variables that you have set up along with details of the characteristics of the variables.

The first thing that we need to do to set up a new data file is tell SPSS about the variables that we are going to enter. To do this we need to click on the variable view tab and then you will be presented with the view shown in Screenshot 2.6.

You will notice here that we again have a number of cells. The information that we insert in the columns represents the characteristics of variables. You should note that each row on this sheet refers to one variable and the columns represent characteristics of variables. For example, the first column contains the name of the variable, the second column tells us what sort of variable it is (e.g. Does it contain labels of some kind or is it numerical data?) and the fifth column contains the proper name for the variable (we will describe these characteristics of variables in more detail soon). OK, then let us set up our first variable in the data file. To do this click on the first cell in the *Name* column and type in 'Age'[2] and then press the return key on the keyboard. You should note that when you type in a variable name there are

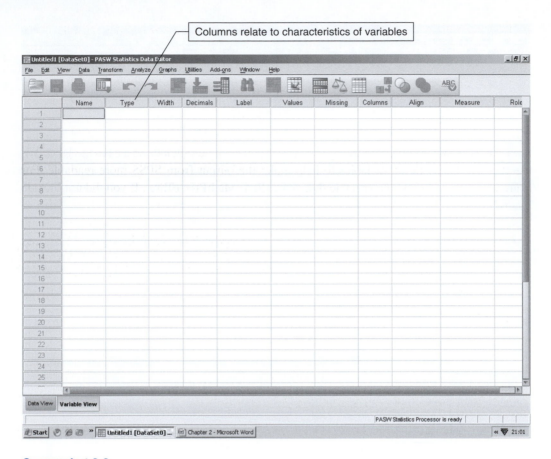

Screenshot 2.6

certain restrictions on the names that you can type in. First of all, variable names should be no longer than 64 characters. Second, they should start with a letter and not a number. Also, you are not allowed to have spaces or punctuation marks in a variable name. Table 2.1 shows examples of valid and invalid variable names. It is a good idea to use short variable names as this makes it easier to see the variables when undertaking analyses using the various dialogue boxes.

Table 2.1

Valid variable names	Invalid variable names
Age_in_years	Age in years
Second_follow_up_measure	2nd_follow_up_measure
Percentage_Of_Correct_Answers	% of correct answers

Once you have entered the variable name you will notice that not only does SPSS fill in the name of the variable it also inserts by default values in many of the other columns (Screenshot 2.7). For example, it sets the data type as *Numeric* (see column 2), the width of the variable as 8 characters (column 3) and the number of decimal places that are displayed to 2 (see column 3). You will notice that for column 5 *Label* SPSS does not insert a value. The purpose of this column is for you to insert a meaningful name for the variable (e.g. 'Age in years'). In this column you are allowed to write the label using normal writing conventions and you can start these with any characters you want and include spaces in the label. We use this characteristic of variables to help make the output from SPSS more readable. For example, suppose you had a variable that you called 'MtchPrimeTarg'. If you did not include a label for the variable your output would contain the variable name (MtchPrimeTarg) to identify output related to this variable. If you save this output and come back to it sometime later you might have trouble remembering what this variable referred to. However, if you used the *Label* characteristic you could type in a more meaningful label for SPSS to include in the output, for example 'Trials with matching primes and targets'. For all the points in the output that include information relating to this variable you would now have a nice clear label which would be much more meaningful for you when you returned to the output at a later time.

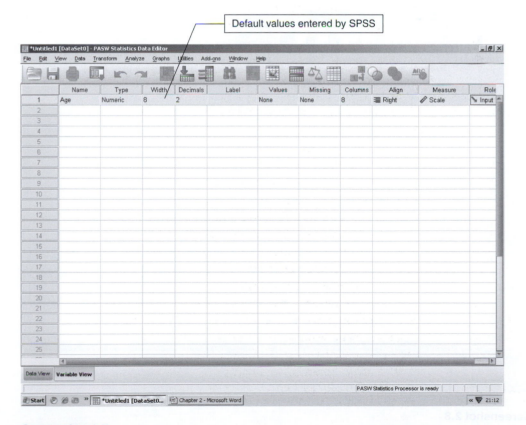

Screenshot 2.7

First rule of data management

Always use the *Label* characteristic to make it clear what each variable refers to.

Let us now enter another variable, this time we want to record the sex of the participants. And so in the row cell in the name column type in 'Sex'. Remember to put in a suitable label too to clarify what this variable is referring to (Screenshot 2.8).

We would now like to draw your attention to the column headed *Measure*. This column indicates what sort of variable we are dealing with. You can see that by default SPSS sets up all variables as *Scale* variables. If you click on the cell in this column for the *Sex* variable you will be presented with a drop-down list containing the *Measure* types (*Scale*, *Ordinal* or *Nominal*) (Screenshot 2.9).

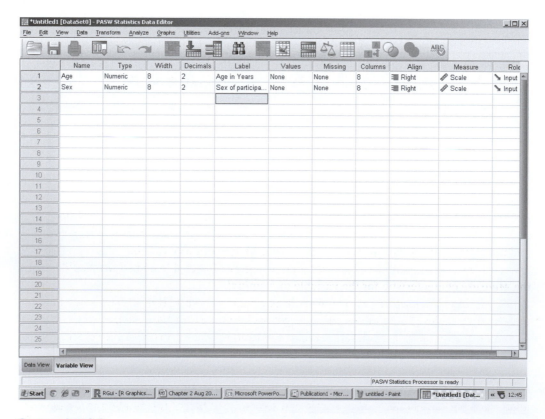

Screenshot 2.8

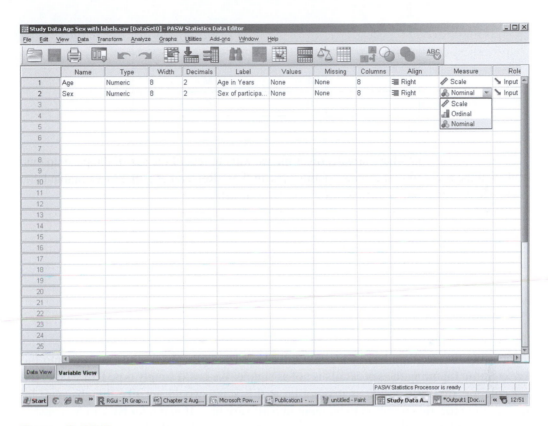

Screenshot 2.9

You should recall that we covered the different levels of measurement in Chapter 1 (see page 8), when we identified four levels of measurement, *Nominal*, *Ordinal*, *Interval* and *Ratio*. You will notice that SPSS only identifies three levels, that is, *Nominal*, *Ordinal* and *Scale*. SPSS treats interval and ratio level data the same in terms of levels of measurement and uses this as the default sort of variable. Returning to our *Sex* variable, it is clear that this is not a scale variable. In fact, it is a nominal (categorical) variable and so we should change the *Measure* characteristic for the variable to *Nominal*.

OK, we have now set up two variables in our data file. We will now enter some data for these two variables. To do this we need to get back to the *Data View* section of the file and so you need to click on the relevant tab in the bottom left-hand corner of the screen. We are going to enter the data in Table 2.2 into the data sheet.

The important point to remember about the *Data View* screen is that columns refer to variables and rows refer to each individual person or case. We have two bits of information about each participant in the above table and so enter two bits of information in the relevant variable columns.

Table 2.2 Example data to be entered into data file

Participant	Age	Sex
1	24	M
2	18	F
3	19	M
4	32	F
5	19	F
6	25	F
7	22	M

Inputting the age data is very straightforward. We simply type in the numbers into the *Age* column. Inputting the sex details is not as simple. We could simply type F or M into the *Sex* column. However, SPSS, as it is set up at this stage, would not like this, because by default it is expecting numbers to be input into all variables. If you refer back to Screenshot 2.9 you should notice that both variable types are *Numeric*. To be able to type letters into a variable you would have to change the variable type to *String*. You would do this by clicking on the variable type cell in the *Data View* screen and selecting the *String* option. We don't want you to do this, however, as this will limit the sorts of analyses that we can conduct on this sort of variable. To overcome this difficulty we need to convert the sex of a person (male or female) into a numeric code for example we can code males as a 0 and females as a 1, or females as 1 and males as 2. It doesn't matter which way around you code these (males as 0 or males as 1) as this is an arbitrary decision on your part. In the following example we have coded males as 0 and females as 1. So you should do the same for now. When you have typed in the data it should look something like Screenshot 2.10.

Now that we have input some data the first thing that we need to do is save the data. To do this you should select the *File, Save* options from the menus or simply click on the floppy disk icon in the menu bar. When you do this you will be presented with the typical save dialogue box (Screenshot 2.11).

Type in a suitable/memorable file name and then click on the *Save* button to save your data. When you are entering a lot of data (as is quite usual) then you should remember to save your data at regular intervals. There is nothing more frustrating than spending hours typing in data only for your computer to freeze before you have had the chance to save your data.

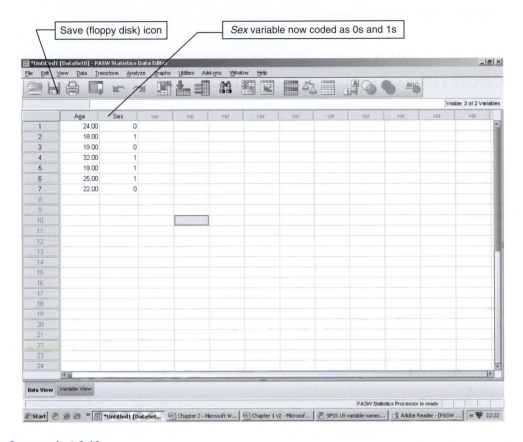

Screenshot 2.10

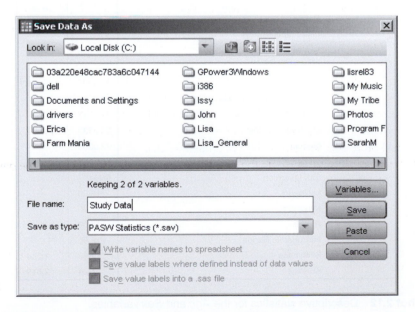

Screenshot 2.11

Second rule of data management

Save your data at regular intervals during input.

Once you have entered your data you will quickly want to get on to the exciting stuff ... running some analyses. We have included some example outputs in Screenshot 2.12 to illustrate what such analyses might look like.

For now we want you to ignore all the statistical detail in this screenshot. We aim to help you make more sense of such output later on in the book. What we want you to notice is that the table is broken down by the *Sex* variable. The problem with this table is that SPSS

Descriptives

Sex				Statistic	Std. Error
Age	0	Mean		21.6667	1.45297
		95% Confidence Interval for Mean	Lower Bound	15.4151	
			Upper Bound	27.9183	
		5% Trimmed Mean		.	
		Median		22.0000	
		Variance		6.333	
		Std. Deviation		2.51661	
		Minimum		19.00	
		Maximum		24.00	
		Range		5.00	
		Interquartile Range		.	
		Skewness		−.586	1.225
		Kurtosis		.	.
	1	Mean		23.5000	3.22749
		95% Confidence Interval for Mean	Lower Bound	13.2287	
			Upper Bound	33.7713	
		5% Trimmed Mean		23.3333	
		Median		22.0000	
		Variance		41.667	
		Std. Deviation		6.45497	
		Minimum		18.00	
		Maximum		32.00	
		Range		14.00	
		Interquartile Range		12.00	
		Skewness		.892	1.014
		Kurtosis		−.924	2.619

Screenshot 2.12   Descriptive statistics for the *Age* and *Sex* variables.

expects you to remember how you coded up your males and females. Did you code males as 0 or did you code females as 0? It might be easy to remember this now, but imagine that you have entered your data and you don't come back to analyse it again for a couple of months (this often happens in real research). What we need is some way of recording how we have coded our nominal variables. Fortunately, SPSS has such a feature and you can find this in the *Variable View* screen (Screenshot 2.13).

The characteristic of variables that will help us out in this situation is the *Values* feature. If you click on the cell in this column for the *Sex* variable you will be presented with the cell activated with a little button which contains an ellipsis (three full stops in a row (…) (Screenshot 2.14). What the ellipses means is that if you click on the button you get further options to play with.

Once you click on the button your will be presented with a dialogue box (Screenshot 2.15).

What this dialogue box allows you to do is to attach a label for each of the coding categories that you have typed into the nominal variable. To do this you should type the first coding category number that you have (in our case 0) into the *Value* box and then type

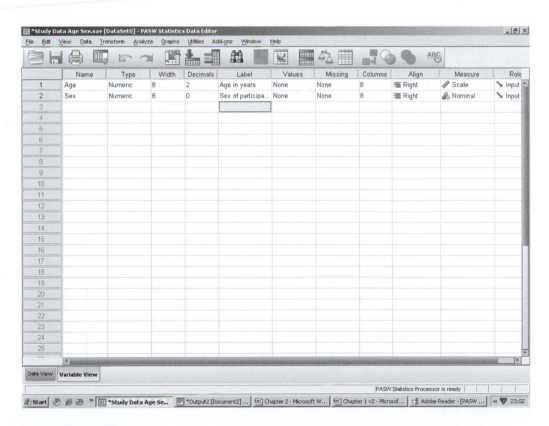

Screenshot 2.13

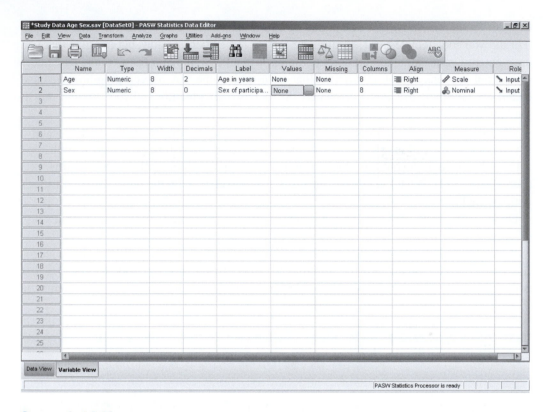

Screenshot 2.14

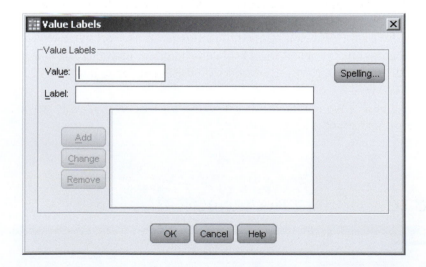

Screenshot 2.15

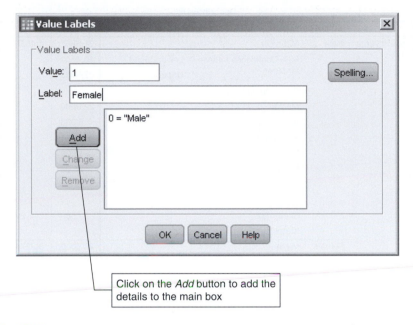

Screenshot 2.16

a label describing what this category refers to (Male) in the *Label* box. You then click on the *Add* button and this will add these details to the large box. You then do the same for the 1 category number and type in the category (Female) before clicking on the *Add* button again (Screenshot 2.16).

Once you have done this, click on the *OK* button and then SPSS will know what labels to printout when this *Sex* variable is included in any analysis. Take a look now at the output in Screenshot 2.17. This is the same analysis as we presented before but this time we have the value labels set up.

You should be able to see from this that it is now much easier to identify which part of the output refers to males and which to females.

Third rule of data management

Always use the *Labels* characteristic to identify how categorical groups have been coded in your data file.

Descriptives

Sex of participants				Statistic	Std. Error
Age in years	Male	Mean		21.6667	1.45297
		95% Confidence Interval for Mean	Lower Bound	15.4151	
			Upper Bound	27.9183	
		5% Trimmed Mean		.	
		Median		22.0000	
		Variance		6.333	
		Std. Deviation		2.51661	
		Minimum		19.00	
		Maximum		24.00	
		Range		5.00	
		Interquartile Range		.	
		Skewness		−.586	1.225
		Kurtosis		.	.
	Female	Mean		23.5000	3.22749
		95% Confidence Interval for Mean	Lower Bound	13.2287	
			Upper Bound	33.7713	
		5% Trimmed Mean		23.3333	
		Median		22.0000	
		Variance		41.667	
		Std. Deviation		6.45497	
		Minimum		18.00	
		Maximum		32.00	
		Range		14.00	
		Interquartile Range		12.00	
		Skewness		.892	1.014
		Kurtosis		−.924	2.619

Screenshot 2.17

Right, we have covered quite a lot of the basics about entering data into SPSS but what we would like to illustrate now is different ways that you would set up your data file when you have a within-groups compared to a between-groups design.

SETTING OUT YOUR VARIABLES FOR WITHIN- AND BETWEEN-GROUP DESIGNS

In the example above, we have already shown you how to input data for a grouping variable. We can call the *Sex* variable a grouping variable as it identifies which category (or group) each person was from. We arbitrarily assigned females as group 1 and males as group 0. Thus, when you have a categorical variable such as *Sex* you can identify which group each person is in, in the same way as we did in the previous example (see Screenshot 2.18).

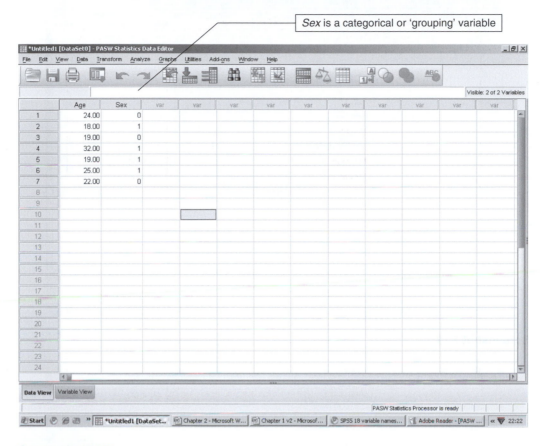

Screenshot 2.18

If you had a grouping variable that had more than one category such as occupation the principle is the same as that used above for *Sex*. For example, let us suppose that we have recorded occupation, we might have a number of different categories here including, lecturers, nurses, consultants and dentists. In such a case we would arbitrarily assign each occupation to a group and then record this information in a variable as above for *Sex*. Let us give the following codes to the occupations (Screenshot 2.19):

- Lecturers = 1
- Nurses = 2
- Consultants = 3
- Dentists = 4

Here we have set up the *Value Labels* to reflect our coding of the occupations. We can then go into the *Data* screen to enter our data. Don't forget to change the *Measure* characteristic for the variable to *Nominal*. Take a look at Screenshot 2.20 for some example data.

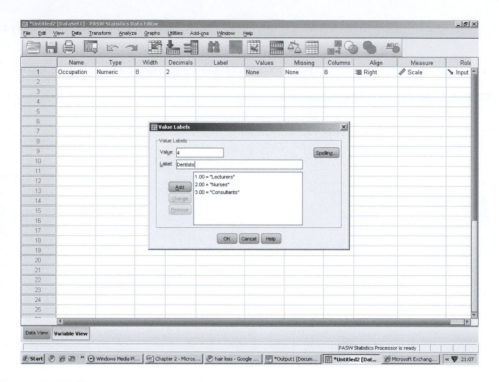

Screenshot 2.19

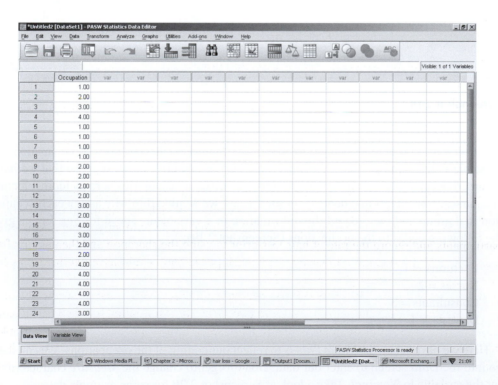

Screenshot 2.20

And Screenshot 2.21 shows the same data when we toggle on the *Value Labels* icon.

Screenshot 2.21

Sometimes though, we have several measures from the same person; that is, we have a within-groups design. Suppose we conducted a study in which we examined the effectiveness of a new shampoo for reducing male baldness. We might randomly select a number of participants and record the rate of hair loss prior to using the shampoo and then again after regular use of the shampoo. In such a study each participant would have two measures for rate of hair loss. For example see Table 2.3.

When setting up this data in SPSS you need to simply remember that each row contains all the details for each participant. We have two pieces of information for each participant, hair loss before and after treatment with the shampoo and so we need to set up two variables in SPSS. You need to go to the *Variables View* window and type in the name of each of the variables. Remember to use the *Labels* feature to give the variable a meaningful name. See Screenshot 2.22.

Table 2.3   Example data for a within-groups design

	No. of hairs lost per day	
Participant	Before using shampoo	After using shampoo
1	166	160
2	182	142
3	194	167
4	321	207
5	190	192
6	258	198
7	124	100

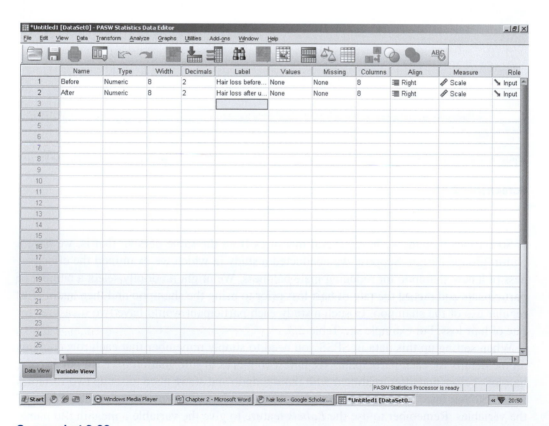

Screenshot 2.22

Once you have set up your variables you can then go back to the *Data View* screen and enter your data as in Screenshot 2.23.

Screenshot 2.23

We have now illustrated how to set up variables and input data for both within- and between-group variables. The principles are the same for most types of grouping and repeated-measures variables that you will come across. and so it is worthwhile spending a little bit of time here ensuring that you understand the difference between them, and how to set them up in SPSS.

To generate the graph that we presented you with earlier in the chapter you should click on the *Graph*, *Legacy Dialogs*, *Scatter/Dot* menus (Screenshot 2.24).

Choose the *Simple Scatter* option and click on *Define*. You can then move the *Before* variable to the *X Axis* box and the *After* variable to the *Y Axis* box (Screenshot 2.25).

Then click on *OK* to generate the graph (Screenshot 2.26).

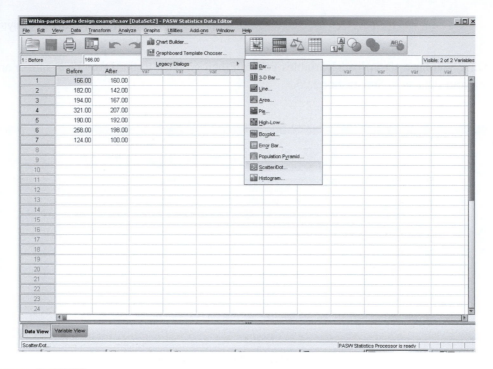

Screenshot 2.24

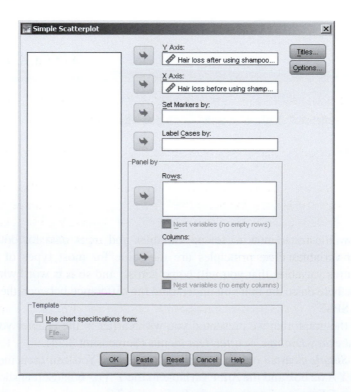

Screenshot 2.25

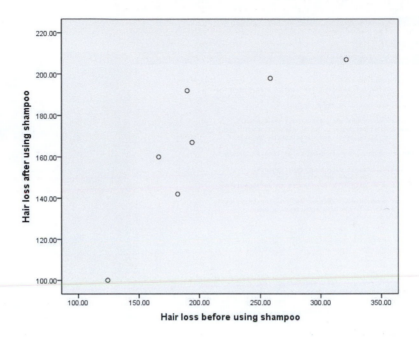

Screenshot 2.26

INTRODUCTION TO R

As we suggested earlier R is different to SPSS in that it doesn't rely on Windows and menus to display data and run analyses. In R you have to type in commands to tell the program what you want it to do.

When you first start the software you will be presented with the *R console* (Screenshot 2.27).

The window that you get is called the *Workspace* and all work in this can be saved by using the *File*, *Save Workspace* options. When you start R you will notice that it tells you the version that you are using in the first line in the *R Console*. We use this *R Console* to communicate with R and tell it what to do (remember you are in charge!). You type in your commands at the command prompt.

The first thing that you will want to do when you start a session is to type in your data. You will notice that when typing data into R we do not use a spreadsheet type window as we do in SPSS. Instead we use the command prompt to enter the data. There are a number of different ways of entering data, but initially we will illustrate a simple single variable means of entering your data. Suppose we refer back to the age and gender example that we used for illustrating data entry in SPSS (see Table 2.2). First of all we will input the age data. To do this we have to combine the data together into one variable name and also assign this a name. We combine the data using the *c* command and assign the name using '<-'. The '<-' symbol

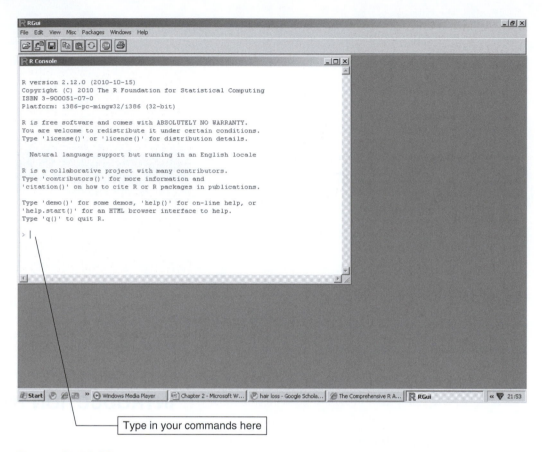

Type in your commands here

Screenshot 2.27

tells R to assign values to an object name. The age data that we want to enter are (24, 18, 19, 32, 19, 25 and 22). Therefore the command to read into R is:

```
Age <- c(24, 18, 19, 32, 19, 25, 22)
```

The important thing to note here is the order. The 'c(…)' tells R to combine the elements in the brackets into a single variable. The elements in the brackets need to be separated by commas. The '<-' command then tells R to name that variable 'Age' (Screenshot 2.28).

We can read in the *Sex* data in a similar way. Remember we arbitrarily categorised males as 0 and females as 1 and so we have done the same in this example. The command for reading in these data is:

```
Sex <- c(0,1,0,1,1,1,0)
```

It is very important that you put the values in the correct order in the brackets because when comparing across your variables (e.g. looking at the age and sex of the third

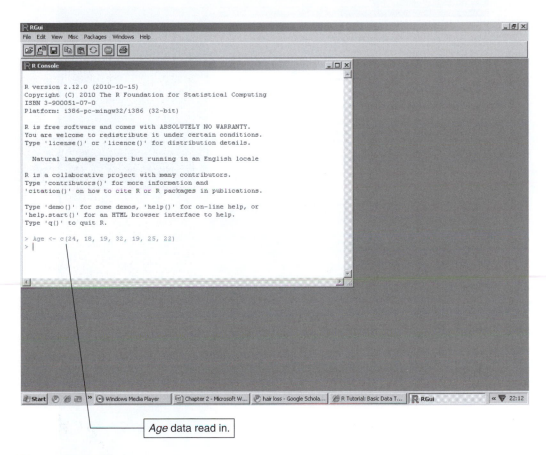

Age data read in.

Screenshot 2.28

person in the list) you need to make sure that the correct values are grouped together (Screenshot 2.29).

Once you have read in some data it is a good idea to save this. To do so simply click on *File*, *Save Workpace*. Once you do this you will see the command for saving the workspace appear in the *R Console* window (Screenshot 2.30).

If you exit from R now your data will be saved for you so that you don't have to read it in again in the future. When you restart R you will be presented with the restored data screen (Screenshot 2.31).

You will notice that R conveniently opens up the last workspace that you saved to prevent you having to doing it. If this is not the workspace you wanted to work on then you can load up the correct one by selecting the *File*, *Load Workspace* menu items.

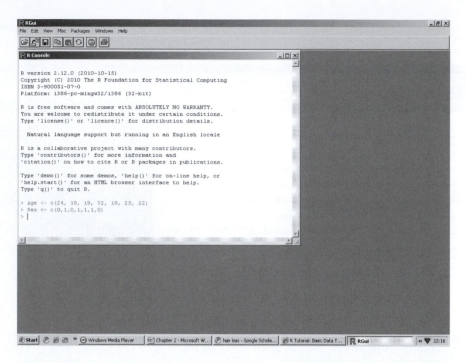

Screenshot 2.29

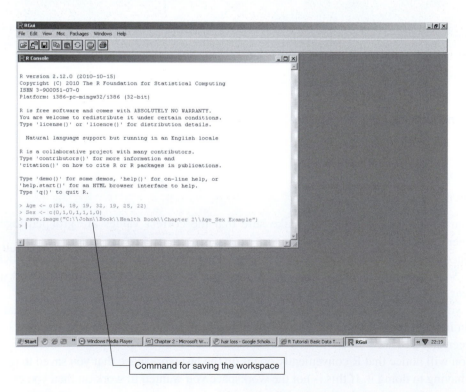

Command for saving the workspace

Screenshot 2.30

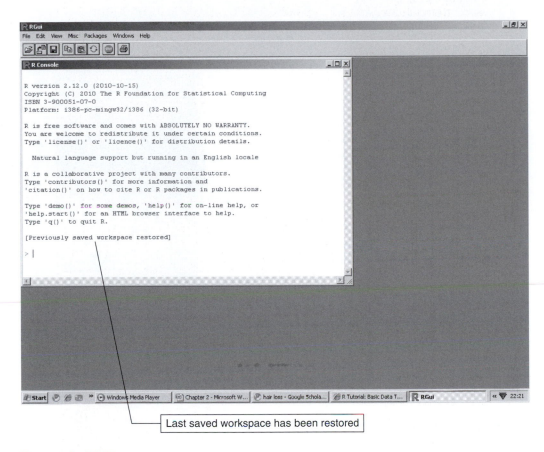

Last saved workspace has been restored

Screenshot 2.31

Let us check that R has kept our data for us. We can do this by simply typing either of the variable names at the command prompt and then pressing the enter key. You need to remember though that names in R are case sensitive, and so you need to type the name in exactly as you originally specified it. Type in 'Age' at the command prompt (Screenshot 2.32).

You should be able to see that R then presents our data for that variable for us. If you type in 'age' you will get an 'Error: object 'age' not found' error message. This is because there is no variable called *age* set up as we originally typed in 'Age'. Type in 'Sex' to list out the *Sex* variable values.

You should recall from the description of SPSS that we were able to indicate to SPSS that the *Sex* variable was a nominal measure and was thus a categorical variable. We can do a similar thing in R by using the *Factor* command. We could indicate that the *Sex* variable is a factor (categorical or grouping) variable by typing in:

```
Sex <- factor(Sex)
```

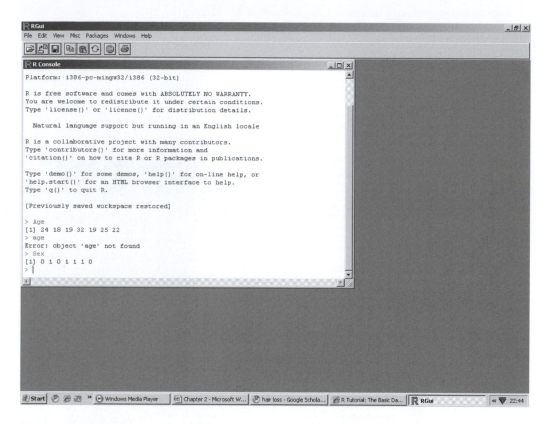

Screenshot 2.32

The 'factor(Sex)' bit of the command converts the variable into a categorical variable and the 'Sex <-' bit assigns this variable the same name as previously.

If you now type in 'Sex' at the command prompt and press enter it will look different to the previous output (Screenshot 2.33).

Now we would like to generate some summary statistics broken down by groups. One thing to note about R is that it is what is called 'Open Source' software. The code for developing routines in R is available to anybody, and as such programmers and statisticians can generate their own modules to analyse data in any way they see fit. Such modules can then be made freely available to anyone else using R. These modules are called *Packages* in R. The version of R that you download and install will only contain a certain number of packages, but as you become more adept with the software and your needs become more complex you might want to install additional packages. We are going to show you how to install a package in R as this will help us generate some summary statistics broken down by group. If you click on the *Packages* menu you can elect to install a new package. Select this option (Screenshot 2.34).

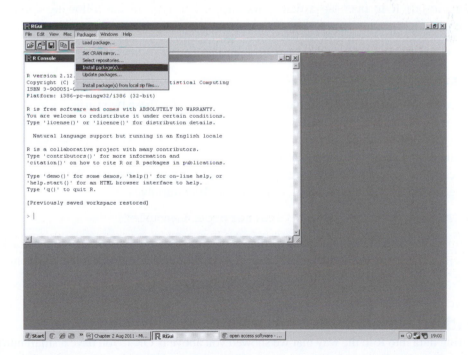

Screenshot 2.33

Screenshot 2.34

You will then be asked to select a *CRAN mirror* which is a website from which you can download the package easily and quickly. Choose the one nearest to you and then click on *OK* (Screenshot 2.35).

You will then be presented with a list of packages that you can install. Scroll down this list until you come to the one called *psych* (Screenshot 2.36).

Click on *OK* and R will install the package. This package was developed specifically for psychology based research but it does have some useful features for displaying some simple statistics.

Once the package has installed you can type in the following two commands to get your summary statistics broken down by age:

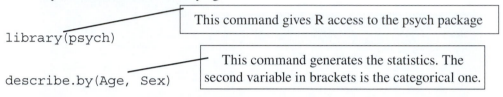

```
library(psych)
```
This command gives R access to the psych package

```
describe.by(Age, Sex)
```
This command generates the statistics. The second variable in brackets is the categorical one.

When you run this you will be presented with the statistics in Screenshot 2.37.

If we wanted to input the two variables for our hair loss example (see Table 2.3) then we would need to open up a new workspace because these are separate data. You will need to restart R to open up a new workspace. Then type in the following commands (Screenshot 2.38):

```
Before <- c(166,182,194,321,190,258,124)
```

```
After <- c(160,142,167,207,192,198,100)
```

We can now generate some simple summary statistics for these two variables by using the 'summary' command. Type this in at the command prompt (note that this is case sensitive and so you need to type 'summary' – lower case 's'). You will be presented with the summary statistics shown in Screenshot 2.39.

We can also generate a simple scattergram using the 'plot' command. We use the following to generate the scattergram for the *Before* and *After* variables:

```
plot(After, Before, main="Scatterplot Example")
```

In this command the variable to be displayed on the *x*-axis is the first listed in the brackets. You will notice that the scattergram is presented in a new window called a graphsheet. Figure 2.4 shows what the plot looks like.

Reading Data into R from a File

Inputting data into R in the way that we showed you above is OK if you have a small number of participants and relatively few variables. If you have quite a large dataset then it is probably best to use some other program to enter your data, like Microsoft Excel. You can then read in the data from Excel into R quite easily. To illustrate this we have typed the Age and Sex data into an Excel worksheet (Screenshot 2.40).

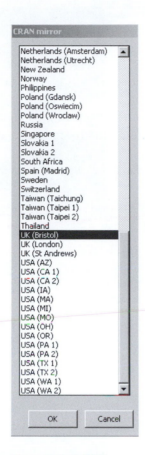

Screenshot 2.35

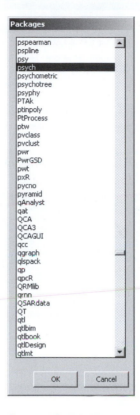

Screenshot 2.36

```
group: 0
  var n  mean   sd median trimmed  mad min max range  skew kurtosis   se
1   1 3 21.67 2.52     22   21.67 2.97  19  24     5 -0.13    -2.33 1.45
------------------------------------------------------------
group: 1
  var n mean   sd median trimmed  mad min max range skew kurtosis   se
1   1 4 23.5 6.45     22    23.5 5.19  18  32    14 0.33    -2.06 3.23
>
```

Screenshot 2.37

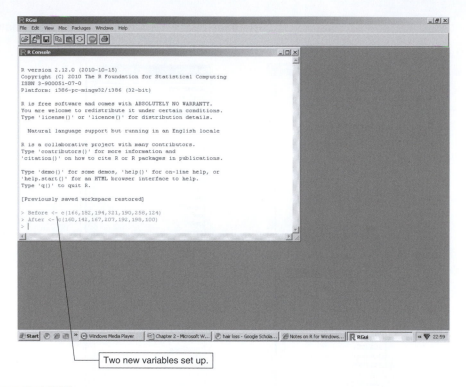

Two new variables set up.

Screenshot 2.38

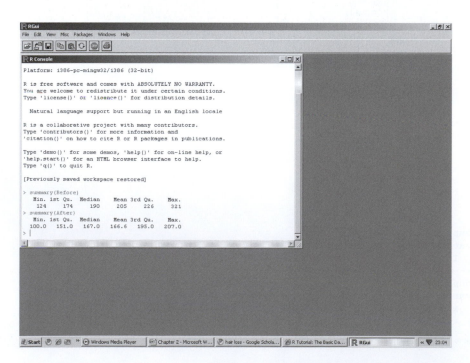

Screenshot 2.39

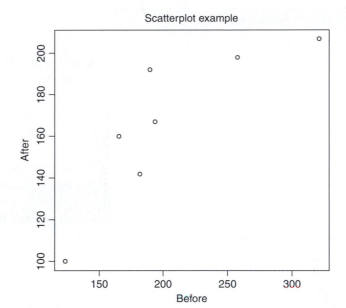

Figure 2.4 Scatterplot generated in R

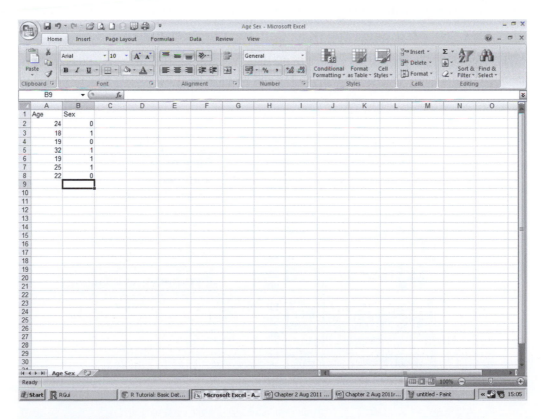

Screenshot 2.40

Notice that we have typed in variable names in the first row of the file. This is important as you can use these names to label the variables when you import the data into R.

If we save this as a traditional Excel file then R won't be able to read it and so you will need to save it in a format called *Comma Separated Values* or *CSV*. To do this simply click on the little Windows icon in the top left corner of the screen and then select Save As (Screenshot 2.41).

In the dialogue box you should type in the filename and then activate the drop-down list in the *Save as type* box and scroll down until you find the *CSV* option. Select this and then save the file (Screenshot 2.42).

You will be presented with a message asking you if you want to keep the file in *CSV* format (Screenshot 2.43). You should answer *Yes* to this and then close down Excel. It will ask you if you want to save your data but there is no need to as you have already done so.

OK, now you have your data in a data file and so we can now read this into R. To do this you will need to first of all change the working folder in R so that it is the same as the folder that you just saved your data to. You do this by clicking on the *File* menu and selecting the *Change dir* option (Screenshot 2.44).

Then select the folder that you want to work from (Screenshot 2.45).

Once you have set up the working directory you can read in the data by using this command:

```
Age _ Sex <- read.csv(file="Age Sex.csv",head=TRUE,sep=",")
```

The 'Age_Sex' simply assigns a name to the data. You can see that in the brackets we have specified the filename that we want to read in and we have used the 'head=TRUE' option to

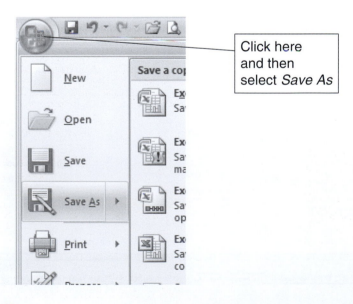

Screenshot 2.41

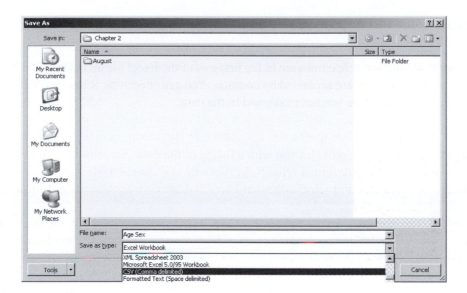

Screenshot 2.42

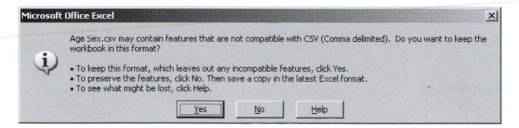

Screenshot 2.43

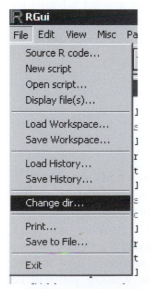

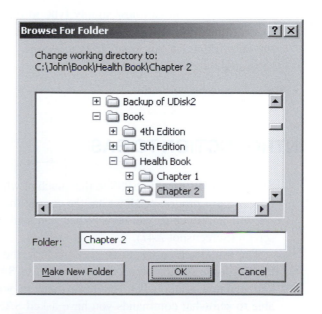

Screenshot 2.44   **Screenshot 2.45**

let R know that the variable names are in the first row of the Excel file and 'sep_","' indicates that the values in the file are separated by commas. You can check that R has read in the data by typing in the the name you have assigned to the data:

```
Age _ Sex
```

You should find that R provides you with a listing of the data (Screenshot 2.46).

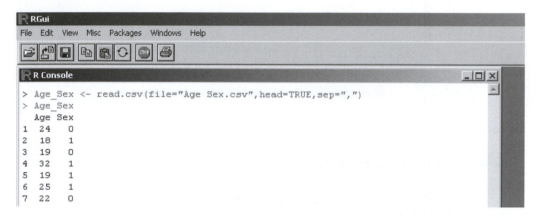

Screenshot 2.46

You should note that when you read in data from a file, R reads it into something called a *data frame*. You can now simply type in the name of the variable and get a listing for that variable. If you want a listing of one particular variable you have to refer to the name of the data frame (in our example that is 'Age_Sex') and then the variable name (these are separated by a $ sign), e.g.:

```
Age _ Sex$Sex
```

INTRODUCTION TO SAS

SAS is very different to SPSS in that much of what you want to do with it will require you to type in mini-programs. However, the core of the system is Windows based and this is what we will introduce to you here. When you start SAS you will be presented with an initial screen (Screenshot 2.47).

The initial screen has three sections to it, the *Explorer*, the *Log* and the *Editor*. We use the *Explorer* section to access and organise SAS files. The *Log* section is used to keep you updated about what you have done in your session. In this window you will be able to see what commands you have asked SAS to run and it will print out any errors in

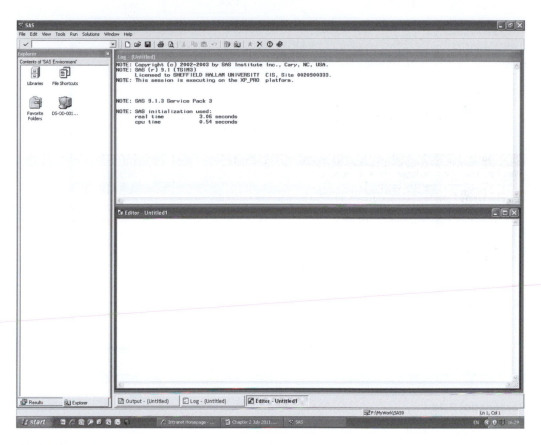

Screenshot 2.47

your commands. If SAS doesn't recognise what you have asked it to do, it will print out an error in the *Log* window. The *Editor* section is where you generate your mini-programs to be run by SAS. You will also notice at the bottom of the screen that there are some tabs that you can click on. These bring up two additional parts of the software; the *Output* window is where the analyses that you get SAS to produce for you will be displayed, and you can then use the *Results* window to navigate through this output swiftly and easily.

Working with Data Files in SAS

SAS data files are stored in *Libraries* and these can be accessed in the *Explorer* window. There are some default libraries shown in the *Explorer* window when you start up SAS but you will probably want to set up your own library so that you know where to find your data files more easily. To set up a library you need to click on the *New Library* icon on the Toolbar (this looks like a filing cabinet, Screenshot 2.48).

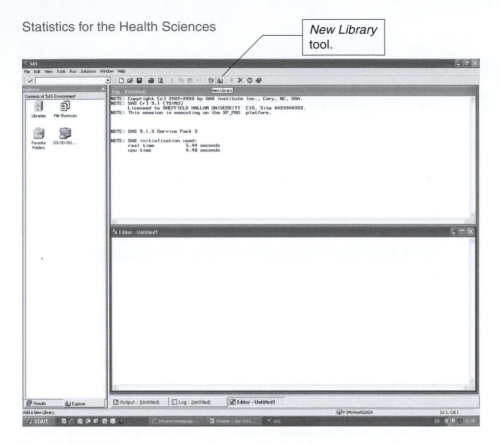

New Library tool.

Screenshot 2.48

When you do this you will be presented with the a dialogue box where you can set up the name and other characteristics of your library (Screenshot 2.49).

You should type in a suitable name for the library but this is limited to eight characters and cannot contain spaces or punctuation. We have called our library 'Data_Lib'.

You should also select the *Enable at startup* option as this will bring the library up in the *Explorer* window automatically when you start up SAS. Finally you should use the *Browse* button to select the folder where you want to store your library and then click on *OK* to create the library. If you now go to the *Explorer* window and double click on the *Librarys* icon you will see your new library created for you (Screenshot 2.50).

Creating a New Data File

It is not obvious from the menus how you create new data files, but once you get familiar with the software it becomes easier. To create a data file you should first double click on the *Library* where you want to keep it. We will store our file in the new 'Data_Lib' library that we have just created. When you double click on this you will get an empty window (Screenshot 2.51).

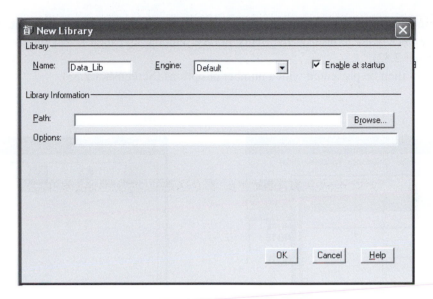

Screenshot 2.49

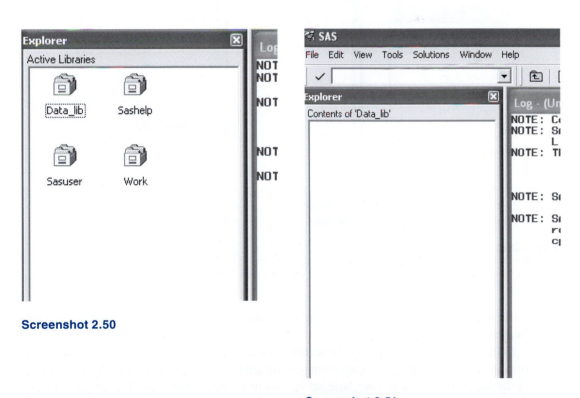

Screenshot 2.50

Screenshot 2.51

This indicates that we have no data files in this library as yet. To create a new data file you can right click your mouse on the blank library window and then select the *New* option (Screenshot 2.52).

You will then be presented with a number of options (Screenshot 2.53).

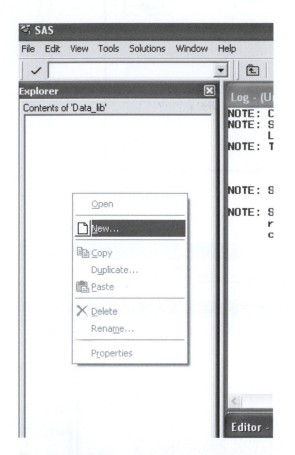

Screenshot 2.52

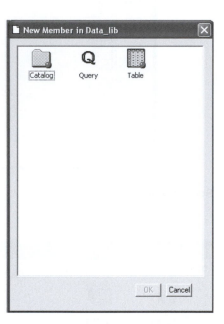

Screenshot 2.53

Click on the *Table* option and you will then be presented with a new data table (Screenshot 2.54).

As in SPSS, each column in the table represents a variable and each row a case (or person). You can change the names of the columns to meaningful variable names by double clicking on the top of each column. We have set up two new variables one for *Age* and one for *Sex* (Screenshot 2.55).

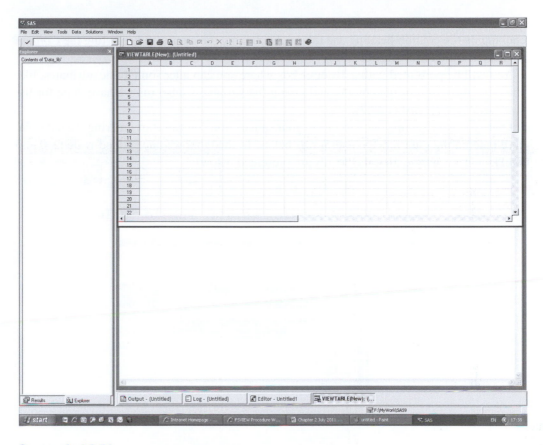

Screenshot 2.54

Screenshot 2.55

As in SPSS we can change some of the characteristics of the variables, and you do this by clicking on the column heading and then right clicking the mouse and selecting the *Column Attributes* option (Screenshot 2.56).

You will be presented with a dialogue box where you can alter some basic attributes, like changing the width of the column and giving the variable a label (as we have done for the *Age* variable, Screenshot 2.57).

Once you have set up your variable to your satisfaction you can start entering the data. We have entered the data for *Age* and *Sex* as below. In the table we have coded male as 0 and female as 1 (as a reminder, the details are presented below).

Age: 24, 18, 19, 32, 19, 25, & 22

Sex: Male, Female, Male, Female, Female, Female, Male

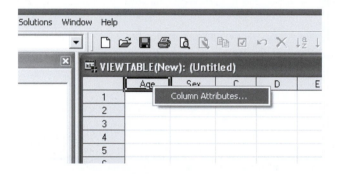

Screenshot 2.56

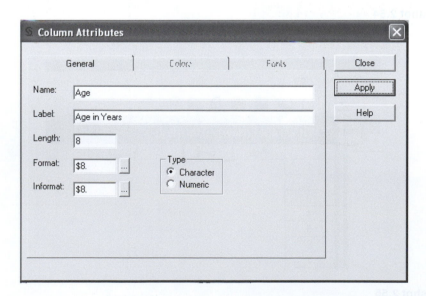

Screenshot 2.57

To type in the data you should click on the first cell of the *Age* column and type in the first age then use the down arrow key to move to the next cell and type in the next age. Do this until you have entered the data for both variables. Your data table should look like Screenshot 2.58.

Now that we have entered the data we should save it. To do this you should left click on the icon in the top-left corner of the data table and choose the *Menu* option and then from the list of options given choose the *File* option and then select *Save As* (Screenshot 2.59).

You will be presented with a dialogue box where you can specify which library you want to save to and the filename. You need to bear in mind that you cannot have spaces or punctuation marks in the filename. We have selected the 'Data_Lib' library and called the file 'Age_Sex_Data' (Screenshot 2.60).

When you click on *Save* you will see that the table is saved in the 'Data_Lib' library. If you want to access the table again you can then simply double click it from the *Explorer* window.

We are now ready to run some basic analyses on the data. You should note that we have to type in the commands to run the analyses in the *Editor* window. First of all we will create

Screenshot 2.58

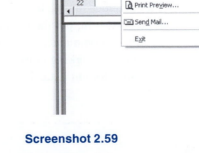

Screenshot 2.59

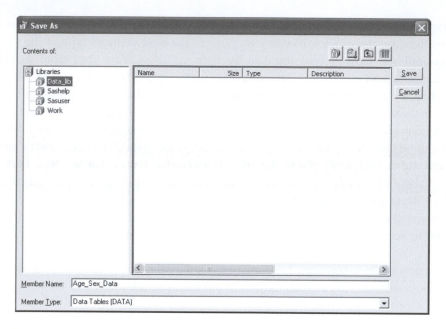

Screenshot 2.60

some simple descriptive statistics for the *Age* variable. SAS handles data files in a different way to SPSS. Just because you have a data file open doesn't mean that SAS will run an analysis on it. You need to generate a working copy of the data file for SAS to work with. This has a major advantage, as it means that all changes within that analysis session are made to the working copy rather than the original, and so if something goes wrong you should easily be able to go back to the original. To set up a working copy of the data file you should type the following command in the *Editor* window. Don't forget to include the semi-colon (;) at the end of each line as this tells SAS that this is the end of that particular command:

```
data working; set Data _ Lib.Age _ Sex _ Data;

run;
```

It is always a good idea to type the 'run' command at the end of a mini-program like this. When you have typed it in, put the cursor after the 'run;' command and then click on the *Submit* icon to run the commands (Screenshot 2.61).

You will now have a working copy of the data to work with. We want to now generate some simple statistics for our data. To do this you can type the following:

```
Proc means;

run;
```

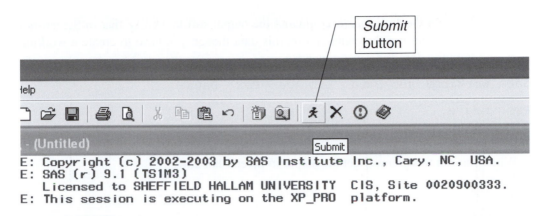

Screenshot 2.61

and then click on the *Submit* button. You will be presented with the output shown in Screenshot 2.62.

Screenshot 2.62

You will notice that this gives you a table with a range of simple statistics (we cover these in Chapter 3). Remember, *Sex* is a categorical variable but the way we have it set up currently is as a numerical variable. As it is set up as a numerical variable you will get summary statistics for it. To ensure that SAS recognises your variable as a categorical one you can, when you enter the data into new data sheet, type in labels, e.g. 'male' and 'female'. And so instead of typing in 1s and 0s you would type in the labels. The data file would then look like Screenshot 2.63.

Screenshot 2.63

Now if you run the *Proc means* command the output still looks like that in Screenshot 2.62. Before you can run the command on this data though you have to create a working copy of it with the *data* and *set* commands:

```
data working; set Data _ Lib.Age _ Sex _ Data;

Proc means;

run;
```

When you run this you will get the output in Screenshot 2.64.

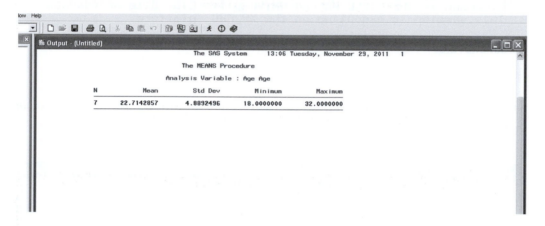

Screenshot 2.64

Now we only get the summary statistics for the *Age* variable. As *Sex* is now a category variable we don't get the statistics. Ideally, what we really want is the summary statistics for *Age* broken down by sex. We can do this by including the *by* command just after the *Proc means* command. However, SAS is a little quirky and it will only do this if you sort the data first and we need also to include a *sort* command. The mini-program should look like this:

```
Proc sort; by Sex;

Proc means; by Sex;

run;
```

You will be presented with the output in Screenshot 2.65.

Now the statistics have been broken down by sex. This is OK, but it would be better if you could get these details in one table. You can, but instead of using the *by* command after the *proc means* command you have to use the *class* command:

```
Proc sort; by Sex;

Proc means; class Sex;

run;
```

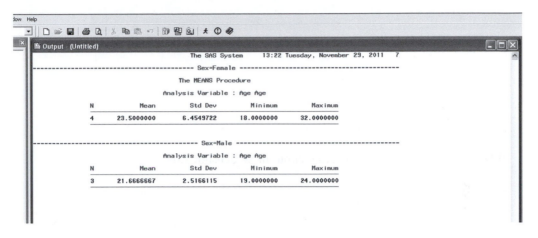

Screenshot 2.65

You will then be presented with a neater table (Screenshot 2.66).

Screenshot 2.66

OK, we have now looked at between-groups designs, how about our hair loss within-groups design? Open up a new data file and type in the data from Table 2.3. You should have two columns, you can label one as 'Before' and the other 'After' (Screenshot 2.67).

Don't forget to save this to your library. We can now generate some simple summary statistics for these two variables. Remember you will have first to make a working copy of the file using the *data* and *set* commands and then you can use the *Proc means* command to generate the summary statistics:

```
data working; set Data _ lib.Hairloss;

Proc means;

run;
```

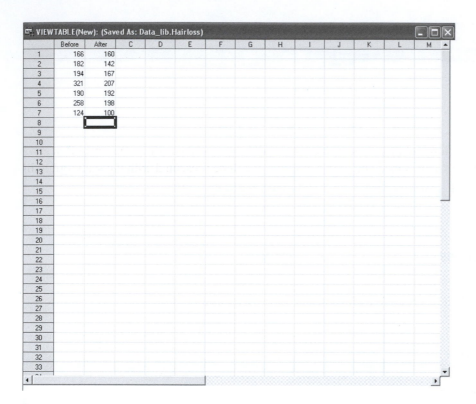

Screenshot 2.67

When you run this you will be presented with the table shown in Screenshot 2.68.

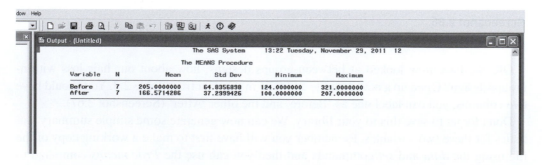

Screenshot 2.68

Finally for this introduction to SAS we will generate a simple scattergram. To do this we have to use the *Gplot* procedure and then the *plot* command. The mini-program will look like this:

```
Proc Gplot;

plot After*Before;

run;
```

In the *plot* command the first variable listed will be presented on the *y*-axis and the second variable on the *x*-axis. Once you have run this you will be presented with the scattergram in Figure 2.5.

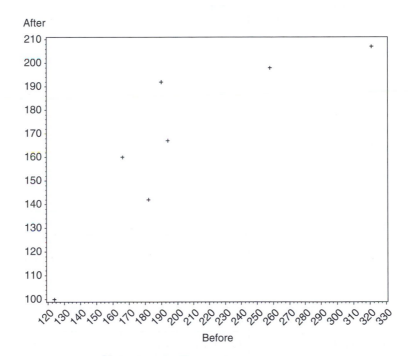

Figure 2.5   Scatterplot generated in SAS

Summary

We have now introduced you to three different statistical software packages. We have shown you how to enter data into all three packages and how to generate some simple numeric and graphical statistics. As you work through the book you will be able get more practice using SPSS, but if you prefer SAS or R we have given guidance on the companion website to show you how to do the same analysis using those packages.

SPSS EXERCISE 1

A researcher is interested in comparing the stress levels of nurses, junior doctors and consultants in a busy city centre hospital. They have asked a sample of each occupation to complete a stress questionnaire where higher scores indicate higher levels of stress. Have a go at entering the data presented in Table 2.4 into SPSS and produce some summary statistics broken down by occupation.

Table 2.4   Stress scores for nurses, junior doctors and consultants

Occupation	Stress
Nurse	32
Nurse	28
Nurse	22
Nurse	35
Nurse	29
Nurse	27
Nurse	26
Junior doctor	31
Junior doctor	23
Junior doctor	29
Junior doctor	34
Junior doctor	26
Junior doctor	24
Consultant	19
Consultant	16
Consultant	11
Consultant	22
Consultant	20
Consultant	17

R EXERCISE 1

Enter the data in Table 2.4 into R and run some summary statistics broken down by occupation.

SAS EXERCISE 1

Enter the data in Table 2.4 into SAS and run some summary statistics broken down by occupation.

SPSS EXERCISE 2

A researcher has conducted a study and collected in-patient satisfaction ratings (where a higher score equals higher satisfaction) and has also recorded the length of time the patients had been in hospital in days. The data are presented in Table 2.5. Input the data into SPSS and produce some summary statistics and a scattergram.

Table 2.5   Patient satisfaction and time spent in hospital data

Patient satisfaction	Time in hospital
7	14
4	12
6	6
3	1
2	3
2	6
5	8
6	6
7	9
2	1

R EXERCISE 2

Enter the data in Table 2.5 into R and run some summary statistics for both variables and produce a scattergram.

SAS EXERCISE 2

Enter the data in Table 2.5 into SAS and run some summary statistics for both variables and produce a scattergram.

Notes

1 You can run SPSS like an SAS or R command interface by using SPSS syntax. This is simply a set of commands you type to run each of the analyses in SPSS. In fact, what SPSS really does is use the menus and dialogue boxes in order to build up the commands to run the analyses. Many people advocate converting the menu/dialogue box orders into syntax as a way of keeping a record of the analyses you have conducted.
2 Quite often when you have conducted a study you may have allocated specific numbers to each participant. When you have done this it is good practice to use the first variable in the data file to record the participant number.

Descriptive Statistics

3

Overview

In this chapter we will introduce you to some simple ways of summarising and describing data. We will highlight the importance of these data analytic techniques for a proper understanding of the results of your own research and the research presented by others. This will include:

- Describing the typical score in a sample (measures of central tendency)
- Describing the variability or dispersion of scores in a sample
- Presenting data graphically including:
  - Bar charts
  - Line graphs
  - Histograms
  - Box-plots
- Running these analyses using SPSS

In order to get the most from this chapter you should make sure that you have read and understood Chapter 1 and that you have read through the introduction to SPSS that we gave in Chapter 2.

ANALYSING DATA

In Chapter 1 we gave an overview of the research process along with different ways of conducting research (research designs). In this chapter we are going to move on a stage and explain some of the simple statistical techniques available to researchers for analysing data. These techniques are used for exploring and describing data, they are called *descriptive statistics*. As you progress through this book you will come to learn that there are generally two different types of statistical techniques that researchers can utilise. One set of techniques are used to simply describe research data, and the other set are used to help us as researchers generalise from our study to the wider population. The former techniques are descriptive statistics and the latter are called *inferential statistics*. In due course you will come to understand the distinction between the two as well as the appropriate uses for them. You will notice that most of this book (and indeed the vast majority of other statistics books) is devoted to explaining inferential statistics. You should not though take this to mean that such techniques are more important. In fact an argument could be made that descriptive statistical techniques are at least as important (and perhaps are more important). A seminal book by Tukey in 1977 called *Exploratory Data Analysis* is devoted entirely to descriptive statistics (all 688 pages of it … wow!), as Tukey felt their importance had been overlooked by mainstream researchers.

Why are descriptive statistics so important? Have a think about this analogy. You are going on a blind date and you are very nervous about doing so. Let us suppose that you are meeting outside a particular restaurant and you decide to wait around the corner so that you can get a sneaky look at your date before you meet them. When you first see your date you will mentally examine them much in the same way a data analyst might examine their data. You might ask yourself a number of questions. Are they good looking or attractive? Are they smartly dressed? Are they carrying a gift (flowers or chocolates)? Are they tall? Do they look nervous? Do they look like a psychopath? These questions all relate to important characteristics of your date and may determine whether or not you cross the road to meet them. As you progress through your meal you will be constantly examining your date and asking more questions. Are they funny? Are they intelligent? Do they let you get a word in? Do they listen to you? Do they eat like a pig? Much of your dinner would be devoted to getting to know each other and you would each ask questions in order to do this. So you might ask them what they do for a living. What are their hobbies? What sort of music, books or films do they like? All these questions will help you get to know your date. This is similar to the initial analyses of our data in research. We conduct descriptive statistical analyses in order to better get to know our data. The other purpose of descriptive statistics is so that you can describe your data to someone else. If you think about the blind date example there are again similarities here. When you see your best friend the next day you would want to tell them all about your date, and you would use the answers to the questions that you asked and your analysis of what they looked like to describe them to your friend.

This process of examining or exploring is exactly what researchers should do in order to better understand their data and how they can use it to address important decisions that they have to make. Is the data telling you anything worthwhile? Is it worth carrying on analysing the data? Do you need to collect more data? It is through exploring your data that you will gain an intimate knowledge of it and better understand what you can do with it in order to address your research aims.

DESCRIPTIVE STATISTICS

Let us start by describing an example research study. Assume that we are interested in discovering whether there are differences between stroke patients and heart attack patients in their ability to come to terms with their illness. Let us say that we have run a study where we have given a group of patients with each illness a questionnaire that measures how well they are coping after they have left hospital. Let us assume that the higher the score on the questionnaire the better the patient is coping. Some hypothetical data for this study are presented in Table 3.1.

Table 3.1   Coping scores for stroke and heart attack patients

Stroke		Heart attack	
39	27	27	27
26	1	29	23
26	25	27	26
9	23	27	35
14	23	33	25
28	40	22	32
21	9	29	32
26	13	23	22
23	13	29	25
18	21	30	30

Activity 3.1

Take a look at the scores in Table 3.1 for the stroke patients. How would you describe these to a friend who couldn't see them?

You might have noticed from Activity 3.1 that it is quite difficult to describe data. You might have said that the lowest score is 1 and the highest is 40. You might have said that most people had scores in the twenties, but some had scores in the teens or lower and only two had scores above 30. You might be a little more precise in your description by saying that there were three scores below 10, four between 10 and 19, eleven scores in the twenties, and two scores above 30. These verbal descriptions might give your friend a good idea of the scores in your dataset, and this is exactly what we do with descriptive statistics. We would describe the data using standardised techniques in order to convey to other people what our data look like. Usually, when we publish research in a journal we do not include all of our data and so we need to describe to the reader what our data look like. We also use standardised descriptive techniques to give ourselves a better understanding of our data. Quite often in research we study a lot more than 20 patients. It is not that uncommon in research to include hundreds (and indeed thousands) of people in the study. In such cases it would be very difficult for you to 'eyeball' the data as we have done here and provide a description of them. Another problem with describing data using 'eyeballing' is that your description of the data might differ from ours. Thus standardised techniques allow for much greater consistency in describing data and provide a shared understanding of the characteristics of the people we included in our study.

NUMERICAL DESCRIPTIVE STATISTICS

There are a number of different ways that you can explore and describe your data. In this section we are going to show you the standard ways of describing your data using numbers. The techniques that we will explain here are essentially similar to the descriptions we gave earlier for the stroke patient data. If you look again at those descriptions you can see that we used numbers to describe the whole dataset. When we do this we often say that we are summarising our data, and these techniques are sometimes called summary statistics. These techniques are a bit like a review of a film. In a review you might summarise the film in a few words, e.g. 'The film adaptation of Statistics for the Health Sciences was jaw-droppingly good'. Or you might use a single number to describe the film, e.g. four out of five. We can do similar things to describe our data.

The 'Typical Score' – Measures of Central Tendency

Activity 3.2

Take a look back at the data for stroke patients in Table 3.1. What single number do you think best represents the data?

We would say that 23 might be a good single number to describe the whole dataset. No doubt you might have come up with a different single number, and this is why it is better to use standardised descriptive statistics.

The Mean

One way of summarising the data is to try to identify the typical score in the dataset. There are a number of different ways of doing this but perhaps the most common of these is the *mean*. The mean is what many people think of as the 'average' and they may have been taught about this in school. The mean is effectively the value that is numerically closest to all the scores in the dataset. We can calculate the mean quite easily by adding up all the scores in the dataset and then dividing this 'sum' by the number of scores that you have. So for the stroke patients we have 20 scores in the dataset and if we add them all up we get 425. If we now divide 425 by 20 (the number of scores in the dataset) this would give us 21.25 which is the mean. Another example might help to consolidate this concept. Let us take a look at the heart attack patient data. To calculate the mean for this you need to add up (or sum) the scores in the dataset this gives us a value of 553. You now need to divide this by the number of patients in the sample which is 20. Thus 553 ÷ 20 = 27.65. The mean for the heart attack patients is 27.65. We can now, if we wanted, compare the mean for the stroke patients with that for the heart attack patients. You should be able to see that the stroke patient mean of 21.25 is quite a bit smaller than that for the heart attack patients (27.65).

The mean is the most commonly reported measure of central tendency and is usually the statistic of choice when you want to present descriptive statistics. The mean can though be rather misleading in terms of how it represents the whole dataset. Take a look at the following data:

27	29	27	27	33	22	29	23	29	30	27
23	26	35	25	32	32	532	25	30		

This is the same data as for the heart attack patients above but has one score changed. Have a go at calculating the mean for these new data. When you add up the scores the answer is 1063, and when you divide this by 20 you get a mean of 53.15. You can see that this mean is a good deal larger than the one we calculated earlier (27.65) and yet we have changed only one of the scores. Also, saying that the typical score in this data set is 53.17 is rather misleading as the vast majority of scores are between 25 and 35. Thus, the mean in this case does a poor job of describing our dataset. This example highlights one of the problems associated with the mean. Because it uses the actual values of all of the scores in the dataset it can be heavily influenced by extreme scores like the score of 532 in the last example. We therefore have to be careful when using the mean to ensure that it is truly representative of the data from our sample.

The Median

A measure of central tendency that is not biased by extreme scores in a dataset is the *median*. The median is the middle score in a dataset after you have put them in ascending order. And so, whereas the value of each score is used in the calculation of the mean, it is not used for the calculation of the median. This means that very high or very low scores have minimal impact on the median. As an illustration of how to calculate the median take a look at the following example of scores (these are the first five scores from Table 3.1 for the stroke patients):

    39   26   26   9   14

The first thing we need to do is to rearrange the scores so that they are in ascending order. This is called 'ranking' the scores or putting them in 'rank order'. The scores in rank order are:

    9   14   26   26   39

Once we have rearranged the scores we need to locate the score that is in the middle of the list. This is quite easy to do when you have an odd number of scores in the sample as we have here. We have five scores and so the middle score is the third one in the list (there are two scores below and two scores above this score). Thus the median in this sample of scores is 26 (the middle score – bold in the list below).

    9   14   **26**   26   39

We have now added a few more scores to the list (we have taken the first nine scores from the stroke data in Table 3.1):

    39   26   26   9   14   28   21   26   23

To calculate the median put the scores in ascending order (rank them):

    9   14   21   23   **26**   26   26   28   39

We now need to find the middle score. In this case as we have nine scores in the sample the middle one is the fifth score (it has four scores above and four below it). Thus the median for this sample of scores is again 26. Finding the median when you have an odd number of scores in your sample is relatively straightforward as there will always be a score in the middle. It is slightly more difficult when you have an even number of scores, for example:

    39   26   26   9   14   28   21   26   23   18

When these scores are ranked they look like this:

    9   14   18   21   **23**   **26**   26   26   28   39

Now we do not have a single score that is directly in the middle of the ranked list. There are effectively two scores and the middle of the list falls halfway between them. What we have to do to calculate the median is work out which number falls halfway between these two numbers. We can do this by adding them up and dividing by two. In this case 23 + 26 = 49 and dividing this by 2 gives us a median value of 24.5.

An interesting point about the median is that unlike the mean it is not influenced by extreme scores. For example, take another look at these scores:

9   14   21   23   **26**   26   26   28   39

Here the median is 26. Now let us change the highest score to 532 (as we did in the example for calculating the mean):

9   14   21   23   **26**   26   26   28   532

The median is still 26 because, as the 532 is still the highest score, it doesn't impact upon the value of the score in the middle once they have been ranked. Now look at this:

9   14   21   23   **26**   26   26   28   500,000,000

We have changed the highest score so that it is much more like a banker's bonus. However, this still has no impact upon the median. It is the median's insensitivity to extreme scores that makes it a useful descriptive statistical technique when we have such scores in our sample data. For information, the means for the previous three sets of scores are 23.56, 78.33 and 55,555,574.78. Thus whilst the median remains unchanged the mean varies dramatically from one sample to the next.

Activity 3.3

Have a go at calculating the median scores for the whole sample of stroke patients and also for the heart attack patients.

The Mode

The final measure of central tendency that we will be presenting in this book is perhaps the least used and it is called the *mode*. The mode is simply the most frequently occurring score in the sample. Thus for each sample you simply look for the score that occurs most often. A useful way of working this out if you have a lot of data is to rank the data first. For the heart attack patients data in Table 3.1 you should be able to see that the most frequently occurring score is 27 and so the mode is 27. It is slightly trickier for the stroke patient scores because there are two scores that occur equally most frequently, and these are 23 and 26. Thus, for some samples of data there might be two or more modes. In such cases using the mean as a measure of the typical score might be inappropriate as we have two different typical scores.

Activity 3.4

Have a go at calculating the mean, median and mode for the following data:

| 21 | 21 | 26 | 18 | 25 | 12 | 20 | 17 | 9 | 23 |

And the following:

| 12 | 17 | 21 | 9 | 20 | 15 | 7 | 20 | 23 | 13 |

CHOOSING A MEASURE OF CENTRAL TENDENCY

Given that there are three different measures of central tendency, which one should you use? The measure you choose is dependent upon the type of data that you have and scores in the dataset. The measure of choice is the mean, but strictly speaking you should only use this if you have no extreme scores in your dataset. We explained previously that the mean is heavily influenced by extreme scores in your dataset and so you should be wary of using the mean if you have such scores. The median is great when you have extreme scores. The mode is perhaps most useful when you have nominal or categorical data. These usually consist of frequency counts, e.g. the number of people in a sample who are lawyers. When you have such data you cannot use the median or mean as it makes no sense to order or rank the categories in terms of magnitude. You have no choice but to use the mode in such cases to give an indication of the typical score.

MEASURES OF VARIATION OR DISPERSION

We have covered the statistics that help us summarise our data in terms of the typical score; however, simply describing the data in this one single statistic only gives part of the picture. It would be like watching a film at the cinema and standing one metre away from the very middle of the screen. You would have a clear idea what was happening in the centre of the screen but you probably would not be able to tell what was happening towards the edges. You would probably miss important aspects of the film. Describing data is the same; you don't want to focus only on what is happening at the centre, you need to take account of what is happening elsewhere in your data set. One important characteristic of a sample of scores is how much variation there is between them. Take a look at the scores for stroke and heart attack patients in Table 3.1. You should notice that there is much greater variability in the scores for the stroke patients than there is for the heart attack sufferers. We have represented the scores from the table in a graph in Figure 3.1.

You should be able to see from Figure 3.1 that the heart attack patients' scores seem to be bunched together between 20 and 35 whereas the stroke patients' scores are much more spread out and range between about 1 and 40. The variability in, or dispersion of, the data is an important characteristic of a sample and needs to be explored alongside the measures of central tendency. As you would expect with statisticians, there are a number of ways

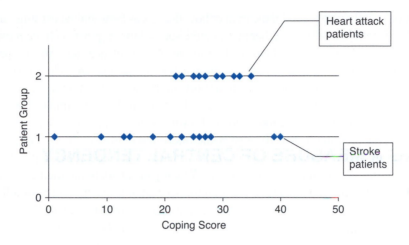

Figure 3.1   Coping scores for the stroke and heart attack patients

of examining the variability in the data and we will cover the most commonly used ones here.

The Range

Perhaps the simplest indication of how much the scores vary in a sample is to look at the minimum and maximum scores. For example, the minimum score for the stroke patients is 1 and the maximum is 40, whereas the minimum for the heart attack patients is 22 and the maximum is 35. It thus appears from these values that there is greater variability in the stroke patient sample. The *range* tells us what the difference is between the minimum and maximum scores in a sample, and is simply the maximum score minus the minimum score. And so the range for the stroke patients is 40 − 1 = 39. The range for the heart attack patients is 35 − 22 = 13.

Quartiles and the Interquartile Range

Whilst the range gives us a rough-and-ready guide to how much variability there is in the data, we often require a more fine-grained measure of the variability. The range is useful for telling us the variability in our sample from each of the extremes but it doesn't tell us much about how the scores vary between these extremities. Take a look at the following two sets of scores:

2	7	8	8	9	9	10	10	10	11	17	23	23	24	26
2	11	12	12	12	13	13	14	15	15	15	15	16	16	26

You can see that both sets of scores have the same range (26 − 2 = 24); however, in between these extremes the top set of scores are much more evenly spread out whereas the bottom set of scores are quite closely clustered between 11 and 16. Another problem with the range that might be apparent from the above two data sets is that it is influenced by extreme scores (in much the same way that the mean is). You should be able to see that for the bottom set of scores the extremes don't really give a good indication of how the scores between the extremes are spread out. Usually we might assume that there is not quite such a large gap between the most extreme scores and the ones adjacent to them in the sample. A way of dealing with the problem of extreme scores like this is to report a *trimmed range*. So, for example, in each sample you would remove the top and bottom scores and the report the range of the remaining scores, which would be 24 – 7 = 17 for the top sample and 16 – 11 = 5 for the bottom sample. These trimmed ranges give a much more realistic indication of how the scores vary within each sample.

A useful version of the trimmed range is the *interquartile range*. To understand this you first need to know how to calculate *quartiles* for a dataset. A good starting point for understanding quartiles is to think about the median. When you calculate the median you rank the scores in order of magnitude and then you find the score that is exactly in the middle. Half of the scores in your dataset are below the mean and half are above the mean. The median thus splits the dataset exactly in two. Quartiles do a similar job, but they split the dataset into four with equal numbers of scores in each quartile. The first step in working out the quartiles is to find the median. You then take the set of scores below the median and find the median of this set of scores – this would be your first quartile score. You next take the set of scores that fall above the median of the whole dataset and find the median of that set of scores – this is called the third quartile. The median of the whole dataset is now called the second quartile. As an example, let's work out the quartiles for the stroke patients' data from Table 3.1. These data are listed in Figure 3.2 in rank order (which is a necessary first step to finding the median).

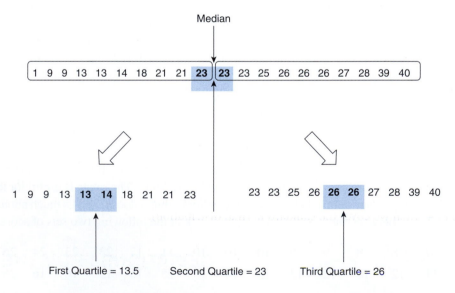

Figure 3.2　Process of calculating quartiles

The calculation of the quartiles is a little different when you have an odd number of participants in your sample. In Figure 3.3 we have taken the last score away from the sample to make it 19 patients rather than 20.

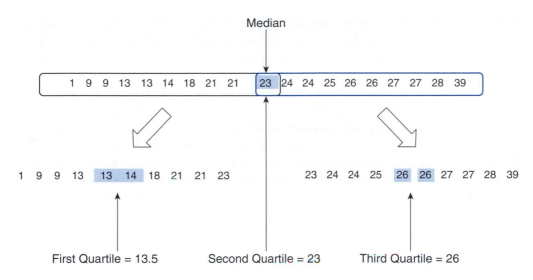

Figure 3.3   Process of calculating quartile when you have an odd number of scores

You should notice here that when we have an odd number of scores in the sample we include the median score in both the lower and upper halves of the sample to calculate the first and third quartiles. Rather surprisingly, there are actually a variety of ways of calculating quartiles and there doesn't seem to be a consensus on which is the best. SPSS uses a more complicated way than we have presented here and so don't worry too much if you notice slight differences between the values that you calculate and those that SPSS does.

When we discussed the range earlier we mentioned that often a better index of variability in your sample is a trimmed range rather than the actual range. Perhaps the most commonly reported trimmed range is the *interquartile range*.

The interquartile range is simply the third quartile minus the first quartile. Thus the interquartile range for the example above would be 26 − 13.5 = 12.5. The interquartile range contains the middle 50% of the scores that are in the sample. This is useful in statistics, as it has been shown for a large number of variables in the health sciences that the majority of the scores fall within the middle region of the sample (this will be explained in more detail in Chapter 4 when we cover the standard normal distribution).

DEVIATIONS FROM THE MEAN

The measures of variation and dispersion that we have covered so far tend to be based upon the distance between one score in a sample and another. Thus the range is the maximum score minus the minimum score, and the interquartile range is the score that cuts off the top 25% of scores minus the score that cuts off the bottom 25% of scores. An alternative way of thinking about variation and dispersion is to think about how much the scores in a sample cluster together. Examples of this sort of measure are the *variance* and the closely related *standard deviation*. Both of these statistics provide us with an indication of how closely the scores in a sample cluster around the middle of that sample, that is, how closely they cluster around the mean. These are both measures of deviation from the mean and are the most widely reported measures of variation. How do we calculate the variance and standard deviation? There is a mathematical formula for this but we will illustrate the calculation in a step-by-step fashion without referring to this formula here.

The first step in calculating the variance is to calculate the mean for a set of scores. We then subtract the mean from every score in the sample. This informs us how great or small the difference is between each score and the mean. It tells us how far each score *deviates* from the mean. What we want is some sort of average of these deviation scores, as this will give us an indication of the average amount by which the scores deviate from the mean. This is potentially useful as, if we have a small average deviation, then we know that the scores are clustered quite close to the mean, and if we have a large value, then it tells us that the scores in the sample are spread out a lot from the mean. OK then, the average of the deviations would be useful and so we could calculate this. There is a problem with this however. Whenever you calculate the deviations from the mean and add them up the total will be zero. Wow, isn't that interesting! Let us demonstrate this with the first ten scores from our data from the stroke victims in Table 3.1 (the mean for this is 23). These are presented in Figure 3.4.

Because the sum of the deviation scores for any sample is zero we cannot calculate a traditional mean for these deviation scores. Remember, when calculating a mean you add up the scores and then divide by the number of scores in the sample. When you add up deviation scores you always get zero and it is a mathematical impossibility to divide into zero, and so we cannot calculate a mean deviation score. The way that statisticians have solved this problem is to introduce an extra step before averaging the deviation scores. You have to square the deviation scores first, which removes any negative numbers from the deviation scores (because squaring any number gives you a positive number, Figure 3.5).

We can then calculate the mean for these scores, which is 61.4. This mean of the squared deviations from the mean is called the *variance* and it gives us an indication of how much the scores vary around the mean. The problem with this statistic is that it is not in the same units of measurement as the original scores. It is in the units squared. It would be better to have a measure of deviation which was in the original units of measurement. To get

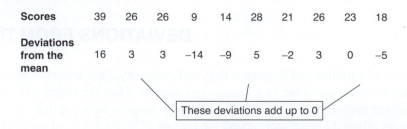

Figure 3.4   Illustration of deviations from the mean (mean = 23)

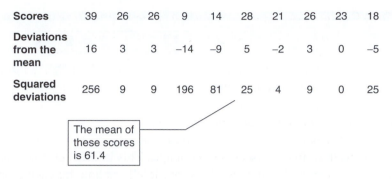

Scores	39	26	26	9	14	28	21	26	23	18
Deviations from the mean	16	3	3	−14	−9	5	−2	3	0	−5
Squared deviations	256	9	9	196	81	25	4	9	0	25

The mean of these scores is 61.4

Figure 3.5   Illustration of deviations and squared deviations

such a measure we can simply take the square root of the variance. This brings us back to the original units of measurement and the statistic is called the *standard deviation*. Thus if we take the square root of 61.4 we get a standard deviation of 7.84. We can say then that on average the scores in the sample deviate from the mean by about 7.84 units. The standard deviation is the most commonly reported measure of variation or dispersion reported by researchers, and so it is very important that you understand what it means. Whenever you report a mean it is good practice to also report the standard deviation. If you report a median then the standard deviation is not really appropriate (because it uses the mean not the median in its calculation) and so you should report either the range or the interquartile range.

Earlier in this chapter we mentioned the difference between descriptive and inferential statistics. Remember inferential statistics are where we want to draw conclusions about a population from our sample and descriptive statistics are where we are simply describing our sample. The standard deviation is a descriptive statistic and it gives us an indication of the variability in our sample. Often we want to report a standard deviation figure that is a better estimate of the variability in the population. Statisticians have found that the sample standard deviation that we have just illustrated tends to be an underestimate of the variability in the population and have found a simple way to correct this. When we calculate the average of the squared deviation scores (the step that leads us to the variance) we should divide the total of the squared deviations by the number of people in the sample minus 1, instead of by the number of people in the sample. When we make this adjustment to the calculation we get a standard deviation of 8.26 and this is probably a better estimate of the variation in the population than the sample standard deviation that we calculated earlier.

NUMERICAL DESCRIPTIVES IN SPSS

In SPSS, to obtain the descriptive statistics that we have covered here you need to click on *Analyze*, *Descriptive Statistics*, *Frequencies* (Screenshot 3.1).

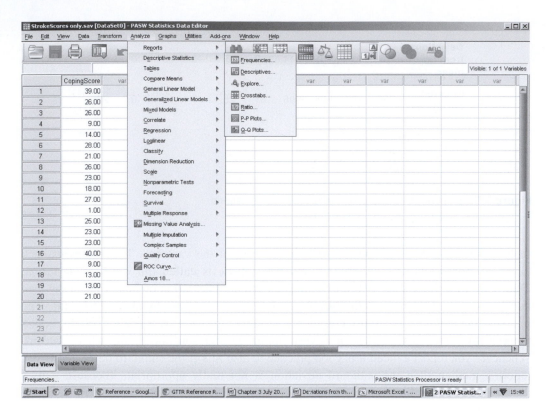

Screenshot 3.1

You will then be presented with a dialogue box (Screenshot 3.2).

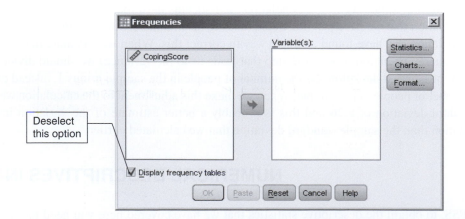

Screenshot 3.2

Highlight the variable that you want to calculate descriptive statistics for and click on the arrow in between the two boxes. This will move the variable across to the *Variable(s)* box. You should also deselect the *Display frequency tables* option as you don't need this for now. You will then need to tell SPSS what descriptive statistics you want to calculate. You do this by clicking on the *Statistics* button and this will open up another dialogue box (Screenshot 3.3).

Select all the descriptive statistics that you want SPSS to generate by clicking on the relevant tick boxes. You can see that we have requested the quartiles, mean, median, mode, standard deviation, variance, range, minimum and maximum. Then click on *Continue* and *OK* to run the analysis. You will be presented with the output in Screenshot 3.4.

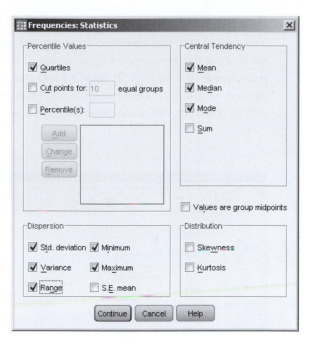

Screenshot 3.3

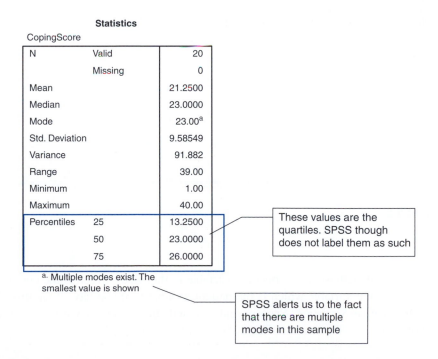

Screenshot 3.4

Frequencies

You should note that there are other ways of getting SPSS to calculate descriptive statistics for you but the *Frequencies* menu is one of the better ways. When you have two groups of participants like we have in Table 3.1 and you want descriptive statistics for both groups you can use the *Analyze*, *Descriptive Statistics*, *Explore* option. Before selecting this you should set out your data file in the same way as we have in Screenshot 3.5.

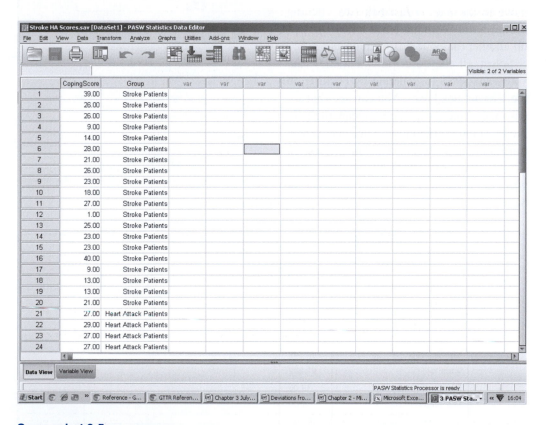

Screenshot 3.5

You can see that we have one dependent variable in this study which is the coping scores and one independent variable which is the patient group. Once you have done this click on *Analyze*, *Descriptive Statistics*, *Explore* and you will be presented with a dialogue box (Screenshot 3.6).

As the coping score is the dependent variable you need to move this to the *Dependent List* box by highlighting it and then clicking on the arrow button to the left of the *Dependent List* box. The *Group* variable is the independent variable and this needs to move to the *Factor List* box (we are sorry but SPSS has a bad habit of being inconsistent with the naming of the options in its dialogue box; independent variables are often called 'factors'). Once you have done this, click on the little circle to the left of the *Statistics* option in the *Display* section of the dialogue box. You can then click on *OK* to run the analyses (Table 3.2).

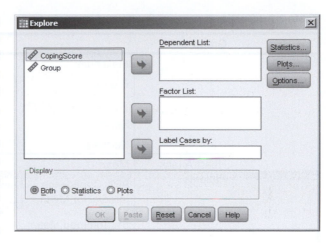

Screenshot 3.6

Table 3.2

Explore

Case Processing Summary

	Group	Cases					
		Valid		Missing		Total	
		N	Percent	N	Percent	N	Percent
Coping Score	Stroke Patients	20	100.0%	0	.0%	20	100.0%
	Heart Attack Patients	20	100.0%	0	.0%	20	100.0%

Group

Descriptives

	Group			Statistic	Std. error
Coping Score	Stroke Patients	Mean		21.2500	2.14338
		95% Confidence Interval for Mean	Lower Bound	16.7639	
			Upper Bound	25.7361	
		5% Trimmed Mean		21.3333	
		Median		23.0000	
		Variance		91.882	
		Std. Deviation		9.58549	
		Minimum		1.00	

Table 3.2   Cont'd

Group			Statistic	Std. error
	Maximum		40.00	
	Range		39.00	
	Interquartile Range		12.75	
	Skewness		−.030	.512
	Kurtosis		.338	.992
Heart Attack Patients	Mean		27.6500	.83122
	95% Confidence Interval for Mean	Lower Bound	25.9102	
		Upper Bound	29.3898	
	5% Trimmed Mean		27.5556	
	Median		27.0000	
	Variance		13.818	
	Std. Deviation		3.71731	
	Minimum		22.00	
	Maximum		35.00	
	Range		13.00	
	Interquartile Range		5.00	
	Skewness		.163	.512
	Kurtosis		−.662	.992

You can see that the sizeable table gives us a large number of descriptive statistics for each of our patient groups including the main ones that we have covered in this chapter so far. It is always useful here to check the *Minimum* and *Maximum* values as these often flag up when you have made an error in typing in your data.

GRAPHICAL STATISTICS

Think back to the analogy that we presented you with earlier about the blind date. Suppose you were trying to describe your date to a friend. A quick way of enabling your friend to know what your blind date looks like is to show them a picture (perhaps on Facebook). They can probably get a much clearer idea of your date's looks from a picture than from your description of them. The same can be true of certain aspects of data description. We used a picture earlier in this chapter to illustrate the difference between the variability of the stroke and heart attack patient coping scores (Figure 3.1). The first pictures, or as statisticians prefer to call them graphs and charts, that we will demonstrate are those that illustrate measures of central tendency. We will then move on to those which are designed to illustrate the variability in samples.

BAR CHARTS

A relatively simple way of comparing means from different groups is to generate a *bar chart*. Following the adage at the beginning of this section, the best way of explaining what a bar chart looks like is to present one (see Figure 3.6).

In many graphs there are two axes, a horizontal axis which is called the *x-axis* and a vertical axis called the *y-axis*. Usually in a bar chart the groups are identified on the *x*-axis and the dependent variable or score is marked on the *y*-axis. In a bar chart each group mean is indicated by a bar, and the height of the bar indicates the value of the mean. In order for us to work out the value of each mean we have to read horizontally across from the top of the line to the *y*-axis. For example in Figure 3.6 we can see that the mean for the stroke patients is about 21 and the mean for the heart attack patients is about 27. Bar charts can be a good way to illustrate a lot of information about your groups. For example, suppose you measured not only the coping of heart attack and stroke patients but also their stress levels and a self-rating of their physical wellbeing. A bar chart representing this data is given in Figure 3.7.

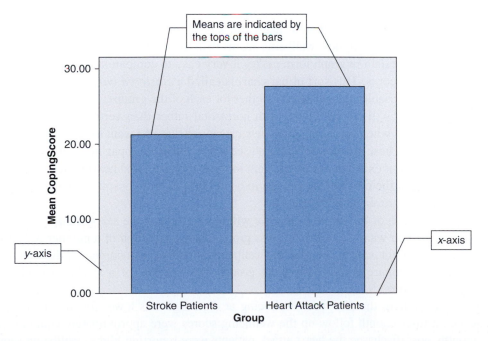

Figure 3.6 Bar chart showing mean coping scores for the stroke and heart attack patients

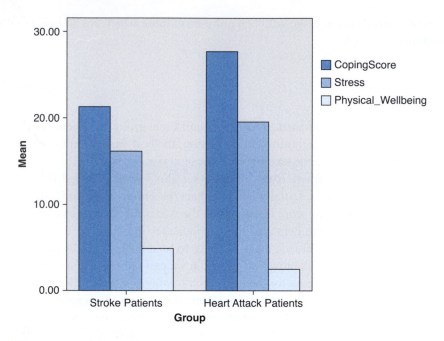

Figure 3.7   Bar chart of the means for stroke and heart attack patients for coping, stress and physical wellbeing scores

We can see from this graph that the heart attack patients had higher coping scores, higher stress scores and lower physical wellbeing scores than the stroke patients. You can see here that presenting the data in graph form makes it very easy to compare across the groups for the three sets of scores. This sort of bar chart is called a *clustered bar chart* as the scores on the different variables are clustered together for each of the groups.

Sometimes you will see bar charts with horizontal rather than vertical bars. These are particularly useful when you have quite a few categories that you want to represent and they have long labels. These are also quite often used when you are comparing groups on a time-related variable. For example, we might want to compare stroke and heart attack patients on the time taken for them to recover enough to be discharged from hospital. The graph might look like the one presented in Figure 3.8.

The final version of the bar chart that we will demonstrate is the *stacked bar chart*. This is useful when you want to compare across groups the contribution of a number of factors. For example, I might want to examine the wellbeing of patients at a number of different time intervals and compare across the patient groups. An example of a stacked bar chart is presented in Figure 3.9.

You can see here that the mean wellbeing at discharge was lower for the heart attack patients. At three-month follow-up the wellbeing scores were approximately equal and by six months post-discharge the heart attack patients were reporting higher wellbeing scores than stroke patients.

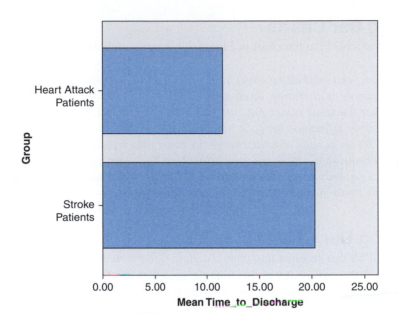

Figure 3.8 Horizontal bar chart showing mean number of days to discharge for stroke and heart attack patients

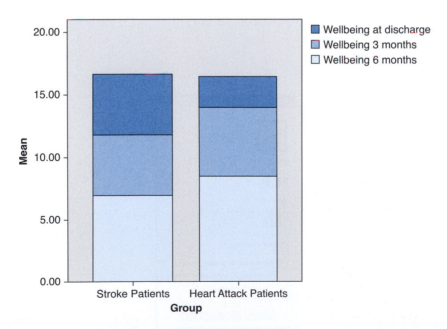

Figure 3.9 Bar chart showing the mean wellbeing of stroke and heart attack patients at discharge and at three and six months post-discharge

Reporting Bar Charts

If you wanted to report the bar chart in Figure 3.9 in a research report you might write:

> *Figure 3.9 shows a stacked bar chart for the stroke and heart attack patients illustrating the wellbeing scores at discharge, three-month follow-up and six-month follow-up. The chart suggests that the heart attack patients had lower wellbeing scores at discharge but that there was little difference between the stroke and heart attack patients at three-month follow-up. By six months after discharge the heart attack patients were reporting slightly higher wellbeing scores than the stroke patients. The chart thus suggests that whilst the heart attack patients have lower feelings of wellbeing at discharge they catch up and even overtake the stroke patients by six months post-discharge.*

Generating Bar Charts in SPSS

All graphs in SPSS can be generated from the main *Graphs* menu. We are going to illustrate the generation of the various bar charts with the data presented in Table 3.3.

To generate bar graphs you need to select the *Graphs*, *Legacy Dialogs* and *Bar* options and you will be presented with the a dialogue box (Screenshot 3.7).

To generate a bar chart for one dependent variable (e.g. coping score) and one independent variable make sure that the *Simple* and *Summaries for groups of cases* options are selected and then click on the *Define* button. You will be presented with another dialogue box (Screenshot 3.8).

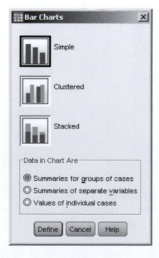

Screenshot 3.7

Table 3.3 Scores for stroke and heart attack patients for coping, stress, number of days to discharge and wellbeing at discharge, three-month and six-month follow-up

Stroke patients						Heart attack patients					
Coping	Stress	Wellbeing at discharge	Time to discharge	Wellbeing at 3 months	Wellbeing at 6 months	Coping	Stress	Wellbeing at discharge	Time to discharge	Wellbeing at 3 months	Wellbeing at 6 months
39	15	4	18	7	8	27	15	1	11	3	9
26	22	5	21	7	7	29	23	3	5	5	8
26	16	3	7	4	5	27	17	4	4	6	7
9	9	6	17	8	7	27	17	3	15	6	8
14	15	1	19	1	10	33	22	2	15	3	10
28	18	3	16	1	5	22	23	3	9	4	8
21	13	5	20	8	5	29	25	2	13	5	9
26	10	5	24	10	9	23	21	2	9	8	8
23	7	7	28	5	8	29	25	2	14	7	7
18	25	5	22	6	8	30	18	3	19	6	9
27	14	3	24	3	5	27	10	3	12	5	9
1	11	5	10	3	6	23	14	2	8	7	9
25	15	7	15	4	6	26	19	2	13	6	11
23	17	6	16	8	9	35	18	1	12	3	8
23	15	7	22	2	7	25	17	2	11	6	7
40	32	1	27	7	8	32	13	4	16	5	9
9	13	5	13	2	7	32	26	2	13	6	7
13	24	9	24	0	6	22	23	1	13	6	9
13	16	5	32	6	6	25	21	4	17	6	9
21	16	6	32	5	7	30	22	3	2	7	9

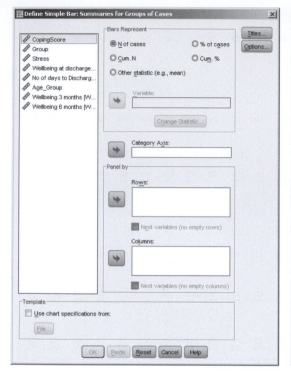

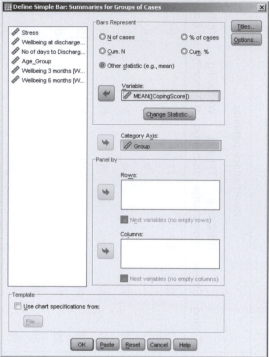

Screenshot 3.8   **Screenshot 3.9**

First you can move the grouping (independent variable) to the *Category Axis* box. Next you need to let SPSS know what the bars represent. We want the bars to represent the mean coping scores and so you should click on the *Other statistic (e.g. mean)* option and then move the coping variable across to the box that become active. The dialogue box should look like Screenshot 3.9.

You should then click on the *OK* button and you will be presented with a bar chart similar to that presented in Figure 3.6.

To generate clustered bar charts you should again select the *Graphs*, *Legacy Dialogs* and *Bar* options and then select the *Clustered* and *Summaries of separate variables* options (Screenshot 3.10).

Click on the *Define* button and then move the Group variable to the *Category Axis* box and the dependent variables that you want to display on the graph to the *Bars Represent* box (Screenshot 3.11).

Once you have done this you should click on the *OK* button to generate the graph. This should look similar to the one presented in Figure 3.7.

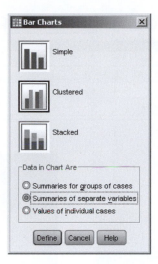

Screenshot 3.10

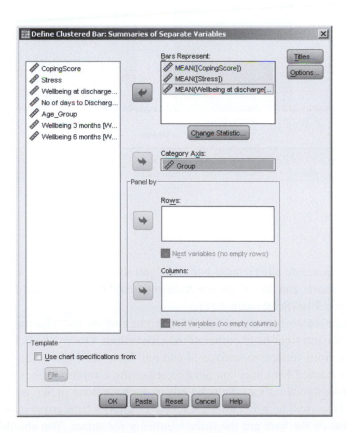

Screenshot 3.11

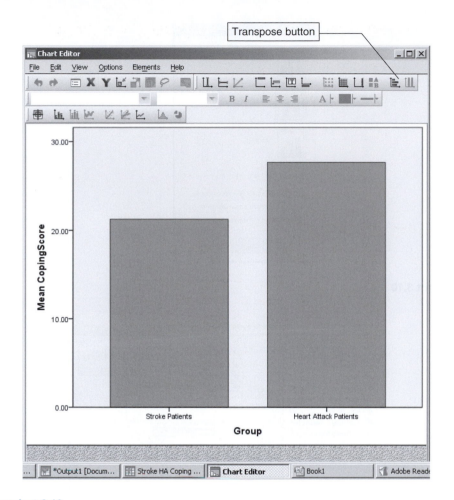

Screenshot 3.12

If you want to generate a horizontal bar chart you should proceed as we suggested for a simple bar chart above, and then when you have generated the bar chart, double click on it to activate the chart editor (Screenshot 3.12).

You can change the orientation of the chart by clicking on the 'transpose' button which can be found in the top right-hand corner of the chart editor. Once you click on this your bar chart will switch from vertical to horizontal and will look like Figure 3.8.

To generate a stacked bar chart you need to select the *Graphs*, *Legacy Dialogs* and *Bar* menus and then set up the options dialogue box as we have done in Screenshot 3.13.

In this analysis we will be generating a stacked bar chart where group is on the *x*-axis and the stacking units of the bars are the three wellbeing measures. You should then click on *OK* and you will be presented with the graph from Figure 3.9.

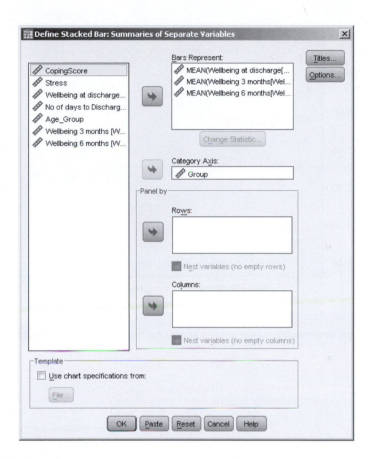

Screenshot 3.13

LINE GRAPHS

Another useful means of representing means is by line graphs. An example of a line graph which is equivalent to the simple bar chart we presented in Figure 3.7 is shown in Figure 3.10.

We have to admit that this is not a particularly good example of a line graph though. Usually we would use such graphs when there is more than one line to present. Figure 3.11 shows a line graph of the wellbeing scores at the three different time points, and this illustrates the value of the line graph more effectively.

If you have a look at Figure 3.11 you will see that at discharge the heart attack patients felt worse than the stroke patients; however, after three months the heart attack patients seem to be improving in physical wellbeing but the stroke patients do not. Both groups have improved substantially at six months but heart attack patients have improved more so. This illustrates

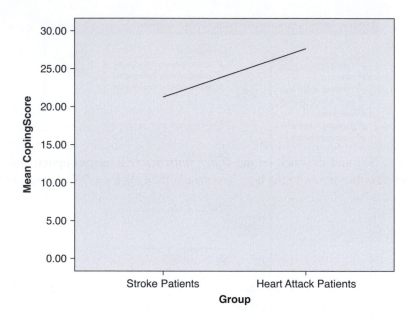

Figure 3.10 Graph to show the mean coping scores for the stroke and heart attack patients

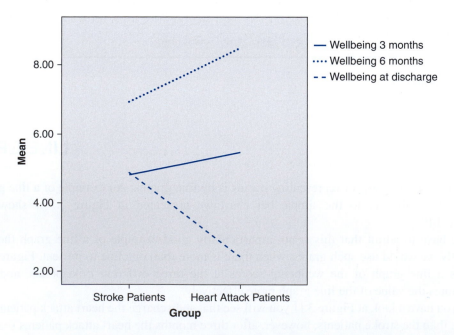

Figure 3.11 Graph to show the mean wellbeing ratings at discharge, three months and six months for the stroke and heart attack patients

the beauty of graphs, as it is pretty easy by looking at this graph to get a good feel for what has happened to both groups over the course of the study.

Generating Line Graphs in SPSS

Generating line graphs in SPSS is similar to generating bar charts. You have to select the *Graphs*, *Legacy Dialogs* and *Line* menus and then choose the *Simple* and *Summaries of groups of cases* options. As with the bar chart, move the grouping variable across to the *Category Axis* box and the click on the *Other statistics (e.g. mean)* option and move the coping score variable across to the box. You should then click on *OK* and you will then be presented with a line graph resembling that presented in Figure 3.10.

Example from the Literature

A nice example of a line graph illustrating a trend across time is presented in a report by Lester et al. (2010). In this study they were interested in assessing the impact of removing financial incentives on some quality of clinical care indicators in hospital and community settings. One of the graphs that they include is presented as Figure 3.12.

This graph showed the impact of financial incentives on the number of adults screened for diabetic retinopathy over a nine-year period. The graph shows that during the first five years of the study, where there were financial incentives to screen, there was an increase in the number of adults screened. The financial incentives for screening then stopped, and in the following four years screening rates fell from about 88% to 80%.

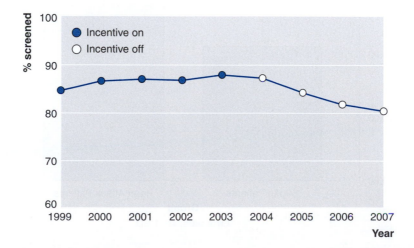

Figure 3.12 Percentage of adults aged ≥31 screened for diabetic retinopathy in relation to financial incentives

INCORPORATING VARIABILITY INTO GRAPHS

The bar charts and line graphs that we have shown have all illustrated the ease with which we can use graphs to present information about group means (we can also generate similar graphs to present median and modes if we wanted to). We can, though, also include information relating to the variability within our groups in such graphs. If we wanted to (and many authors do) we can add a graphical indication of the standard deviations to line and bar charts. Figure 3.13 shows a bar graph where we have included lines which represent the standard deviations for each group.

This chart is similar to the one presented in Figure 3.6 but we have added lines to each bar which represent the standard deviations. The lines within each bar give us a good indication of how much variability there is in the data. The longer the lines the greater the variability within the sample. We can see from Figure 3.13 that there is a lot more variability in the stroke patients' data than there is in the heart attack patients' data. We can present the same information if we wish in a line graph (Figure 3.14).

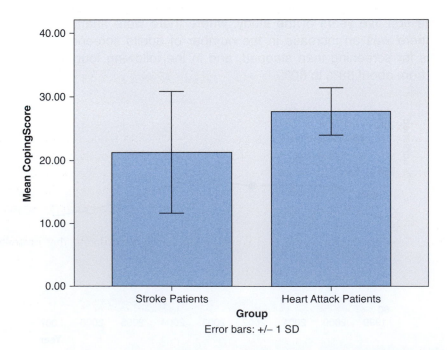

Figure 3.13 Bar chart showing the means and standard deviations of coping scores for heart attack and stroke patients

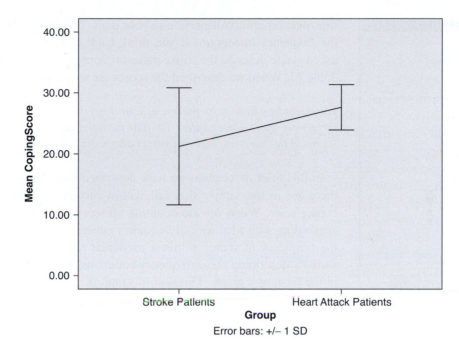

Figure 3.14 Line graph showing the means and standard deviations of coping scores for heart attack and stroke patients

GENERATING GRAPHS WITH STANDARD DEVIATIONS IN SPSS

To include the standard deviation in a line graph (this is what you would have to do to include standard deviations on bar charts too) follow the instruction given earlier for generating a simple line graph. Before you finish and run the analysis you should click on the *Options* button and then click on the *Display error bars* option. Once you have done this you need to select the option and change the multiplier to '1'. The dialogue box should be set up as in Screenshot 3.14.

Click on *Continue* and then *OK* and you will get a graph similar to that presented in Figure 3.14.

GRAPHS SHOWING DISPERSION – FREQUENCY HISTOGRAM

So far we have described graphs that are used to illustrate measures of central tendency. In this section we will introduce you to two graphical techniques that have been developed to

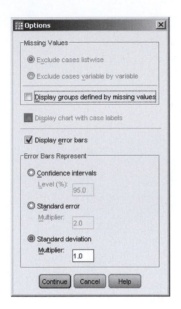

Screenshot 3.14

illustrate variability/dispersion in your data. The first of these is the frequency histogram. If you think back to Activity 3.1 we asked you to describe the stroke patients coping data presented in Table 3.1. When we described the scores we wrote the following

You might be a little more precise in your description by saying that there were three scores below 10, four between 10 and 19, eleven scores in the twenties, and two scores above 30.

In this brief description we have described how many scores there are in the sample that fall within certain values on the coping scale. When you are counting up scores in this way you are dealing with what we call *frequency counts*. We are counting the frequency of scores within a particular range. Rather than verbally describing these frequency counts we can present these in the form of a graph. This sort of graph is called a *frequency histogram*. At its basic level a frequency histogram is a graph of the frequency of each score within a sample. In Table 3.4 we have re-presented the stroke patients' coping scores.

To generate a frequency histogram we need to count up how many times each score appears in the sample dataset. And so we have one score of 1, two scores of 9, two scores of 13, one score of 14, one score of 18, two scores of 21, three scores of 23, one score of 25,

Table 3.4　Coping scores for the stroke patients

Stroke patients	
39	27
26	1
26	25
9	23
14	23
28	40
21	9
26	13
23	13
18	21

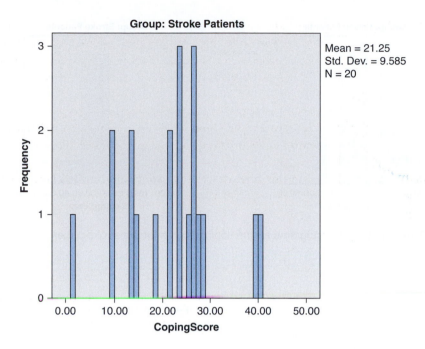

Figure 3.15   Frequency histogram of the coping scores for the stroke patients

three scores of 26, one score of 27, one score of 28, one score of 39 and one score of 40. We can represent these in graph form by generating a bar chart which has the scores on the *x*-axis and the frequency of occurrence on the *y*-axis. The histogram representing the stroke patients' coping scores is presented in Figure 3.15.

The height of each bar represents the number of times each score appears in the sample. Where there is no bar this means that there were no scores of this value in the sample. The highest bar in the histogram gives us an indication of the mode. You can see from Figure 3.15 that there are two bars that are equally the highest, and this suggests that there are two modes. We can vary the way we count up the scores for displaying on the histogram. Usually, we can make the graph neater by trying to remove the gaps between bars. To do this we might count up the number of scores falling within a range of values on the variable of interest. So for example we might break the scale up into intervals of five units and count how many scores fall within that range. Specifying the range within which we are counting the scores is called 'binning' and we can vary the 'bins' in a histogram to ensure a more concise presentation of the frequency of occurrence of scores. For the graph in Figure 3.16a we have used intervals of five scores (i.e. 1–5, 6–10, etc.) and in Figure 3.16b we have used intervals of ten scores (i.e. 1–10, 11–20, etc.).

You should be able to see that when we increase the width of the 'bins' the frequency histograms become neater. You can easily adjust the bin widths in SPSS and will learn by experience how best to present your frequency histograms. The histogram in Figure 3.15 is

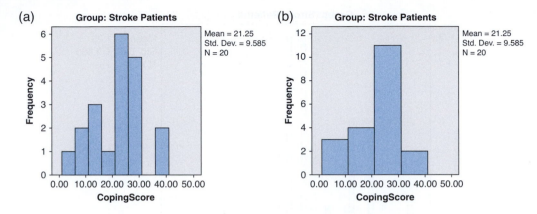

Figure 3.16 Frequency histograms for the coping scores for the stroke patients with 'bin' widths of five and ten

not particularly good as it has far too many spaces between bars. The histograms in Figure 3.16 are much better and we would probably settle on the one with bin widths of five (Figure 3.16a).

You can see from the histograms in Figure 3.16 that we have more scores in the mid-range (between 20 and 30) than we do in either of the extremes of the scale. This is a common feature of data that we collect in the health sciences and we will come back to this in Chapter 4.

Generating Frequency Histograms in SPSS

You can generate frequency histograms through the *Graphs* menu in SPSS. Click on the *Graphs*, *Legacy Dialogs* and *Histogram* menus and you will be presented with a dialogue box (Screenshot 3.15).

You need to highlight the variable that you are interested in and then move it across to the *Variable* box. You can see that we have moved across the *CopingScore* variable. You can then click on *OK* to generate the histogram. When you do this you will be presented with the graph given in Figure 3.17.

SPSS tries to work out the best bin width to display the histogram. You might want to change this, and if you do you need to double click on the graph to start the graph editor. Then double click on one of the bars and it will bring up a dialogue box (Screenshot 3.16).

To change the width of the bins click on the *Binning* tab and then select the *Custom* option. Click on the *Interval width* option and type in the bin width that you wish to display. We have chosen a bin width of five. You can also change the point where the first bar will start from (this is called the anchor). We have changed the anchor to 1. Click on *Apply* and then close the graph editor and you will now have your histogram customised to how you want it.

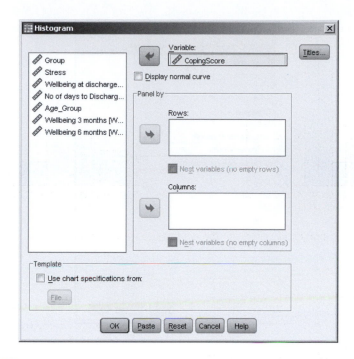

Screenshot 3.15

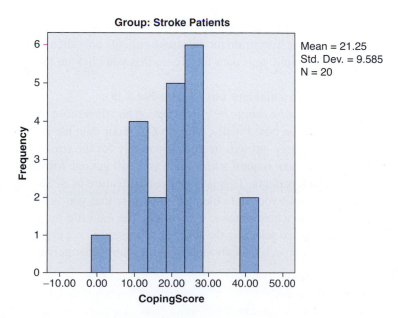

Figure 3.17

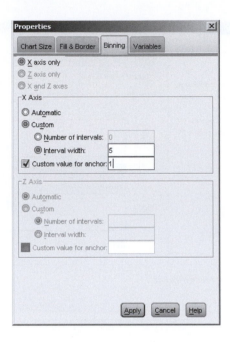

Screenshot 3.16

We should note here that we have glossed over a little issue with regards to generating the histogram for the stroke patients only. If you follow the instructions above you will get a histogram which includes all the participants (both stroke and heart attack patients) mixed together. If you want to get the histogram for the stroke patients only then there are two ways of doing this. The first is to split your data file. To do this you click on the *Data*, *Split File* options (Screenshot 3.17).

You will be presented with a dialogue box (Screenshot 3.18).

You should select the *Organise output by groups* option and then move the *Group* variable across to the *Groups Based on* box. Finally, click on *OK*. Your data file is now split in two. All analyses that you now carry out will be done separately for the stroke patients and the heart attack patients. If you now request a histogram you will get one for the stroke patients and one for the heart attack patients. This is a very useful feature of SPSS, but you have to remember when you have split your data file and make sure that you 'unsplit' it when you want to run analyses on the whole dataset. You unsplit the data file by going back to the *Data*, *Split File* option and then selecting the *Analyze all cases, do not create groups* option. We will cover the second approach to analysing the two groups separately in the next section on box-plots.

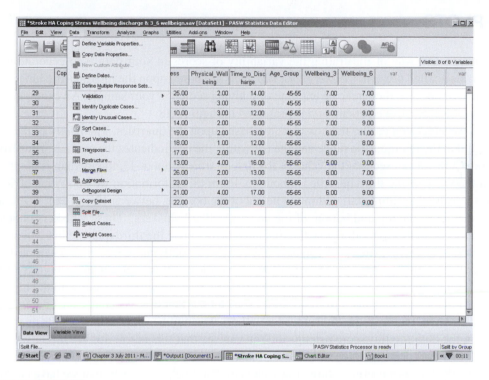

Screenshot 3.17

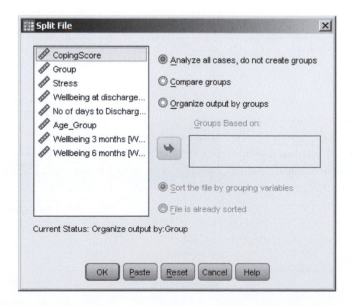

Screenshot 3.18

BOX-PLOTS

An alternative way of illustrating the variability of scores in your data is to generate *box-plots*, also called *box and whisker plots*. Box-plots are based upon the interquartile range and are useful because they indicate extreme or outlying scores in your sample. An example of a box-plot for the stroke patient data is presented in Figure 3.18.

As we suggested earlier the box-plots are based upon the quartiles. The height of the box is equal to the interquartile range and the bar within the box indicates the median. Thus from Figure 3.18 we can see that the value of the first quartile is about 13, the median is about 23 and the value of the third quartile is about 26. From this information we know that 50% of the scores in the sample fall within the height of the box (i.e. between 13 and 26). The lines coming out of the top and bottom of the box are called 'whiskers'. These whiskers indicate the range of scores that fall below the first quartile or above the third quartile but which are not classed as being extreme. If you have any extreme or outlying scores in your sample then these will be displayed on your box-plot. An illustration of this is presented in Figure 3.19.

The data represented in Figure 3.19 is the same as that in Figure 3.18 but with the highest score in the dataset changed from 40 to 62. You can see that this extreme score is now indicated by an 'o' on the graph ('o' stands for outlier). The number next to the 'o' tells us which row in the data file this score belongs to. You can see that this is row 16. We might want to check this data point to make sure that we have not made an error when we entered the data into SPSS. This is a useful feature of box-plots in that it helps us verify that we have entered the data correctly.

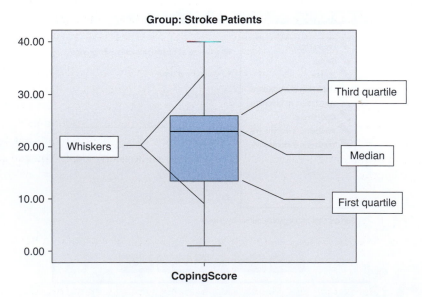

Figure 3.18   Box-plot of the coping scores for the stroke patients

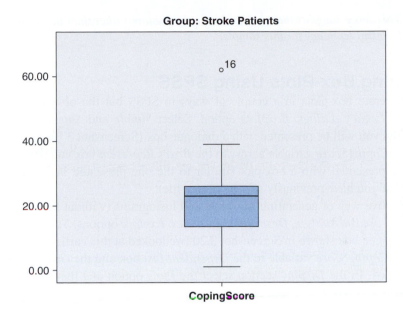

Figure 3.19   Box-plot illustrating an outlying score in the dataset

There is another reason why we would want to identify outliers. If you think back to the discussion of the mean earlier in the chapter you will recall that we said that the mean is heavily influenced by extreme or outlying scores. This is true of many of the statistical techniques that we cover in this book and so you need to check your data for such outliers. The box-plot is a useful way of doing this. The box-plot identifies outliers as those that are more than one and a half times the interquartile range above or below the edges of the box. The interquartile range for the box-plot in Figure 3.19 is 12.75. One and a half times this is 19.13, and so an outlier is a score that is greater than 19.13 + 26 (which is the third quartile) or a score that is less than 13 (the first quartile) – 19.13 . All such outliers will be displayed on the graph. If you have any scores in your data that fall outside the edges of the box but are not outliers then these are within the length of the whiskers on the graph. The highest score above the box but which is not an outlier marks the end of the whisker and is called an 'adjacent score'. In the same vein, the lowest score below the box but which is not an outlier marks the end of the lower whisker and also is called an adjacent score. You can see from Figure 3.19 that we have adjacent scores of 1 and 40.

Reporting Box-Plots
If you were to include the box-plot in Figure 3.19 in a research report you might present it like this:

Figure 3.19 shows a box-plot for the stroke patients' coping scores. This box-plots shows that 50% of the scores fall between 17 and 26. It also shows that there is one outlying score

of 62. This score suggests that we should use the median rather than the mean as the measure of central tendency for this sample.

Generating Box-Plots Using SPSS

You can generate box-plots in a couple of ways in SPSS but the obvious way is to use the *Graphs*, *Legacy dialogs*, *Boxplots* option. Select *Simple* and *Summaries of separate variables* and you will be presented with a dialogue box (Screenshot 3.19).

Move the *CopingScore* variable across to the *Boxes Represent* box and then click on *OK*. You will be presented with a box-plot similar to the one presented in Figure 3.18 above (this is only if you have previously split your data file).

An alternative way of generating box-plots and histograms (without having to split your data file) is to use the *Analyze*, *Descriptive statistics*, *Explore* options. You will be presented with the dialogue box shown in Screenshot 3.20 (we looked at this earlier in the chapter).

Move the *CopingScore* variable to the *Dependent List* box and the *Group* variable to the *Factor List* box. In the *Display* section select the *Plots* option and then click on the *Plots* button. You will be presented with another dialogue box (Screenshot 3.21).

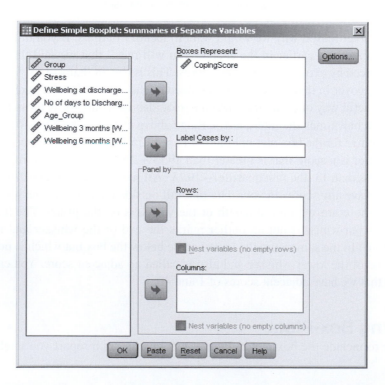

Screenshot 3.19

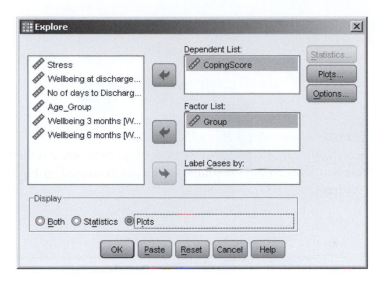

Screenshot 3.20

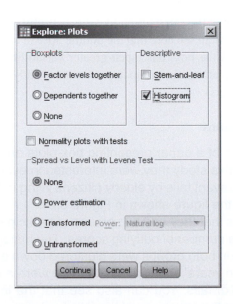

Screenshot 3.21

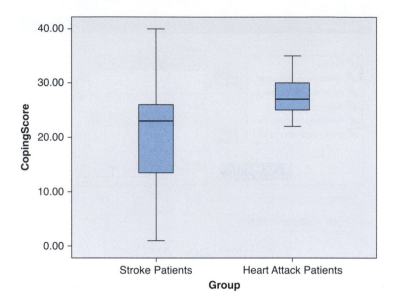

Figure 3.20

Deselect the *Stem-and-leaf* option and select the *Histogram* one and then click on *Continue* followed by *OK*. You will be presented with separate histograms for the two groups as well as a box-plot graph which contains the box-plots for both groups side-by-side (Figure 3.20).

Presenting the box-plots in the same graph like this is useful, as it allows you to compare across your two groups. We can see here that the middle 50% of scores for the stroke patients (indicated by the height of the box) has much greater variability than for the heart attack patients. We can also see that neither group has extreme or outlying scores (there are no 'o' markers beyond the whiskers).

Example from the Literature

There is a nice example of a paper presenting box-plots and histograms written by Logan et al. (2010). In this study they were interested in evaluating a service which was designed to help prevent falls by elderly citizens living in the community. In their results they presented the figure shown in Figure 3.21.

You can see from this that they had two groups of participants and in both groups the box-plots illustrate a number of outlying scores. The histograms suggest that the majority of participants in both groups were clustered down at the bottom end of the 'Rate of falls per person years' scale, although there were a number of participants who experienced a lot of falls. You can also see that the intervention group were more tightly clustered at the lower end of the falls scale.

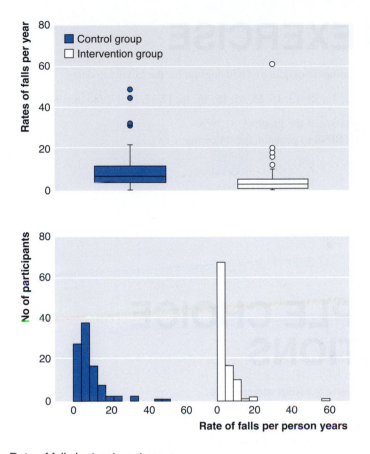

Figure 3.21 Rate of falls by treatment group

Summary

In this chapter we have started to get to grips with analysing data. We have covered a range of statistical techniques that helps you get to know your data really well. If you use these techniques appropriately you will have a really good understanding of the meaning of your data, and you will be able to present meaningful descriptive statistics when you present your data in a research report. In the next chapter we will start to explore what our sample data might say about the wider population.

SPSS EXERCISE

Have a go at generating a box-plot and a histogram for the following data:

12, 13, 13, 13, 15, 15, 15, 15, 16, 16, 17, 17, 17, 17, 18, 18, 19, 20, 32

Give your interpretation of the graphs.
Additionally, get SPSS to generate the following:

- Mean
- Median
- Mode
- Range
- Standard deviation
- Variance
- Quartiles

MULTIPLE CHOICE QUESTIONS

1. Why are descriptive statistics so important?
   a) They allow us to get to know our data
   b) They allow us to assess our blind dates
   c) They allow us to describe our data to others
   d) Both a) and c) above

2. Which of the following is not a measure of central tendency?
   a) Mean
   b) Range
   c) Mode
   d) Median

3. If you wanted to plot the frequency of occurrence of the scores in your sample which of the following would you use?
   a) Box-plot
   b) Line graph
   c) Histogram
   d) None of the above

4. In a box-plot the length of the box is equal to which of the following:
   a) Variance
   b) Range
   c) Interquartile range
   d) Standard deviation

5. What could you do with a bar chart if the category labels on your *x*-axis were too long?
    a) Use fewer categories
    b) Use a line graph instead
    c) Don't bother graphing the data
    d) Change the orientation to a horizontal bar chart

6. What percentage of the scores in a sample fall between the first and third quartiles?
    a) 25%
    b) 50%
    c) 75%
    d) 100%

Questions 7, 8 and 9 relate to the following box-plots:

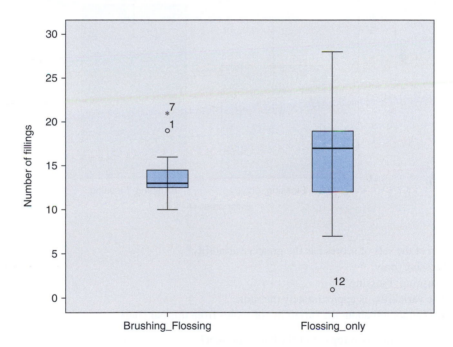

7. Which condition has the greater variability in terms of number of fillings?
    a) Brushing_Flossing
    b) Flossing_only
    c) The variability is roughly the same
    d) We can't tell anything about the variability of scores from this box-plot

8. From which rows in the data file do the outlying scores come from?
    a) 1, 5, 30
    b) 3, 5, 8
    c) 1, 7, 12
    d) We can't tell from the box-plots which rows the outliers are from

9. Which set of scores has the highest median?
   a) Brushing_Flossing
   b) Flossing_only
   c) The medians are equal
   d) We can't tell about the medians from this box-plot

Questions 10 and 11 relate to the following bar chart

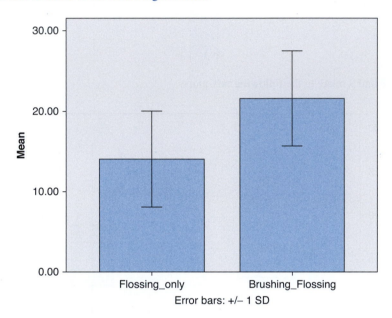

Error bars: +/– 1 SD

10. Which of the sets of scores has the greater variability?
    a) Flossing_only
    b) Brushing_Flossing
    c) The variability is approximately the same
    d) We cannot tell about the variability of scores from this bar chart

11. What do the lines coming out of the bars represent?
    a) The mean
    b) The interquartile range
    c) The standard deviation
    d) None of the above

Questions 12, 13 and 14 refer to the following graph:

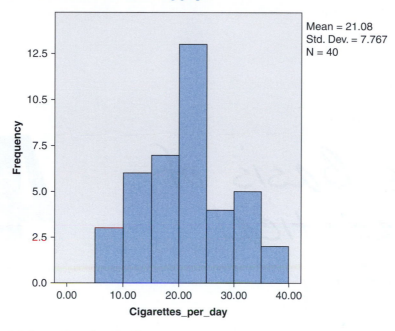

Mean = 21.08
Std. Dev. = 7.767
N = 40

12. What is this form of graph called?
    a) Histogram
    b) Bar chart
    c) Box-plot
    d) None of the above

13. What is the bin width for this graph?
    a) 1
    b) 2
    c) 5
    d) 10

14. What are the least frequently occurring scores?
    a) 5–10
    b) 10–15
    c) 20–25
    d) None of the above

15. What are the mean, median and mode of this set of scores:
    6, 5, 7, 9, 11, 15, 17, 5, 8
    a) 6.5, 11, 17
    b) 9.22, 8, 5
    c) 7.45, 15, 11
    d) None of the above

The Basis of Statistical Testing

4

Overview

In this chapter we will be explaining the concepts important for an understanding of null hypothesis significance testing. Although we won't be teaching you the formulae for the statistical tests that we cover in the book, we think that it is important that you understand the rationale behind the approach taken by the majority of researchers when analysing their data. Thus in this chapter you will learn about:

- Samples and populations
- Sampling error
- Using probabilities in statistical testing
- Null hypothesis significance testing
- Statistical significance
- Normal and the standard normal distribution
- Power
- Confidence intervals

In order to understand the concepts that we present in this chapter you need to make sure that you have understood the features of research that we highlighted in Chapter 1 and the descriptive statistics that we covered in Chapter 3.

INTRODUCTION

In Chapter 1 we described some of the important features of research, including different types of variables and different ways of designing studies (e.g. between-participant versus within-participant designs). In Chapter 3 we started showing you how we can analyse the data that we have obtained in our research. The sorts of analyses that we covered were descriptive statistics and were techniques that we use to get to know what our sample data are telling us. We suggested in Chapter 3 that there were other types of statistical techniques that we can use, and which help us draw conclusions about the wider populations from which our samples were selected. These are called inferential statistics. In this chapter we will be explaining some fundamental ideas which will allow you to understand the purpose of and rationale for inferential statistics.

Before moving on to the meaty stuff we will describe a hypothetical study which we will use to illustrate the important concepts underlying inferential statistics. Let's assume that we are interested in the impact of hearing aids on a person's social anxiety. There is some evidence that hearing impairment seems to be related to social anxiety (e.g. see Knutson and Langsing, 1990) and so we might expect that if we can improve a person's hearing ability then we may reduce their fear of social situations. We might identify everyone in the country who is on a waiting list for their first hearing aid (of course, this would be relatively easy if the UK National Health Service had a centralised computer system that worked properly). We could then randomly select, say 40 people, from these hearing impaired patients, and randomly assign them to either a group where they get a hearing aid immediately or to a group who have to wait a little while before they can get their hearing aid (this is called the *waiting list control group*). Here we have one intervention group (getting a hearing aid) and one control group. We could then measure social anxiety using a questionnaire (e.g. the Social Avoidance and Distress Scale; Watson and Friend, 1969). We would do well to measure social anxiety at two time points for both groups. We would measure social anxiety before the patients received their hearing aids and then at some time later, say at one-month follow-up. We would also measure the social anxiety of the control group at similar times. We might hypothesise that the hearing aid group would have lower social anxiety scores than the waiting list control group at one-month follow-up. The design of the study would thus look like Figure 4.1.

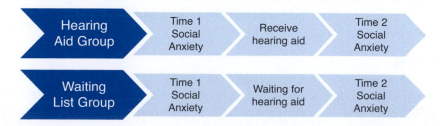

Figure 4.1   Design of the social anxiety and hearing aid study

This is a typical sort of design in the health sciences and is called an experimental design. We introduced this sort of research design in Chapter 1. If you adhere to certain strict design considerations whilst carrying out the study (e.g. random allocation of participants to conditions) you could also call the design a randomised control trial (RCT). We cover these sorts of design further in Chapter 14.

SAMPLES AND POPULATIONS

The description of the hearing aid study highlights two fundamental concepts for statistics, *samples* and *populations*. A population could refer to everyone in a particular country, e.g. the population of Scotland, or it could refer to everyone in a particular village, e.g. the population of Creswell in Derbyshire (UK). In statistical terms, however, a population refers to everyone in a specified target group rather than a specific region. For example, all those people who have a hearing impairment and are waiting for a hearing aid, or all those people who have a particular disease (e.g. cholera). Actually, strictly speaking, in statistics 'populations' needn't even refer to people, and so if we were marine biologists we might be interested in the population of bottlenose dolphins or the population of great white sharks. Populations can even refer to inanimate objects such as the population of widgets used in cans of Guinness.

A sample refers to a selection of individuals from the population. And so I might select a sample of 15 Scots, or 15 people from Creswell in Derbyshire. I might select a sample of 40 people who have a hearing impairment but who are waiting for a hearing aid or 100 people who have cholera. These would all be selections of people from wider populations, they are all samples. In the health sciences the vast majority of research that is published involves samples rather than populations. Why might this be? Samples are convenient to work with for a number of reasons, but among these are:

a) They are cheaper than investigating populations
b) They are quicker to test than populations
c) They are easier to recruit than populations

Although samples are convenient to work with, researchers are usually much more interested in what happens in the population as a whole rather than just their samples. They usually want to try to generalise from their sample to the wider population.

Sampling

There are many ways of selecting people from the wider population to take part in our research. We will introduce a few of the more common sampling strategies here. Most of the statistical tests that we cover in this book assume that you have randomly selected participants from your population of interest. To do this you would need to identify all the people in your target population and then randomly select the number that you need for your research. This approach to selecting samples is called *simple random sampling*. Each member of the target population has an equal chance of being selected.

Although random sampling is a fundamental assumption underlying the use of many inferential statistical tests, this is rarely used in practice. Why is this so? It is rarely used because it is extremely difficult and can be time-consuming and very expensive. First of all you have to have identified all of the individuals in your population. Can you imagine trying to pull together a list of all of the people in the UK who currently have influenza? This would be extremely difficulty. Another problem is that for many studies we cannot simply randomly select participants and assume that they will definitely take part in our study. Research ethics stipulate that it is extremely desirable that human participants are given the opportunity to decline to participate in research. Thus, even though we may have randomly selected participants from the population, not all of those selected may take part, and this undermines the assumption of random selection.

A useful way around the problem of having to identify everyone in a particular population is to use a technique called *cluster sampling*. In this approach we would identify clustering units in the population. For example, we might look at boroughs in England, or UK National Health Service (NHS) primary care trusts (PCTs). We would then randomly select one or several of these smaller units, and then randomly select from the people within these smaller units. We could even refine this further by using *multistage clustering*. Here we would randomly select a small number of NHS PCTs, and then from within these PCTs we would randomly select a small number of primary care centres (e.g. family doctor surgeries), and from these centres randomly select individuals to be invited to participate in the study.

In practice, a large number of researchers do not seem to worry about this fundamental assumption of statistical tests and select their samples through means other than random sampling.

Opportunity Sampling

Opportunity sampling refers to selecting participants who just happen to be available at the time and the place that you are conducting your research. Thus if you were working in a particular hair loss clinic and you were interested in conducting an experimental study on the effectiveness of a new treatment for baldness you might ask all the patients that come to your clinic at the time you are conducting your study (they would of course have the opportunity to decline to take part).

Snowball Sampling

Snowballing is where you ask the people who have taken part in your study to refer you to other people that they know, so that you can also ask them to participate. This is a useful technique when you have limited contacts yourself.

Volunteer Sampling

Volunteer sampling is where you might advertise your study and wait for people who have read your advert to come forward to take part.

You should be able to see that these three ways of selecting participants are all non-random. If you or any researcher that you have read about has used such methods to select participants then you need to be aware of the increased problems in trying to generalise from your sample to your population. If we use non-random sampling then we really need to be sure that the sample that we have selected is representative of the population of interest. For example, if you recruited a sample of dementia patients with an average age of 95 this would not be an accurate representation of all the people who have dementia, the average age of whom is likely to be much lower than 95. Because this sample isn't representative of the wider dementia population we would need to be wary of generalising from our sample to the population. We discuss further issues relating to selecting representative samples later in this chapter and in Chapter 5.

How Generalisable Are Data?

Generalising from samples to populations is something that we all do quite naturally. Think about a group of people who have something in common, for example, scientists. We quite often have a view on what the typical person from this group (i.e. the typical scientist) is like. We might think of them as dull studious types who spend far too much time in their white coats in their laboratory. We do this 'stereotyping' quite often, and the process by which our views of groups of people come about can be the result of our experiences with only a few of those individuals. We generalise from a few individuals to all individuals of a particular group. Think about some common stereotypes; for example, all Englishmen have a stiff upper lip, all Yorkshiremen are careful with their money, all computer programmers are geeks, all bankers are … well you know what we mean! Drawing conclusions from samples to populations is a bit like this. We want to examine how our samples respond and then generalise this to the typical member of the target population. We like to think though that in health and medical research we do this in a more scientifically rigorous and appropriate way than would happen with normal social stereotyping!

Let us now return to our hearing aid intervention study. For the coming explanation we are going to focus on the data collected for both groups before the members of the intervention group were given the hearing aids. Some hypothetical data for both groups are presented in Table 4.1. These scores were all randomly selected from a population which has a mean social avoidance and distress score of 14.5; however, we usually don't know the population mean from which our samples have been selected.

We would like to know whether these scores are generally representative of all those patients who have a hearing impairment and are waiting for a hearing aid. Remember, we suggested that we might have identified all of these people from their medical records and randomly selected 20 for our intervention condition and 20 more for our waiting list

Table 4.1 Social avoidance and distress scores for the hearing aid and waiting list control groups before the intervention

Hearing aid group	Waiting list group
14	9
12	15
19	14
25	17
14	10
21	13
2	23
23	7
20	14
12	12
21	22
12	16
10	19
13	15
12	9
10	11
13	16
12	13
19	14
15	20

control condition. Because we have randomly selected participants from the wider population of those who are hearing impaired and waiting for a hearing aid (HIWHA), we do not really know whether the people we have chosen are representative of everybody in the HIWHA population. Another way of putting this is: Are the typical scores in these samples approximately the same as the typical scores in the HIWHA population? When we think about the typical score, we are generally talking about measures of central tendency and so here we will focus on the mean (we explained the mean in Chapter 3). Are the means for our sample approximately equal to the mean from the population? We are going to focus our attention in the forthcoming discussion on the score for the hearing aid group, but you need to bear in mind that what we explain is equally relevant to the waiting list control group.

The mean for the hearing aid group is 14.95. This is quite close to the mean from which these scores were randomly selected (14.5), and so we might conclude that these data are reasonably generalisable to the wider HIWHA population. The mean for the waiting list control group is an even better estimate of the wider population mean because it is 14.45. So here we have two samples which appear to be reasonably representative of the wider population. This needn't be the case though. Take a look at the data in Table 4.2.

Again, these scores were randomly selected from a population whose mean was 14.5. Here the mean for the hearing aid group is 11.9 and that for the waiting list group is 15.95. Neither of these means are as close as those in the previous table and you would perhaps

Table 4.2   A second sample of social avoidance and distress scores for the hearing aid and waiting list control groups before the intervention

Hearing aid group	Waiting list group
12	6
8	16
19	6
15	17
9	28
16	14
12	21
8	23
10	16
4	14
20	14
7	11
19	21
13	12
4	16
14	26
12	15
14	17
15	17
7	9

suggest that these samples might not be as representative of the underlying HIWHA population. We should emphasise here that the differences between the means of all of these samples and the underlying population are randomly generated differences. There is no systematic reason for these to be different from the population mean of 14.5. They are different because we have randomly selected them from the population. Because of this random factor in our sampling we are likely to get samples that are not exactly representative (in terms of the typical score) of the wider population. One of the difficulties we face in real world research is that we usually don't know what the typical score is in the wider population, and so we do not know how close our sample means are to the population means. We will return to this problem later in this chapter.

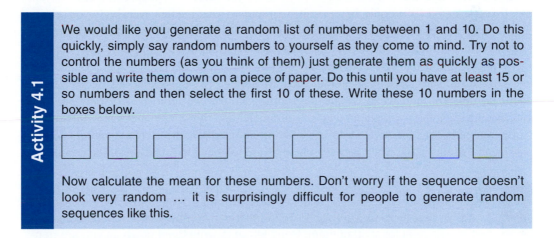

Activity 4.1

We would like you generate a random list of numbers between 1 and 10. Do this quickly, simply say random numbers to yourself as they come to mind. Try not to control the numbers (as you think of them) just generate them as quickly as possible and write them down on a piece of paper. Do this until you have at least 15 or so numbers and then select the first 10 of these. Write these 10 numbers in the boxes below.

Now calculate the mean for these numbers. Don't worry if the sequence doesn't look very random … it is surprisingly difficult for people to generate random sequences like this.

If you randomly generated an infinite array of numbers from 1 to 10 you would have a population of such numbers. You would find that the mean of this population is 5.5. You have thus effectively randomly chosen 10 numbers from this population. How close is the mean of your randomly generated sequence to the population mean of 5.5? Chances are that there is a least a little difference between your mean and 5.5. Much like the differences we observed earlier for our randomly generated social anxiety scores.

Sampling Error

The point that we are trying to get across here is that the samples that we select for our research are not necessarily truly representative of the wider population, and we need to bear this in mind when conducting our statistical analyses. Indeed we would expect samples to be slightly different to the whole population in at least some characteristics and these differences are the result of *sampling error*. Thus we would more often than not find that a random sample from a population will have a different mean score on the variable that we are interested in than the mean for the population. The difference between the sample mean and the population mean reflects sampling error. If you look back at the data in Tables 4.1 and 4.2

you will see that there are differences between each sample mean and the population mean. These differences all reflect sampling error.

It turns out though that if you randomly select enough people from a population, then you tend to get quite good estimates of the population statistics (like the population mean) that you are interested in. Thus, when designing research using samples you should ensure that you have enough participants so that you get an accurate reflection of the population that you are interested in. It has been shown by statisticians that the degree of sampling error is directly related to the number of people that you are sampling. This is quite logical when you think about it. Imagine that you were interested in the mean age of people who choose to have botox injections. If you randomly selected two people from the population of those who have had botox injections, it could be that by chance you select two people who are 100 years old. If you selected 100 people, however, it is difficult to imagine that everybody you selected would be 100 years old and thus the mean age that you calculate for the 100 people is likely to be a better estimate of the population mean age than that of the sample of two people.

We should point out here that statisticians have different labels for population statistics and sample statistics. Strictly speaking, when we are describing populations we need to talk about *parameters*, and when we are describing samples we refer to *statistics*. So, again strictly speaking, the population mean is a parameter and the sample mean is a statistic. It is worth remembering this when you are reading about research, as often authors refer to parameter estimates and when they say this they are referring to estimates of the population.

Activity 4.2

As in Activity 4.1 we asked you to generate a sequence of random numbers between 1 and 10. This time we want you to generate these numbers until you are confident that you have at least 50 of them. Don't forget to write them down as you are generating them. When you are sure that you have more than 50 please stop and then work out the mean of the first 50 of the numbers that you generated.

How does this compare to the mean for the 10 numbers that you generated in Activity 4.1? For most of you, the mean of the 50 numbers will be closer to the population mean of 5.5 than that of the 10 numbers. We should though stress that these are random occurrences and so for a small number of you the mean of the 10 numbers will be closer to the population mean than that of the 50 numbers. In general though, we tend to find that the larger the samples we have the closer to the population parameter your sample statistics will be. That is, there will be less sampling error.

If you want to see a demonstration of this then please go to the companion website where we have provided an Excel file which randomly generates samples from the population numbers from 1 to 10. You should see from this demonstration that larger samples tend to have means that are closer to the population mean of 5.5.

We have discussed here the influence of sampling error when estimating population parameters from sample statistics. There is another more subtle influence of sampling error on our research which we will now discuss. Let us return to the hypothetical study that we described earlier about hearing aids. Remember we had two groups of participants, where those in one group were given hearing aids and those in the other were put on a waiting list for hearing aids. One month after the first group of participants received their hearing aids all participants in the study were required to complete a social anxiety questionnaire. Some hypothetical data for this follow-up measure are presented in Table 4.3.

Your should recall we hypothesised that the hearing aid group would have lower social anxiety scores at follow-up than the waiting list control group. The means for the two groups of scores in Table 4.3 are 11.90 and 15.20 for the hearing aid and waiting list control

Table 4.3 Social avoidance and distress scores for the hearing aid and waiting list control groups one month after the intervention

Hearing aid group	Waiting list group
7	9
15	17
17	12
14	16
12	14
6	10
12	27
4	8
4	22
12	24
20	19
21	4
7	14
15	17
3	7
10	12
13	21
11	10
16	20
19	21

groups, respectively. It thus appears as though we have support for our hypothesis. Let us return to the issue of sampling error. Remember we explained that we would get differences between sample means and population means simply because of sampling error. The same is also true of two sample means. We can get random differences between two samples that we select from a population. Think back to the data presented in Table 4.2. Here we randomly selected two samples of data from a population which had a mean of 14.5 on the social anxiety scale, yet there was quite a large difference between the two means. Indeed the difference between the two means from Table 4.2 is larger than the difference between the two means from Table 4.3. How then do we know that the difference we have observed in Table 4.3 represents a genuine effect of receiving a hearing aid on levels of social anxiety?

Table 4.4 was created by randomly selecting two samples of 20 scores from a population of scores with a mean of 14.5, and doing this 50 times. The entries in Table 4.4 are the differences between these randomly selected samples of scores. In this table we have emboldened those differences that seem to be quite large. By quite large we mean a difference of three or more between the two randomly selected sample means. These large differences are interesting because they simply reflect random differences between two samples. There is no systematic underlying reason for these differences; they are simply the result of sampling error. So out of 50 potential studies we would have three of them that would lead to large differences between the samples, even when the populations from which they were selected did not differ (they were selected from a single population). This illustrates the fundamental problem that we as researchers face when trying to interpret our data. That is, do our sample data represent genuine differences between two populations or are they simply the result of sampling error? If they represent genuine differences then we might be able to conclude that

Table 4.4   Differences between 50 randomly generated pairs of samples of 20 scores drawn from a population with a mean of 14.5

0.85	2.05	0.95	1.85	1.85
1.60	0.85	2.45	1.20	0.90
0.40	0.80	2.00	0.50	0.50
1.25	2.7	0.75	1.20	1.10
1.3	0.40	2.30	0.65	1.30
3.00	1.85	1.8	1.20	1.00
0.30	1.05	1.15	0.60	0.45
1.05	2.60	0.75	1.25	0.05
2.25	2.90	0.90	1.35	1.25
3.90	2.40	0.15	**3.90**	2.85

something we have manipulated in the study has led to the difference. Thus, in our hypothetical study we might be able to suggest that the difference that we observe in our samples is the result of one of the groups having been given their hearing aids. The main reason that we need inferential statistics is so that we can determine whether any effects (e.g. differences between groups) that we observe in our samples might be due to sampling error, or as some people say due to *Chance*. You should note that there are many factors that might contribute to this sampling error. For example, participants might not follow instructions as you intended, or some participants might experience a traumatic event on the way to the testing session, or they might simply be worried about something and so not concentrate properly on what you want them to do. The problem with sampling error is that for any particular samples we don't know how much differences between them are the result of the factors that contribute to sampling error, and how much represents a genuine difference in the underlying population. We might summarise what we have covered so far in this chapter in Figure 4.2.

In Figure 4.2(a) we have a scenario where there are no differences between the two populations from which we have sampled (e.g. hearing impaired people with hearing aids and

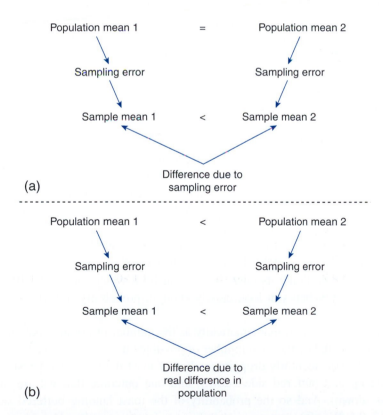

Figure 4.2 Possible explanations when observing differences between two sample means

hearing impaired people without hearing aids) but there is a difference observed between the two samples that we have drawn from these two populations. The difference between the samples in this case is the result of sampling error. In Figure 4.2(b), though, we have a difference between the two populations, and so the difference between the two samples is not the result of sampling error (alone) but reflects the difference in the underlying populations. In research using samples, we don't know which of these two scenarios is the true one and so we use inferential statistics to help us decide. The reason for this is that we don't know what the population means (parameters) are and so we can't know for sure if there is a difference between the populations. When we as researchers conduct studies we have to make a decision as to whether (a) or (b) above is the correct scenario, and we use inferential statistical tests to help us make this decision.

Probabilities

One way that researchers are able to decide between a scenario which indicates no effect in the population (see Figure 4.2(a)) and one that suggests a genuine population difference (see Figure 4.2(b)) for their studies is by using probabilities. If we could work out how likely it is that we would get a pattern of results if the scenario illustrated in Figure 4.2(a) were true, then we might be able to make a decision about the likelihood of this scenario being true. Alternatively, if we could work out the probability of getting a pattern of results if the scenario illustrated in Figure 4.2(b) were true, this also would help us decide between the two scenarios. It turns out that this is in effect what researchers do, and they base their decisions about effects in populations by calculating probabilities associated with the scenario represented by 4.2(a) above. To be able to understand this you will need to understand a little about probabilities.

Many events that happen in life have a probability attached to them. We referred you to a book by Mlodinow (2008) in Chapter 1 which provides quite a thorough account of the way in which chance influences our lives. Think about everyday things that you do and you will come to realise that chance plays a role. What are the chances of the slice of toast landing butter side down when you accidently drop it? What are the chances of a bit of the egg shell falling in the jug when you are making an omelette? What are the chances of you bumping into a friend when shopping in the local supermarket? What are the chances of you catching a cold from a colleague at work? What are the chances of you getting a bunion? What are the chances of a pigeon doing its business on your head when you are on your way to an important interview? When you look closely enough, probability influences us in a great many ways.

Probabilities are expressed mathematically as the number of possible outcomes that you are interested in divided by the total number of possible outcomes associated with an event. For example, when accidentally dropping a slice of toast there are two possible outcomes (buttered side up and buttered sided down) and one outcome that we are interested in (buttered side down). And so the probability of the toast landing buttered side down is $1 \div 2$, which is 0.5. We often express probabilities as fractions such as ½, and we can express probability as a percentage. To calculate the probability as a percentage we simply multiply the decimal probability by 100. Thus the probability of the toast landing buttered side down would be 0.5×100 or 50%.

When dealing with probabilities in statistics you will most often come across them in their decimal form. In this form probabilities can range from 0 to 1, where 0 means that the event of interest will definitely not occur and 1 means that the event definitely will occur. The closer to 1 that a probability expressed as a decimal is, the more likely the event of interest will occur. Here are some examples of probabilities expressed as decimals:

- Probability of selecting a Club from a pack of cards: $13 \div 52 = 0.25$
- Probability of winning the national lottery in the UK: approximately $1 \div 14{,}000{,}000 = 0.00000007$
- Probability of rolling a six on a die: $1 \div 6 = 0.167$
- Probability of rolling an even number on a die: $3 \div 6 = 0.5$

The first and last examples above are interesting, as they illustrate cases where we have multiple events of interest. For example, in a pack of playing cards there are 52 cards in total and 13 of them are Clubs. We want to know the probability of selecting a Club, and there are 13 possible ways of selecting a Club and so 13 possibilities of the event of interest. Thus the numerator (first number) in the division is 13 and the denominator (second number) is 52: $13 \div 52$. In the last example there are three even numbers on a die and so there are three ways of obtaining the desired event and six possible outcomes, thus the calculation is $3 \div 6$.

Activity 4.3

Have a go at calculating the probabilities associated with the following events of interest (work out the percentages for each one too – the answers are at the back of the book):

- Rolling a number greater than two on a die
- Selecting an ace from a pack of cards
- Getting tails when tossing a coin
- The probability of selecting a red ball from a bag which contains four red balls, five blue balls, seven green balls and four white balls
- The probability of obtaining a difference of three or greater from the data in Table 4.4

Using Probabilities to Generalise from Samples to Populations

Let us now return to the problem of working out whether the differences we observe between two samples is the result of sampling error or represents a genuine difference in the population. One potential means of establishing the probability of randomly selecting samples with differences as large as the ones we observe in our research is to follow the process we did in generating the data in Table 4.4. What we did for Table 4.4 was generate a series of random samples and then count up how many differences between the samples were as large as the one that we had in our research. Table 4.5 illustrates this point. In this table we have continued from Table 4.4, and generated a total of 100 pairs of samples which have been drawn from populations with a mean of 14.5 (i.e. there is no difference between the populations). We have emboldened all the differences between means that are at least a large as the difference between the means that we found in Table 4.3. The difference between the two means from Table 4.3 (11.90 and 15.20) is 3.30. The number of times differences of this magnitude or larger appear in this table is only three. So only three out of 100 times would we be likely to get a difference as large as the one we have observed in Table 4.3. Expressed as a probability this is .03 or 3%. This is quite a small probability, and so we might suggest that because this is so unlikely to occur because of sampling error then perhaps the pattern of data in Table 4.3 represents a situation more akin to Figure 4.2(b) than to Figure 4.2(a).

Table 4.5 Differences between 100 randomly generated pairs of samples of 20 scores drawn from a population with a mean of 14.5

0.85	2.05	0.95	1.85	1.85
1.60	0.85	2.45	1.20	0.90
0.40	0.80	2.00	0.50	0.50
1.25	2.7	0.75	1.20	1.10
1.3	0.40	2.30	0.65	1.30
3.00	1.85	1.8	1.20	1.00
0.30	1.05	1.15	0.60	0.45
1.05	2.60	0.75	1.25	0.05
2.25	2.90	0.90	1.35	1.25
3.90	2.40	0.15	**3.90**	2.85
0.35	0.55	0.70	0.25	0.40
2.90	0.45	2.45	0.30	0.30
0.50	0.05	2.25	1.20	0.20
1.10	1.15	1.45	1.75	0.20
1.60	0.60	0.25	0.10	1.35
0.50	0.45	2.80	0.20	0.00
1.60	2.30	0.00	2.05	0.9
0.75	0.55	0.15	0.15	1.95
0.50	1.45	2.75	0.25	0.75
0.85	0.60	0.85	**3.60**	0.85

For illustration, let us take a look at the difference between the means from Table 4.1. Here the mean for the hearing aid group was 14.95 and that for the waiting list control group was 14.45. Thus, the difference between them was 0.50. Looking at Table 4.5 we can see that there are many more cases where we have randomly generated differences between means which are at least as large as 0.50. In fact there are 75 occurrences of differences of 0.5 or above in Table 4.5. That means that 75 in every 100 occurrences we would be likely to get a difference between two sample means as large as 0.50 if they were drawn from populations which had equal means. Represented as a probability this would be 0.75 or 75%. This is a highly likely occurrence and thus we would likely conclude that our data best represent the scenario in Figure 4.2(a).

Null Hypothesis Significance Testing

What we have described in the previous few sections is essentially the process we go through when conducting inferential statistical tests. This process is represented in Figure 4.3.

The way that most research in the health sciences is carried out is through the process of *null hypothesis significance testing* or *NHST*.[1] We derive a research hypothesis, and from this we can generate something called a *null hypothesis*. The null hypothesis is central to this whole approach to conducting research. The null hypothesis states that there is no effect in the population of interest. For example, if we hypothesised a difference between hearing aid

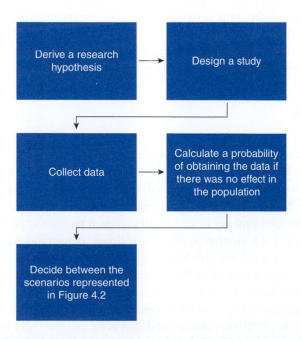

Figure 4.3   Illustration of the process of null hypothesis significance testing

and waiting list control patients in terms of their social anxiety, then the null hypothesis would be that there is no difference between these in the population Thus the null hypothesis stipulates that there is zero effect (e.g. zero difference) in the population. We then design and carry out a study to collect the data necessary to test our hypothesis. We calculate the probability that we would obtain our pattern of data if there were no effect in the population, i.e. if the null hypothesis was true. If this probability turns out to be large, it suggests that there is a high probability of obtaining our data if the null hypothesis were true (similar to Figure 4.2(a)) and then we would conclude that there is probably no effect in the population. If the probability we calculate is small, it suggests that there is only a small chance of obtaining our data if there is no effect in the population and we might conclude that there is a genuine effect in the population (similar to Figure 4.2(b)). This is the process of NHST.

The tricky part of NHST is the calculation of the probability of obtaining your pattern of data if the null hypothesis were true. Statisticians have come up with numerous ways of doing this, and these are called inferential statistical tests. The majority of the remainder of this book is devoted to explaining these inferential tests. You will find that the majority of the statistical techniques that we cover present you with a probability value or *p-value*. This is simply the probability of obtaining your pattern of data if the null hypothesis is true. This is a special kind of probability called a *conditional probability*. It is the probability of an event occurring if certain conditions are met. Thus the *p*-value is the probability of you obtaining your pattern of results *if* the null hypothesis is true.

When we used Table 4.5 to calculate the likelihood of obtaining large differences between groups by sampling error alone, the probability we calculated was a conditional probability. It was the probability of obtaining differences between the means from two samples of data at least as large as the one we observed in our study *if* we selected them randomly from populations which themselves had equal means, i.e. there was no difference in the populations. This is effectively the process underlying null hypothesis significance testing.

DISTRIBUTIONS

This all seems quite simple so far. If you have followed the explanation above, then you will have a good understanding of the principles underlying NHST. However, there are difficulties that we have not explained yet, and we will do this in the remainder of this chapter.

Imagine a population of numbers, e.g. the numbers shown in Figure 4.4.

In Figure 4.4 there are numbers from 1 to 10 and each number appears in the population with equal frequency. Each number appears four times. If we randomly selected numbers from this population each number would have an equal chance of being selected. In the real world, however, the populations of numbers (scores on variables) that we are interested do not always appear with equal frequency. Think about the number of teeth that you have filled at the dentist. According to the UK Adult Dental Health Survey from 1998 (Kelly et al., 2000) the mean number of fillings that an adult has is seven (see also Pine et al., 2001). The proportions of adults with filled teeth in this survey is presented in Figure 4.5.

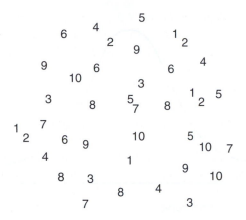

Figure 4.4   Population of numbers ranging from 1 to 10

Let us assume that this distribution of fillings is representative of all the adults in the UK (this survey was based upon over 3800 adults and so should be representative). You can see from this that a large proportion of adults have between six and 11 filled teeth and the vast majority have between one and 11 filled teeth. We have much lower proportions with no filled teeth or with 12 or more filled teeth. You should be able to see from this that if we randomly selected individuals from the population then we are much more likely to select someone with 6–11 fillings than someone with more than 12 fillings. Thus when we randomly select from such populations we do not have an equal opportunity of selecting each value on the variable of interest. The graph in Figure 4.5 represents the distribution of numbers of fillings in the population. This shape of distribution of scores is typical of many variables that we might be interested in in the health sciences. Statisticians have a name for this sort of distribution, and it is called a *normal distribution*.

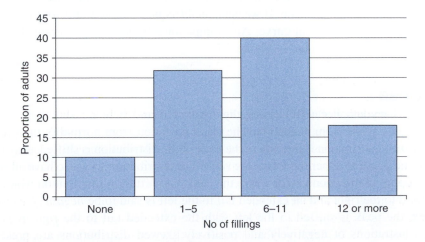

Figure 4.5   Proportions of adults with fillings

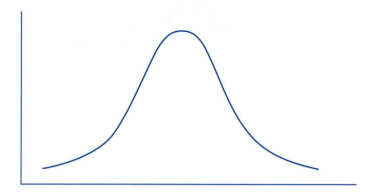

Figure 4.6   Illustration of a normal curve

The Normal Distribution

The *normal distribution* is a distribution of scores similar to that presented in Figure 4.5 and has the following characteristics:

- It is bell-shaped
- It is symmetrical about the peak in the middle
- It tails off approximately equally at both sides of the distribution
- The tails meet the *x*-axis at infinity, that is they will very slowly get closer to the *x*-axis on each side of the distribution but will not actually touch the *x*-axis until an infinite distance away on both sides

The normal distribution looks like the curve shown in Figure 4.6.

If we plotted the distributions of many variables in the population (e.g. height, number of filled teeth, number of visits to the family doctor each year) they would be distributed in a shape similar to that in Figure 4.6. If we generated frequency histograms for these variables they would look like a normal curve. An example of a frequency histogram illustrating a normal distribution is presented in Figure 4.7.

Skewness

Not all data that you collect will be normally distributed, and there are a number of ways that such data can deviate from normality. The usual deviation from normality involves *skewness*. A skewed distribution is one where the peak of the distribution is shifted away from the middle of the graph to either the left or the right. The distribution will also have an extended tail in the opposite direction to that where the peak has shifted. A distribution which has the peak shifted to the right and an extended tail to the left is said to be *negatively skewed* and one where the peak is shifted to the left with the extended tail to the right is *positively skewed*. Illustrations of negatively and positively skewed distributions are presented in Figure 4.8.

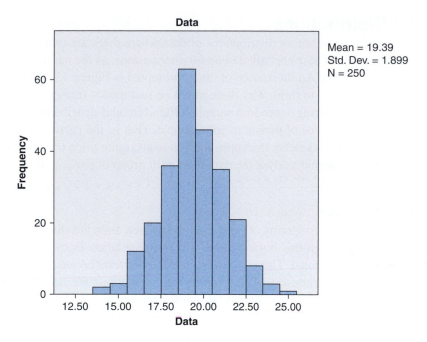

Figure 4.7   Histogram illustrating a normally distributed sample

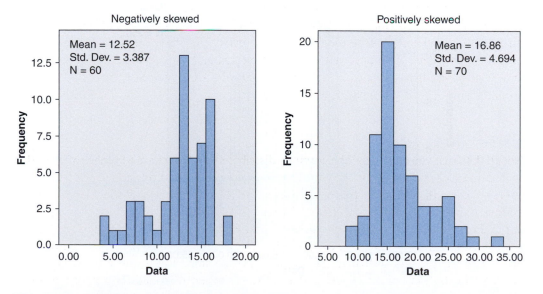

Figure 4.8   Negatively and positively skewed distributions

Bimodal Distributions

Sometimes you will come across distributions of data where there are two clearly identifiable peaks to the graph. These are called *bimodal distributions*; as the name suggests, there are two modes in the data. An illustration of this is presented in Figure 4.9. When you come across such data you need to think why there might be two modes (remember the mode is the most frequently occurring score in a sample. Often bimodal distributions suggest that you have more than one type of person in your sample. That is, the participants have been drawn from two populations rather than one, and you would quite often try to identify these two different populations and analyse the data from each group of participants separately.

Parametric Tests

It is important to check histograms of your data to see how they are distributed as many statistical tests presented in this book assume that the population from which scores are drawn are normally distributed. These are called *parametric tests* because they are making assumptions about the parameters of the underlying population. We don't usually know whether the distribution of the population is normal for any given variable and so it is usually

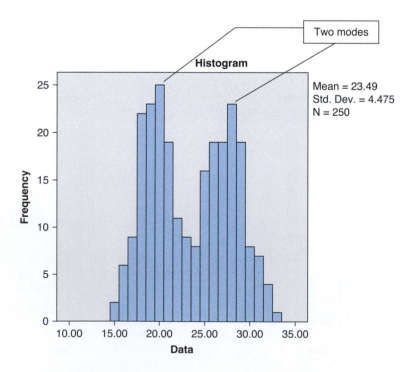

Figure 4.9   A bimodal distribution

recommended that you check to make sure that your sample is approximately normally distributed. There is quite a lot of leeway here, but you should at least check the histograms to ensure that your data are approximately normally distributed.

When considering the use of parametric tests you need to know that many of these tests make use of the mean and standard deviation. You therefore need to ensure that your samples do not include any outliers or extreme scores. If you think back to Chapter 3, we explained that the mean is heavily influenced by extreme scores, and so if you have extreme scores in your sample this will lead to biases in your statistical tests if you use the parametric ones. Always use box-plots to check for outliers and extreme scores.

Why worry about these assumptions? The reason is that parametric tests are usually the most sensitive tests that we can use. They are the most powerful tests and are the ones that will most likely help us detect an effect in the population. Examples of parametric tests that we cover in this book are the *t*-tests and ANOVAs. If your data do not meet the assumptions for parametric tests all is not lost, as there are *non-parametric tests* and other techniques that we can use. These sorts of tests (e.g. Wilcoxon's or Friedman's tests) do not have strict assumptions about the population distributions, but they tend to be less likely to detect an effect that exists in the population of interest. We will explain both parametric and non-parametric tests in a number of the remaining chapters in this book.

The Standard Normal Distribution

There is a special kind of normal distribution called the *standard normal distribution* (SND). This is what we call a probability distribution. It is a normally distributed set of scores where we know the probability of randomly selecting scores from any part of the distribution. The scores that are distributed in this special distribution are *z-scores*. If you have a sample of data, e.g. the hearing aid sample from Table 4.1, then you can convert any or all of the scores from the sample into *z*-scores. You do this by first calculating the mean and standard deviation for the sample. You then subtract the mean from the score that you want to convert and divide the resulting number by the standard deviation:

$$z = \frac{\text{score} - \text{mean}}{\text{standard deviation}}.$$

So, using this formula, let us convert the first score in the hearing aid sample in Table 4.1 to a *z*-score. The calculation will be:

$$z = \frac{14 - 14.95}{5.47}.$$

The calculated *z*-score is −0.17. This is a negative *z*-score, which tells us that the actual score is below the mean. When you get a positive *z*-score the actual score is above the mean. *z*-scores are calculated so that they are in standard deviation units. And so the *z*-score of −0.17 tells us that the score of 14 is 0.17 standard deviations below the mean. Let us take a different score from the hearing aid sample in Table 4.1. The fourth score down has a value of 25, which when converted produces a z-score of 1.84. This tells us that this score is nearly two standard deviations above the mean. When we convert a set of scores into z-scores this is called *standardising*. We are converting them into scores that are represented in standard deviation units. You should note that this standardising does not change the shape of the distribution of scores in your sample, it merely converts them to a different scale of measurement. This is rather like converting temperature from Fahrenheit to Centigrade. It doesn't actually change the temperature in a room, just the scale on which you are measuring it.

The SND is thus the distribution of z-scores and, as we suggested earlier, statisticians have been able to calculate the probabilities associated with randomly selecting scores from any part of the distribution. The SND is illustrated in Figure 4.10.

Figure 4.10 shows the standard normal distribution divided into standard deviation units. The middle of the distribution is the mean and this has a value of 0 in the SND. A score from a sample that gets a z-score of 0 is exactly equal to the mean of the sample (there is no difference between the score and the mean). A positive z-score will fall on the right of the SND whilst a negative z-score (a score in the sample that falls below the mean) will fall on the left of the graph. We suggested earlier that we know the probability of any score being randomly selected from any part of the SND. It has been calculated that the probability of selecting a score from the region of the graph between −1 and +1 z-scores is approximately 68% (see Figure 4.11).

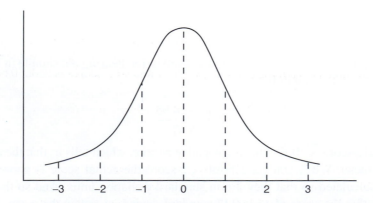

Figure 4.10 The standard normal distribution

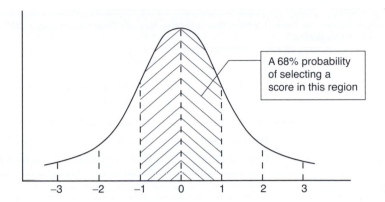

Figure 4.11   Probability of selecting a score between −1 and +1 standard deviations in the SND

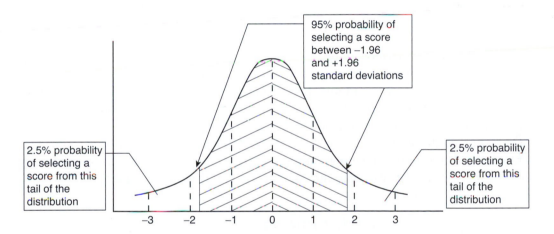

Figure 4.12   Probability of selecting a score between −1.96 and +1.96 standard deviations in the SND

One interesting feature of the SND is that the area beneath the curve between any two points gives us the probability of randomly selecting a score between those two points. The proportion of the area beneath the curve between −1 and +1 z-scores is about 0.68 or 68%. It has also been shown that there is a 95% probability of selecting a score from between −1.96 standard deviations and +1.96 standard deviations from the mean (see Figure 4.12).

Example from the Literature

Quite a nice example of the use of z-scores is a study reported by Vermeer et al. (2003). In this study they examined the association of 'silent' brain infarcts in the elderly with dementia and cognitive decline. They used magnetic resonance imaging (MRI) to detect the brain infarcts and used a number of tests of cognitive

Table 3. Association between the Presence of Silent Brain Infarcts on Magnetic Resonance Imaging in 1995–1996 and Subsequent Cognitive Decline.*

Variable	Silent Brain Infarcts		
	All	Thalamic	Nonthalamic
		decline in z score (95% CI)	
Memory performance	−0.01 (−0.16 to 0.15)	−0.50 (−0.87 to −0.13)	0.06 (−0.10 to 0.23)
Psychomotor speed	−0.19 (−0.34 to −0.04)	−0.11 (−0.36 to 0.13)	−0.20 (−0.36 to −0.05)
Global cognitive function	−0.15 (−0.27 to −0.02)	−0.28 (−0.50 to −0.06)	−0.13 (−0.26 to 0.001)

* Values are the mean differences in the z scores between follow-up and base line, with 95 percent confidence intervals (CIs) between those with and those without silent brain infarcts, adjusted for age, sex, level of education, and interval between neuropsychological tests. A positive value indicates an increase in the z score.

Figure 4.13 Table showing association between performance and silent infarct. From Vermeer et al. (2003)

function at baseline and follow-up. In their preparation of the data for analysis they converted their cognitive function tests scores for each participant into z-scores and then used these z-scores to formulate a composite measure of cognitive function at baseline and at follow-up. They presented the differences between z-scores at baseline and at follow-up in a table (Figure 4.13).

They concluded from their analysis that silent brain infarcts in the thalamus were associated with greater decline in memory performance, whereas as silent infarcts elsewhere were associated with greater decline in psychomotor speed.

Other Probability Distributions

The standard normal distribution is but one example of mathematical distributions of scores where we know the probability of selecting a score within any region of the graph. All of the inferential statistical tests that we cover in this book make use of these probability distributions. Thus, in this book you will come across tests which use the chi-square distributions, the binomial distribution, the t-distributions and the F-distributions. We won't describe these here, but all you need to know is that they have similar properties to the SND in that we know the probability of randomly selecting scores from within any region of the respective graphs.

Calculating the *p*-Value

We can use probability distributions such as the standard normal distribution to help us calculate the probability of obtaining our pattern of scores if the null hypothesis were true (see the section on null hypothesis significance testing, NHST, above). Remember as a part of the process of NHST we calculate the probability of obtaining our pattern of data if there were no difference between our groups (or no relationship between our variables) in the population. We use inferential statistical tests to calculate this probability and the probability is presented as a *p-value*. The way statisticians (and statistical packages like SPSS, R and SAS) calculate this *p*-value is by converting our data into scores from probability distributions like the SND or the *t*-distribution. We then work out the probability of obtaining such a score or greater by chance, and this then tells us how likely it would be for us to obtain our pattern of data if the null hypothesis was true. For example, suppose we used the SND and converted some data from a study into a score from this distribution, we might find that it produces a *z*-score of 1.96. We would look to the SND distribution to see how likely it is that we would obtain a *z*-score this large or greater, and this would be the *p*-value (probability value) associated with our statistical test. We know that 95% of the scores fall between −1.96 and +1.96 on the SND, and so we can see that 2.5% of scores must be equal to or greater than 1.96. Thus, the probability of obtaining our pattern of data through sampling error, if there were no difference in the population between hearing aid wearers and those waiting for a hearing aid, is 2.5%. This is rather a small probability and so we might suggest that the null hypothesis in this case is implausible. In statistical terms we state that we reject the null hypothesis and accept the experimental or research hypothesis that there is a difference between the two groups in social anxiety score in the population.

One- and Two-Tailed Hypotheses

You will quite often see that researchers refer to their hypothesis as being one- or two-tailed. Or they might indicate that their statistical tests were one- or two-tailed. In order to understand what such statements mean, you need to think about both the specifics of the hypotheses and the nature of the probability distributions that we base our inferential statistical tests on. There are a number of ways of framing a research hypothesis. For example, in our hearing aid study we might predict that there will be a difference between the hearing aid and waiting list control group in social anxiety scores. You will notice here that we have only predicted a difference between the two groups. We haven't predicted which group will have the higher social anxiety scores after the intervention. This is called a *bi-directional* or a *two-tailed* hypothesis. Because we haven't predicted a direction for the difference, the difference could go in either direction (hearing aid patients' scores greater than waiting list controls, or waiting list controls' scores greater than hearing aid patients). We might have been more specific in our prediction by suggesting that after getting their hearing aids these participants would have lower social anxiety scores than the waiting list control participants. Here we have specified a direction to the difference between the two groups, and thus we have generated a *directional* or *uni-directional hypothesis* (also called a *one-tailed hypothesis*).

When you have a two-tailed hypothesis, then you should use a two-tailed inferential statistical test to calculate the probability (the *p*-value) that you would obtain your data if the null hypothesis were true. Similarly, if you have a one-tailed hypothesis you should use a one-tailed inferential test to calculate this *p*-value. Why are these 'tailed' terms used?

Take a look back at the section on normal distributions. You will notice that when describing such distributions we used the term 'tails' to describe the way that the frequency of occurrence of scores tends to get lower as we move away from the centre of the distribution. The distribution is said to tail off as we move to both the left-hand side of the distribution and also the right-hand side. Now look at Figure 4.12. In this figure we indicated that the probability of selecting scores from the middle of the distribution is high. This means that the probability of selecting scores from either edge of the distribution must be quite low. When we use such probability distributions to help calculate our p-values, if we obtain a value in either of the extreme tails of the distribution then this suggests that such a pattern of scores has a low probability of occurrence if the null hypothesis is true. Thus, in order for us to 'reject the null hypothesis' and conclude that we have a genuine effect in the population we want to obtain scores in the tails of the distributions. Now, it turns out that if you have a two-tailed hypothesis it doesn't matter which tail of the distribution your calculated score comes from. If, however, you have a one-tailed hypothesis then you are making an explicit prediction about which end of the distribution your calculated score will come from. A concrete example might help. We hinted in our description of the hearing aid study that we thought that introducing hearing aids would lead to lower levels of social anxiety. We would thus have specified which tail of the distribution the calculated score will come from. If we found that the score came from the opposite side of the distribution, this would negate our hypothesis because it would show that introducing hearing aids led to higher levels of social anxiety.

You will find, when we explain certain inferential statistical tests in later chapters, that some allow us to conduct one- or two-tailed tests. This is important, as one-tailed tests tend to be more sensitive, that is, they are more likely to confirm an effect in the population if one actually exists. If you have a one-tailed hypothesis then you should use a one-tailed test.

Type I and Type II Errors

Another distinction that you need to understand is that between *Type I* and *Type II* errors. To understand what we mean here you need to cast your mind back to our explanation of null hypothesis significance testing (NHST). NHST can be conceptualised as a competition between two hypotheses, the null hypothesis and the research or experimental hypothesis. Remember, when the research hypothesis states that there is a difference between two groups or two conditions then the null hypothesis states that there is absolutely no difference between the two groups in the population. We carry out NHST in order to calculate a p-value which helps us decide which of the two hypotheses (research or null) is the more plausible. On the basis of the p-value that is calculated we will decide either to reject or accept the null hypothesis. However, we are making decisions based upon incomplete information, on the basis of a probability judgement. Thus, we might find that we obtain a small p-value, and so we quite reasonably decide that the research hypothesis is more plausible and thus our data indicate that there is an effect in the population. It might be, however, that we are incorrect. There might be no effect in the population (i.e. the null hypothesis is true), but we have

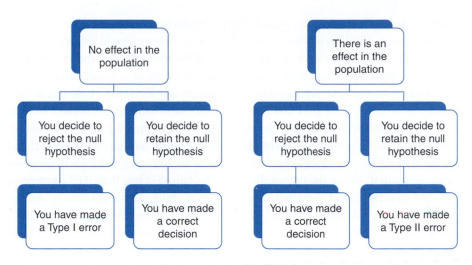

Figure 4.14 Illustration of the circumstances under which we make Type I and Type II errors

been unlucky to obtain a set of data which are highly unlikely. If we reject the null hypothesis in this case it is clear that we have made a mistake. This sort of mistake is called a Type I error.

There is another sort of mistake that you can make in NHST. You might conduct your research and calculate a *p*-value which is quite high, and thus this is telling you that your pattern of data is highly likely if the null hypothesis were true. In this situation you would probably reasonably conclude that there is no evidence of an effect in the population and thus retain the null hypothesis. It could be though that the research hypothesis is true, but due to a variety of reasons your study has not found enough evidence to support it. If you retain the null hypothesis in this case you have again made a mistake and this sort of mistake is called a Type II error (see Figure 4.14). Thus:

- A Type I error is when you reject the null hypothesis when it is in fact true
- A Type II error is where you fail to reject the null hypothesis when it is in fact false

The way we design our research and conduct our statistical analyses are all to some extent trying to balance the probabilities of making Type I and Type II errors.

The probability of making a Type I error is often denoted by the Greek symbol α (alpha) and the probability of making a Type II error is often denoted by the Greek symbol β (beta).

STATISTICAL SIGNIFICANCE

We have so far been rather vague when discussing the use of probabilities to help us decide between the null and the research hypothesis. We have suggested that we use probability distributions to help us calculate the probability of obtaining our pattern of results if the null hypothesis were true. If this probability is small enough, then we would suggest that that null hypothesis is implausible and thus reject it in favour of the research hypothesis. This begs the question of how small does the probability value have to be for us to be able to reject the null hypothesis and retain the research hypothesis? Traditionally in NHST there has been a cut-off value of 5%. That is, if we find that the probability of obtaining our pattern of results if there was no effect in the population is less than 0.05 or 5%, then we would be able to con-fidently reject the null hypothesis. Conversely, if the probability value that we calculated was greater than 0.05 (5%), we would not feel confident in rejecting the null hypothesis and would instead retain it. When the probability value (p-value) is less than 0.05, then research-ers often state that they have a *statistically significant* result. If the p-value is above 0.05, then it is said to be *non-significant*. These are terms that are used very widely in the litera-ture and so please do take some time to ensure that you follow what we have said in this section.

Why do we use the 0.05 probability value as our cut-off for statistical significance? The use of this *criterion for significance* dates back to the early days of NHST and stems from concern to try to balance the probability of making a Type I error with the probability of making a Type II error. To illustrate this we will discuss the use of different criteria for sig-nificance. Let us assume that we have conducted some research into the effects of hearing aids and unbeknownst to us there is a real effect of using hearing aids on social anxiety in the population. We have collected some data and the p-value that we calculated using our statistical test is 0.04. If we used the traditional criterion for significance we would correctly reject the null hypothesis and thus avoid making a Type II error. If, however, we had decided that we would only reject the null hypothesis if our p-value was less than 0.01, then with our calculated p-value of 0.04 we would not reach this cut-off and thus would not reject the null hypothesis. In this case, as there is a genuine effect in the population we would be making a Type II error. So you can see that the lower we set our criterion for significance the higher the chances are that we will make a Type II error. Let us now assume that hearing aids do not help to reduce social anxiety (the null hypothesis is true). Let us also assume that we have conducted a study and have calculated a p-value of 0.07. If we stick with the traditional criterion for significance, we would decide that as our calculated p-value is greater than 0.05 we would not feel comfortable rejecting the null hypothesis, and so we would instead retain it. In this case this would be correct. Let us suppose we decided before the study that we were going to use a more liberal criterion for significance of 0.10. As our calculated p-value of 0.07 is less than this we would reject the null hypothesis when it is in fact true and we would have thus made a Type I error.

You should be able to see that shifting the criterion for significance around has an impact on the probability of us making a Type I or II error. It has been argued that the 0.05 cut-off provides the best balance between making a Type I and a Type II error. Therefore, unless you have specific reason and good justification to alter the criterion for significance you should routinely use the standard cut-off of 0.05.

CRITICISMS OF NHST

Effect Size

Although NHST is very widely used in the health sciences, it is an approach that has its critics. We do not have space here to present a full discussion of the criticism of NHST, but we wanted to alert you to some of these criticisms as they provide a useful link into some of the other concepts that we aim to explain in this chapter. We recommend that you read some of Jacob Cohen's papers on the subject as they are very accessible (e.g. Cohen, 1990). One of the chief criticisms of NHST is that there is far too much attention given to the p-value. Obtaining a p-value of less than 0.05 becomes the sole focus of the research rather than the focus being the strength of the effect in the population. One of the interesting properties of the p-value that we calculate is that it is directly related to sample size, and so generally the larger the sample you have the lower the p-value that your statistical tests will give you. This means that you are more likely to reject a null hypothesis if you have large samples. Therefore, we should focus a lot of attention not only on the p-value but also on the actual strength of the effect that we are investigating. This is called the effect size. It seems logical that this should be of utmost importance to researchers, but it is very often neglected in the literature.

The effect size simply refers to the size of the difference between two or more groups or conditions in your study or the strength of a relationship between two or more variables. In this book we will demonstrate a number of different ways of calculating standardised effects sizes which allow us to compare the strength of the effects that we have found across different studies. Examples, of standardised effect sizes that we cover are Cohen's d and r^2 (these are covered in Chapters 7, 8, 10 and 11). It is good practice to present effect size measures when reporting the findings from your statistical analyses. Many of these measures of effect size come with guidelines from people like Cohen as to what constitutes a small effect, a medium effect and a large effect (e.g. Cohen, 1992). These are useful guidelines but should be used with much caution, as what might be considered a small effect in one field might be considered a large effect in another field.

Statistical Power

Another criticism of NHST is that it has led to researchers to focus too much on the probability of making a Type I error. In order to design appropriate studies and to draw appropriate conclusions from our inferential statistical tests then we need to also pay attention to Type II errors. What we ideally want to do in our research is design studies that are sensitive enough to detect real effects in the underlying population. The ability of studies to detect real effects is called *statistical power*. If there is a genuine effect in the population (i.e. the null hypothesis is false) then we should be designing research which will allow us to reject the null hypothesis. A focus on statistical power at the design stage is crucial for undertaking studies that will allow you to reject the null hypothesis when it should be rejected. A good deal of important work on statistical power has been presented by Jacob Cohen[2] who has produced books on how to calculate the levels of power associated with studies (e.g. Cohen, 1988). Power is directly related to the probability of making a Type II error. In fact power = 1 minus the probability of making a Type II error (i.e. $1 - \beta$). Power ranges from 0 to 1 where 0 would mean that the study has absolutely no chance of detecting a genuine effect in the population, and 1 signifies that a study will definitely find the effect in the population. Usually, the power of studies vary between these two extremes. Why should we pay attention to power? Power is particularly important in medical research as we do not want to waste the time of sometimes very ill participants in a study that is never likely to be able to detect the effect that it is looking for. Designing such research is essentially unethical. This has been discussed nicely in a paper by Halpern et al. (2002) in which they highlight the widespread use of underpowered randomised control trials in medical research. They give a very good discussion of the ethical dimensions of underpowered research, suggesting that there are very few circumstances where underpowered studies are ethically justifiable. Cohen (1988) has argued that a reasonable level of power to aim for in a study is 0.80, which means that we would have an 80% probability of finding the effect if it exists in the population. You should note, however, that researchers often aim for higher power levels than this.

Power is influenced by a number of factors and these are indicated in Figure 4.15. The main factors are:

- Sample size, the larger the samples you have in your study the higher the power
- Effect size, the bigger the effect that you are trying to detect the higher the power of the study (big things are much easier to detect than small things)
- The criterion for significance which is usually set at .05 and which we discussed earlier. If you have a very strict (i.e. low criterion for significance) then you are less likely to reject the null hypothesis (even when it is false)
- Whether you have a one- or two-tailed hypothesis, one-tailed statistical tests tend to be more powerful than two-tailed tests

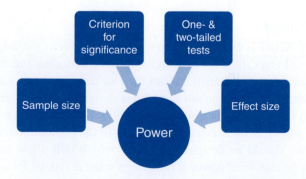

Figure 4.15   Factors influencing statistical power

It is thus very important to pay attention to these factors when designing research, to ensure that you conduct studies that are powerful enough to detect the effects you are looking for. It is also important to bear these factors in mind when you are reading others' research, particularly if they do not reject their null hypothesis. If researchers have failed to reject the null hypothesis they might argue that there is no effect to detect in the population. If, however, they have an underpowered study (e.g. if they have a small sample size) then we don't know if they have correctly accepted the null hypothesis or whether they have made a Type II error.

Power Calculations – Estimating Samples Sizes

When designing studies researchers are advised to think about power from the very beginning. They are advised to conduct what we call *a priori* power calculations. The term *a priori* as used in statistics indicates that we make decisions about our statistical analyses prior to running the study. Essentially, what we do in such power calculations is to work out how many participants we would need to ensure that we had adequate power to reject the null hypothesis if it was false. There are a number of software packages that can help us with such calculations but one of the most commonly used and widely available is a program called 'GPower'. You can download it from this website: http://www.psycho.uni-duesseldorf. de/aap/projects/gpower/

It is quite a simple little program but you will need to read the excellent guide to using it to figure out exactly which options you need to select in order to run an *a priori* power analysis. It is not appropriate to give you detailed guidance on this here as it requires that you understand the different inferential statistical tests before you can use it. Instead, here we will give you a broad overview of what such calculations involve. Let us return to the hearing aid and social anxiety example presented earlier in the chapter. To perform an *a priori* power calculation for this study we would need some idea of the effect size that we think will be in the population. How large will the difference in social anxiety be between the hearing aid participants and the waiting list control participants? This does seem a strange thing to ask, because if you knew the size of the effect then you probably wouldn't need to conduct the research in the first place. If you knew that there was a specific difference between hearing aid wearers and non-wearers in terms of their social anxiety, then you wouldn't need to run the study. Thus, you are probably designing the study to establish the existence of such a difference. So, we don't know the size of the difference in the population (it could be zero or it could be large) but we can use our knowledge of previous research in the area to suggest the value of the effect size. If there is no basis on which to estimate the effect size then the recommendation is to assume that you are looking for a medium effect size (this is the default option in GPower). We will go with this medium effect size.

Other information that we need is the level of power that we wish to achieve in our study. Cohen recommends that we should aim for at least 0.80 and we will stick with this advice here. You might want to increase this to a higher level if you want to be more certain of detecting an effect. Also, you will need to know your criterion for significance. This should be set at the usual 0.05 level unless you have a very good reason to alter it. Finally, you need to know whether you have a one- or two-tailed hypothesis. We have a one-tailed hypothesis, as we are predicting that receiving a hearing aid will reduce the social anxiety in a hearing impaired group when compared to the waiting list control group. Thus the information that we need to input into GPower is:

- Medium effect size
- Power = 0.80
- Criterion for significance 0.05
- One-tailed test

When we put this information into GPower it tells us that we need 51 participants in each group (Screenshot 4.1). This is considerably more than we have included in our examples above.

Confidence Intervals

A further criticism of NHST is that it leads us to focus too much on the samples themselves. There is too much emphasis on sample means and standard deviations, and this leads to a neglect of what the effects might be in the underlying populations. Let us go back to the hearing aid example and look at the data in Table 4.3 (the post-intervention social anxiety scores). The mean social anxiety score for the hearing aid participants is 11.90.

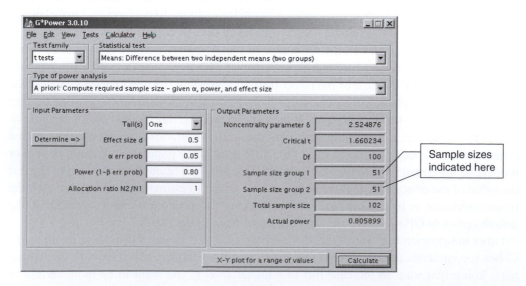

Screenshot 4.1

Think about this and write your answer on a sheet of paper before reading any further. How close is the sample mean (11.90) for the hearing aid group to the population mean for such individuals?

As we do not know the population mean social anxiety score for hearing impaired individuals who have hearing aids we cannot provide an answer to the question posed in Activity 4.5. The population mean could be a long way below the sample mean, or it could be a good deal larger than the sample mean, or it might be exactly the same. We simply do not know. This is problematic for us as researchers as we are trying to generalise from the samples to the populations. If we don't know how close our sample statistics might be to our population parameters then this might seem like a completely unenlightening exercise. This is where *confidence intervals* come to the rescue. Take a look at Figure 4.16.

We know that the minimum and maximum value on the Social Avoidance and Distress Scale (SADS) are 0 and 28 respectively, and so we can be 100% confident that the population means for the hearing impaired people with hearing aids is within these two limits. These are what we call 100% confidence limits. This though is not really that helpful. It turns out that if you allow yourself to be slightly less confident where the population mean might lie we can start to narrow the confidence limits. The usual confidence intervals that researchers calculate are 95% intervals. Thus, we are allowing ourselves to be slightly less confident, but take a look at Figure 4.17 to see what effect this has on the range of scores we think the population mean will fall within.

You should notice that now the range of scores within which we think the population mean will fall has dramatically narrowed. And so we can say that we are 95% confident that the population mean will be between 9.39 and 14.44. The interesting thing about confidence intervals is that they are directly related to sample size, and so the more people you have in your samples the narrower the intervals become.

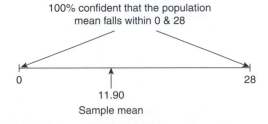

Figure 4.16   Diagram illustrating where we are 100% confident that the population mean lies in relation to the sample mean

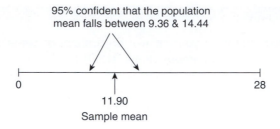

Figure 4.17   Diagram illustrating 95% confidence intervals

Let us now look at the waiting list control participants from Table 4.3. The mean for these participants is 15.20 and the 95% CIs are 12.29 to 18.11. If we put both sets of confidence intervals into the same diagram we get a very interesting picture (see Figure 4.18).

You can see from Figure 4.18 that there is very little overlap between the two sets of confidence intervals. We are 95% confident that the population mean for the hearing aid group falls between 9.36 and 14.44, and for the waiting list control group between 12.29 and 18.11. Thus, we might tentatively conclude that in the population the social anxiety for hearing impaired people without a hearing aid is likely to be higher than for those with a hearing aid. We might tentatively suggest that we have support for our research hypothesis.

Confidence intervals have an almost magical quality because they get us focussing on the populations rather than our samples. It is very easy in research to get absorbed by your sample data and forget to relate these back to the wider populations. Confidence intervals grab our attention and focus it back where it should be focussed – on the wider populations.

GENERATING CONFIDENCE INTERVALS IN SPSS

The best way of getting confidence intervals in SPSS is through the *Analyze*, *Descriptive Statistics* and *Explore* commands. Set up the dialogue box in the same way as we have done below (Screenshot 4.2) and then click on *OK*. SPSS will present 95% confidence intervals in the output (Screenshot 4.3) (these outputs were created using the data from Table 4.3).

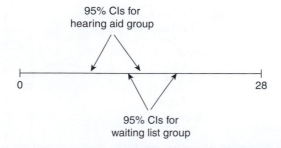

Figure 4.18   Diagram illustrating 95% confidence intervals for both the hearing aid and the waiting list control groups

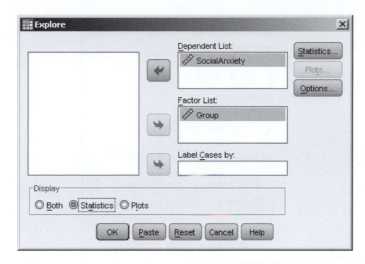

Screenshot 4.2

Descriptives

	Group			Statistic	Std. Error
Social Anxiety	Hearing Aid Group	Mean		11.9000	1.21157
		95% Confidence Interval for Mean	Lower Bound	9.3642	
			Upper Bound	14.4358	
		5% Trimmed Mean		11.8889	
		Median		12.0000	
		Variance		29.358	
		Std. Deviation		5.41829	
		Minimum		3.00	
		Maximum		21.00	
		Range		18.00	
		Interquartile Range		8.75	
		Skewness		-.083	.512
		Kurtosis		-.915	.992
	Waiting List Control Group	Mean		15.2000	1.39095
		95% Confidence Interval for Mean	Lower Bound	12.2887	
			Upper Bound	18.1113	
		5% Trimmed Mean		15.1667	
		Median		15.0000	
		Variance		38.695	
		Std. Deviation		6.22051	
		Minimum		4.00	
		Maximum		27.00	
		Range		23.00	
		Interquartile Range		10.75	
		Skewness		.070	.512
		Kurtosis		-.806	.992

Screenshot 4.3

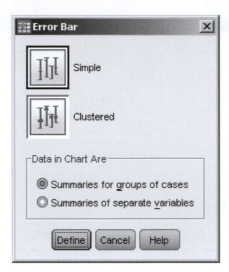

Screenshot 4.4

A useful way of presenting confidence intervals is through *error bar charts*. You can generate these by selecting the *Graphs*, *Legacy Dialogs* and *Error Bar* options. You will be presented with a dialogue box (Screenshot 4.4).

Select the *Simple* and *Summaries for groups of cases* option and then click on the *Define* button (Screenshot 4.5).

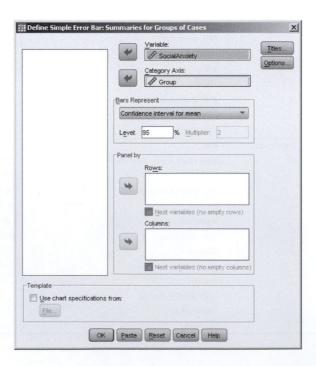

Screenshot 4.5

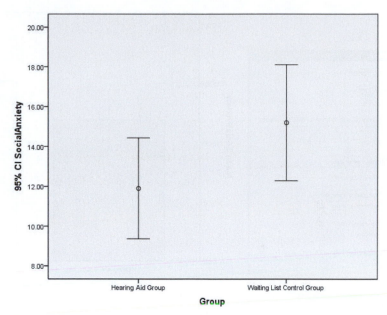

Screenshot 4.6

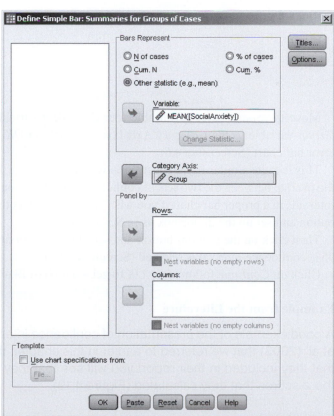

Screenshot 4.7

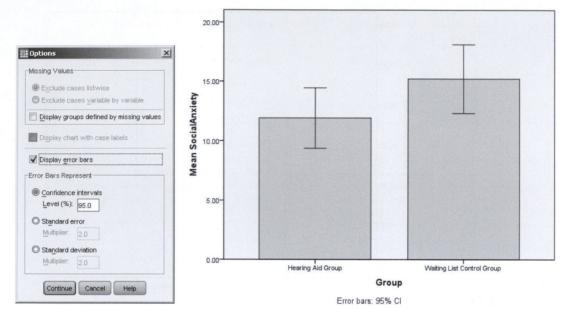

Screenshot 4.8   **Screenshot 4.9**

Move the *Social Anxiety* variable (our dependent variable) to the *Variable* box and the *Group* variable to the *Category Axis* box and click on *OK*. You will be presented with an error bar chart (Screenshot 4.6).

This is quite similar to the illustration we gave in Figure 14.14, and gives an indication of the overlap between the two sets of confidence intervals. You can also include the confidence intervals in a proper bar chart if you wish. To do this select the *Graphs*, *Legacy Dialogs*, *Bar* option and set up the dialog box as in Screenshot 4.7.

Then click on the *Options* button and select the *Error bars* option and make sure that the 95% confidence interval is selected (Screenshot 4.8).

Click on *Continue* followed by *OK* to get a bar chart like Screenshot 4.9.

Example from the Literature

A good example of the presentation of confidence intervals is the paper by Vermeer et al. (2003) that we referred to earlier in this chapter. If you have a look at the table that they included in their report you will see that they have presented 95% CIs for the *z*-scores that they calculated (Figure 4.19).

Table 3. Association between the Presence of Silent Brain Infarcts on Magnetic Resonance Imaging in 1995–1996 and Subsequent Cognitive Decline.*

Variable	Silent Brain Infarcts		
	All	Thalamic	Nonthalamic
		decline in z score (95% CI)	
Memory performance	−0.01 (−0.16 to 0.15)	−0.50 (−0.87 to −0.13)	0.06 (−0.10 to 0.23)
Psychomotor speed	−0.19 (−0.34 to −0.04)	−0.11 (−0.36 to 0.13)	−0.20 (−0.36 to −0.05)
Global cognitive function	−0.15 (−0.27 to −0.02)	−0.28 (−0.50 to −0.06)	−0.13 (−0.26 to 0.001)

* Values are the mean differences in the z scores between follow-up and base line, with 95 percent confidence intervals (CIs) between those with and those without silent brain infarcts, adjusted for age, sex, level of education, and interval between neuropsychological tests. A positive value indicates an increase in the z score.

Figure 4.19

Summary

We have covered a lot of conceptual ground in this chapter but this should give you a firm basis for understanding statistical testing, particularly null hypothesis significance testing. You have learned about the difference between samples and populations, and how we use samples to try to generalise to the populations. You have learned that we use inferential statistical tests to help us do this generalising. We have explained that null hypothesis significance testing (NHST) is the basis for all the main statistical techniques covered in this book. We have described the process of NHST and how it gives us a probability value (*p*-value) which helps us decide whether to accept or reject the null hypothesis. We have explained that we can make errors in rejecting a true null hypothesis (a Type I error) or in retaining a false null hypothesis (a Type II error). We have highlighted some of the criticisms of NHST and suggested that we need to pay attention to issues like power and sample size calculations when designing our research. Finally, you have learned about the magical ability of confidence intervals to draw our attention to populations rather than samples and how to generate these using SPSS.

SPSS EXERCISE

Using the data from Table 4.2 generate confidence intervals for both groups and get SPSS to present these on a bar chart and error bar chart.

MULTIPLE CHOICE QUESTIONS

1. Which of these are characteristics of the normal curve?
   a) Square-shaped
   b) Non-symmetrical
   c) Tails steadily move away from the x-axis
   d) None of the above

2. If your research hypothesis stated that there would be a difference between males and females in the number of teeth they had filled, what would be the null hypothesis?
   a) That females would have more fillings than males
   b) That males would have more fillings than females
   c) That there would be no difference between males and females in the number of fillings
   d) None of the above

3. Referring to the research hypothesis in MCQ2 above, what sort of hypothesis is this?
   a) A null hypothesis
   b) A one-tailed hypothesis
   c) A two-tailed hypothesis
   d) Any of the above is correct

4. Probability distributions are useful because:
   a) We know the probability of randomly selecting a score from any region of the distribution
   b) We know the probability of the tails being equal
   c) We know the probability that the peak of the distribution will be in the middle
   d) Probability distributions are not useful

5. How much of the area under the standard normal distribution falls within −1 and +1?
   a) 50%
   b) 68%
   c) 95%
   d) 100%

6. Which of these are not related to statistical power?
   a) Effect size
   b) Sample size
   c) Computer size
   d) Criterion for significance

7. What is the probability of selecting the Ace of Spades from a deck of cards?
   a) 0.25
   b) 0.019
   c) 25
   d) 19

8. Which of the following is a criticism of NHST
   a) It is too easy
   b) It doesn't give us useful *p*-values
   c) We can't generalise to the population
   d) Too little attention is paid to effect sizes

9. How do we calculate *z*-scores?
   a) Subtract the median and divide by the range
   b) Subtract the mean and divide by the standard deviation
   c) Subtract the standard deviation and divide by the mean
   d) Subtract the mean and divide by the median

10. When you convert a set of scores into *z*-scores what is this called?
    a) A waste of time
    b) Inferential analysis
    c) Descriptive analysis
    d) Standardising

11. If you had confidence intervals for two groups which did not overlap what could you reasonably conclude?
    a) That there was unlikely to be a difference between the means of the two groups in the population
    b) That there was unlikely to be a difference in the variability of two groups in the population
    c) That there was likely to be a difference between the means of the two groups in the population
    d) That there was likely to be a difference in the variability of the two groups in the population

12. In order to run an *a priori* power analysis which of the following do you need?
    a) The power
    b) The criterion for significance
    c) The effect size
    d) All of the above

13. Which of the following is a standardised measure of effect size?
    a) r^2
    b) Cohen's *d*
    c) Criterion for significance
    d) Both a) and b) above

14. If you have a negatively skewed distribution then the extended tail points towards:
    a) The higher numbers
    b) The lower numbers
    c) Neither the high or low numbers
    d) None of the above

15. What is the probability of 0.0125 as a percentage?
    a) 0.0125%
    b) 0.125%
    c) 1.25%
    d) 12.5%

Notes

1 There are other ways of analysing data and testing research hypotheses, such as through the use of Bayesian statistics, but these are beyond the scope of this introductory text.
2 It may look like we are fans of Jacob Cohen, but he has been highly influential in this area and his work tends to be very readable.

Epidemiology

5

Overview

Epidemiology involves studying disease and other health-related factors within specified populations. Epidemiologists are often interested in:

- The prevalence of disease. Prevalence refers to the existing frequency of disease
- The incidence of disease. Incidence refers to onset of new cases of disease within a particular time frame
- Identifying risk factors for disease. Individuals exposed to risk factors are more likely to develop disease. Potential risk factors include a very wide range of things such as age, sex, social factors such as quality of best friendship, and biological factors such as exposure to high levels of testosterone during pre-natal development. Once risk factors that increase the chance of disease are identified, further research is required to understand how/whether the risk factor is involved in disease causation

The term 'epidemiology' might make you think of epidemics where there are unusual increases in the incidence of a particular disease. For example, you might hear in the media about an 'influenza epidemic' during the winter months. The methods of epidemiology are indeed suitable for studying abnormal disease outbreaks of this sort. However, epidemiological methods are more usually applied to diseases that are

(Continued)

(Continued)

present at relatively constant levels (i.e. they are endemic). An important aim is to inform prevention and treatment efforts and to help plan health service provision. We can only scratch the surface of epidemiology in this chapter, as the discipline includes a wide range of research techniques. However, many of the statistical methods covered through this book are applicable in epidemiological studies.

In this chapter you will:

- Learn the ways in which statistical methods can aid the understanding of the distribution and causes of ill-health
- Learn about some basic statistics used by epidemiologists, including estimates of prevalence, incidence, risk ratios and odds-ratios
- Appreciate some of the difficulties in identifying causal relationships
- Develop the skills required to read epidemiological papers in the scientific literature

INTRODUCTION

Some epidemiological studies involve recruiting samples designed to be representative of the general population of a geographical area. The sample might only be observed once (a cross-sectional study) or it might be followed up over time (a cohort study). These designs can be useful for estimating the prevalence of disease and also for identifying underlying risk factors. A case-control design is an alternative approach. In this design participants will be recruited because they have a particular disease (i.e. they are cases). Their characteristics are compared to another group of people who do not have the disease (the control group). This design does not allow prevalence to be estimated but it does allow risk factors to be examined by comparing the histories of the cases and controls. Epidemiologists can also sometimes work with health interventions. For example, epidemiologists could investigate whether a vaccination programme has an effect on disease incidence in a specified population.

Examples of epidemiological findings include:

- Lipton et al. (2011) found that the prevalence of chronic migraine was 1.75% in US adolescents and that this had a severe impact on their everyday functioning. Despite this, only 40% had visited a health care provider during the previous year
- Gabriel (2001) reviewed the epidemiological literature regarding rheumatoid arthritis and found the risk of this disease was higher in a range of groups of people, including smokers and users of oral contraceptives

ESTIMATING THE PREVALENCE OF DISEASE

A common aim of an epidemiological study is to estimate the frequency of a disease or other health-related factor in a specified population at a particular time. The study might examine who has a disorder at the time of the survey or assess whether participants suffered the illness at any time over a specified period (e.g. the last three months) irrespective of whether they have recovered by the time of the survey. Prevalence information is useful to clinicians, as it helps them to decide how likely a patient is to have a particular disease. It is also useful for policy makers, as it informs them how much service provision is required. The prevalence of a disease is simply the proportion or percentage of people in the population with that disease. If you recruit a sample from your population of interest then prevalence can be calculated as the number of people with the disease divided by the total number of people (with disease and without) in the sample. This gives the proportion of the sample with the disease. Multiplying by 100 turns this into a percentage.

For example, imagine you are studying the prevalence of eye-brow rings in your local area. You recruit a sample of 250 people and find that 37 of them have eye-brow rings. You can calculate the prevalence of eye-brow rings by dividing 37 by 250 and them multiplying by 100. This gives you a prevalence estimate of 14.8%.

DIFFICULTIES IN ESTIMATING PREVALENCE

This description might make the process of estimating prevalence sound very easy. Do not be fooled by this! Estimating prevalence can be very difficult.

A large sample that is genuinely representative of the population of interest is required. Samples in epidemiology often include hundreds or thousands of participants. Consequently, large studies are often funded to examine the prevalence of a large number of disorders at the same time. For example the British Child and Adolescent Health Survey was funded by the United Kingdom Office for National Statistics to estimate the prevalence of all common psychiatric disorders in children aged 5–15 from across the UK. The study included a sample of over 10,000 children (Meltzer et al., 2000).

Even with a large sample, accurate population estimates are not possible unless the sample genuinely represents the population of interest. The participants who are invited to take part in the study need to be carefully selected to ensure that they are representative. Even if the invited sample is representative, the achieved sample can become unrepresentative if some participants decline the invitation or cannot be included for other reasons. Unfortunately, it is usually impossible to include the full target sample, and studies that achieve 80% of their target sample are often thought to be doing well. In terms of estimating prevalence this will not be a problem if those with and without the condition of interest are equally likely to decline the study invitation. Sometimes though, the very thing you want to study has a strong bearing on whether someone will participate or not. This introduces a problem of *selection bias*. For example, imagine you are measuring the prevalence of a debilitating illness.

Participation in your study might involve filling in a lengthy questionnaire or attending a clinic assessment that will not offer any treatment benefit. You would not be surprised that people who feel really poorly do not want take part in your study. Therefore, people without the disease are more likely to take part in your study than people with the disease and you will underestimate the true prevalence in the population. There are many other factors related to non-response that might bias the prevalence estimate as well. Epidemiologists and statisticians are working on methods to deal with the problems caused by these missing data. We discuss some of these issues and approaches in Chapters 6 and 11.

A further problem in large-scale studies is that the measurement of disease may not be entirely accurate. For example, in the British Child and Adolescent Mental Health Survey it would have been prohibitively expensive for every participant to attend a full psychopathology assessment with a psychiatrist. Instead, studies often measure disorder on the basis of questionnaire scores or some other brief assessment. Epidemiologists will carefully choose the measures to be as accurate as possible and may carry out validation studies prior to their main data collection. Even the best measures suitable for epidemiological studies will usually not be in perfect agreement with the most effective means of diagnosis available (often referred to as the 'gold standard'). In terms of estimating prevalence, the key question is whether the brief assessment identifies the same number of cases as the gold standard test. If the brief test identifies more, then prevalence will be overestimated; if it identifies less, then prevalence will be underestimated.

At this point in the discussion you might be thinking that the prevalence of disease can never be accurately estimated in a population. It is true that any one study is unlikely to do so perfectly. However, that does not mean the endeavour is futile. Often a number of independent studies will estimate the prevalence of the same disorder in the same target population. Different studies may use different methods of sampling, different approaches to dealing with non-response and different measurement instruments. By looking across these independent estimates we can usually gain a good idea of the range of values within which the true prevalence falls. Also, repeating studies with exactly the same methodology at different times can be very useful in estimating whether the frequency of disease is changing.

Example from the Literature: Estimating the Prevalence of Childhood Psychiatric Disorder in Rural North Carolina, USA

Costello and colleagues (1996) carried out the Great Smoky Mountains Study of Youth to estimate the prevalence of psychiatric disorders in young people. The study sampled children aged 9, 11 and 13 from a largely rural area of the southern USA. The public school records contained 12,000 age eligible children who formed the population of interest. Following a process of participant selection, 1346 were invited to participate in the study from which 1015 took part in the initial data collection. The presence of all common psychiatric disorders over the previous three months was measured. This assessment was carried out by trained staff and involved an in-depth interview with the child and the parent. The interview collected detailed

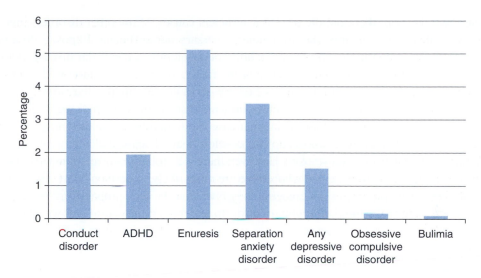

Figure 5.1

quantitative information on the frequency, intensity and duration of the assessed symptoms. A computer algorithm decided whether full diagnostic criteria were met, combining the parent and child reports. Selected prevalence estimates are shown in Figure 5.1.

This study estimates the prevalence of disorder in the target population. The information will be very useful for planning service provision when interpreted in the context of other similar studies. You might, however, be concerned that prevalence may be underestimated because 331 children selected for interview did not take part. If the non-participants were more likely to have disorder than children who did take part, then the prevalence figures will have been underestimated. It is unusual for researchers to be able to test this possibility directly. However, in the Great Smoky Mountains Study the sampling procedure collected a brief measure of psychopathology on an enlarged sample that included the 331 children who were not interviewed. The authors found there were no differences in the brief measure in the excluded children compared to the included sample. This indicates the prevalence estimates were not likely to have been biased markedly by non-response.

BEYOND PREVALENCE: IDENTIFYING RISK FACTORS FOR DISEASE

In some cases a single causal factor is both necessary and sufficient to cause a disease outcome. Huntington's disease is a good example. A disordered copy of a particular gene is necessary for Huntington's disease to develop and no other factors are needed to ensure the disease will develop (therefore the gene is a sufficient cause). Many other disorders involve a large number of risk factors that are neither necessary nor sufficient. Exposure to a risk factor of this type might increase the probability of developing a particular disease, but the disease might also manifest in the absence of the factor, albeit less commonly. Conversely, many people can be exposed to such a risk factor without developing the disease in question. For example, well-documented risk factors in heart disease include smoking, high body-mass index and high blood pressure. In each case these causes are neither necessary nor sufficient. Many people who smoke do not develop heart disease and many people who suffer heart disease have never smoked. However, there is a probabilistic relationship between smoking and heart disease; people who smoke are more likely to develop heart disease than non-smokers. A major purpose of epidemiology is to identify such probabilistic risk factors and to contribute to the multi-disciplinary effort to understand the causal pathways through which they increase risk of disease.

RISK RATIOS

To begin to illustrate how epidemiology approaches this task, we can start by extending the concept of the prevalence estimate that we explained above. We will start by thinking about *cross-sectional* studies, where data are collected from participants at a single time point. Later in the chapter we will consider designs where participants are followed up over time.

As well as calculating prevalence across an entire sample, prevalence may also be calculated separately for particular sub-groups. For example the prevalence might be calculated separately in males and females. The British Child and Adolescent Mental Health Survey mentioned above found that the prevalence of Attention Deficit Hyperactivity Disorder[1] (ADHD) was 2.4% in boys and 0.4% in girls (across the 5–15 age range). In this case, you might think of being male as a risk factor for ADHD. Epidemiologists often talk about comparing individuals who are exposed to a risk factor to those who are not exposed. In this example there is a greater risk of ADHD for someone who is exposed to being male (i.e. they are born male) than for someone who is not exposed to being male (i.e. the females). The extent of the increased risk can be expressed as a *risk ratio*. The probability (or risk) of ADHD in boys is calculated in the same way as the prevalence of ADHD in boys: it is number of boys with ADHD divided by the total number of boys. In the UK Child and Adolescent Mental Health Survey the risk of ADHD for boys is .024 and it is .004 in girls. The risk ratio is calculated by dividing the risk in the exposed group (in this case the males) by the risk in the unexposed group (the females). This gives us a risk ratio of:

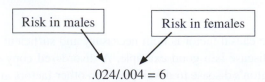

Risk in males   Risk in females

.024/.004 = 6

A risk ratio of six means that a child is six times more likely to have ADHD if they are male than if they are female.

Risk ratios are always positive numbers. A risk ratio of one indicates the risk of the outcome is exactly the same in the exposed and unexposed groups. A risk ratio above one shows that the outcome is more common in the exposed group than in the unexposed group. A risk ratio less than one indicates that the outcome is less common in the exposed group than the unexposed group and therefore exposure is potentially protective against the disease.

Activity 5.1

An epidemiologist might be interested in whether inconsistent parental discipline is a risk factor for conduct disorder (i.e. antisocial behaviour) in children. Inconsistent discipline involves an unclear relationship between child behaviour and parental response. On some occasions the child might be severely punished for doing almost nothing wrong, while on other occasions the parents might leave clearly antisocial behaviour unpunished. In a fictional cross-sectional study the following data might be observed:

	Consistent parenting	Inconsistent parenting	Total
No conduct disorder	8580	920	9500
Conduct disorder	420	80	500
Total	9000	1000	

Calculate the risk of conduct disorder in children with consistent and inconsistent discipline separately and then calculate the risk ratio.

THE ODDS-RATIO

Another statistic that you will need to understand is the *odds-ratio*. Odds-ratios are not as intuitive to understand as risk ratios. However, they have a number of mathematical properties that make them useful in epidemiological studies. It is important for you to understand what odds-ratios are and how the interpretation differs from risk ratios. Odds are calculated as the probability (p) that an event will happen divided by the probability that it will not ($1-p$). The odds-ratio is simply the odds in one group divided by the odds in another. In our ADHD example the odds can be calculated as:

$$\text{Odds in boys:} \quad .024 / (1 - .024) = .025$$
$$\text{Odds in girls:} \quad .004 / (1 - .004) = .004$$

The odds in both girls and boys look very similar to the risks. Odds and probabilities are always similar when the risks are small. The odds-ratio is calculated as follows:

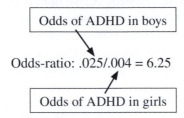

Again the odds-ratio of 6.25 is quite similar to the risk ratio of six calculated above. This is not true when the probabilities are higher, however; differences between the risk ratio and odds-ratio can be much bigger. For example, if a hypothetical disease was present in 80% of males and 20% of females, the risk ratio would be:

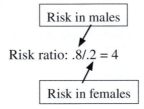

Now we will work out the odds-ratio:

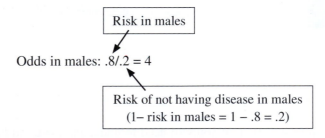

Odds in females: .2/.8 = .25

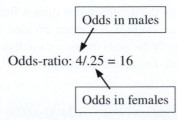

In this example the risk ratio of four and the odds-ratio of 16 are very different.

Odds-ratios may take on any value between zero and infinity. If the odds are equal in the exposed and unexposed groups then the odds-ratio would be one. If the odds of the outcome are greater in the exposed group than the unexposed group then the odds-ratio will be greater than one. If the odds are smaller in the exposed group than the unexposed group then the odds-ratio will be between zero and one.

Inferential statistical tests can be used to test whether differences in odds between exposure groups are statistically significant or whether the difference may be the result of sampling error. We cover methods appropriate to test the significance of the associations we have discussed so far in Chapters 9 and 13. We refer you to these chapters particularly because the variable of interest can only take on one of two values (i.e. diagnosed with ADHD or not). Epidemiologists may also be interested in continuous dependent variables such as body-mass index and blood pressure. Inferential statistical tests to analyse variables of this sort are covered in many of the chapters in this book including Chapters 7, 8, 10, 11 and 12.

ESTABLISHING CAUSALITY

Epidemiologists might study a wide range of potential risk factors for disease. Examples might include age, sex, social class, diet, upbringing, intelligence and exposure to toxins. Which factors are studied depends on the disease outcome in question and the relevant theoretical literature on potential causal agents. For example, studying the genetic factors involved in processing serotonin in the brain would be very useful in a study of depression but may be much less informative in a study of ruptured knee ligaments. If a variable is identified as a significant risk factor in the study designs we have discussed so far, then this demonstrates an association or correlation. It does not necessarily imply that the risk factor plays a causal role in the disease process. For example, in Activity 5.1, the fictional study addressed whether inconsistent parental discipline was a risk factor for antisocial behaviour during childhood. In the activity, it looked like antisocial behaviour was more common in children exposed to inconsistent parenting. It is possible that this association represents a causal relationship; inconsistent parenting leads to the development of conduct disorder. However, as we discussed in Chapter 1, a simple relationship identified in a cross-sectional study of this sort leaves open a number of other possibilities. For example, it might be that highly antisocial children are very difficult to parent consistently because of their extreme behaviour. In this scenario the child's antisocial behaviour causes the inconsistent discipline. It is also possible that there is not a causal relationship between parenting and antisocial behaviour but that one or more other factors are causal to both. For example, poverty might cause both antisocial behaviour in children and inconsistent discipline in parents. In this example poverty is a potential confounding variable (see Chapter 1, page 13) in the relationship between discipline and antisocial behaviour.

Gaining definitive evidence of causality in cross-sectional observational studies is not usually possible. Despite this, there is still much we can learn from studying risk factors in cross-sectional observational studies:

1) Knowing that a risk factor is associated with disease may often be useful in its own right, regardless of whether the relationship is causal. For example, where a clinician is trying to decide on a patient's diagnosis, information regarding the patient's experience of risk factors for disease may be helpful. In this situation it does not matter whether the risk factors have causal effects or whether they simply help to identify vulnerable individuals.

2) Showing that a potential cause is *not* associated with a disease outcome may be interpreted as evidence against causality in many situations (although not all) if this evidence comes from a strong study design.

3) Where risk factors are identified in epidemiological studies, these may then provide the impetus to conduct experimental studies that are able to test causal hypotheses. For example, evidence that smoking was associated with cancer led to experimental studies that showed there was a causal relationship.

Activity 5.2

A researcher wants to know whether wearing high heels is a risk factor for bunions in women. She contacts 2000 women by selecting random phone numbers from the London telephone directory and assesses them for bunions using a standard foot pain and disability index. She recorded the following results.

	Irregular high heel wearers	Regular high heel wearers
Bunion	23	208
No bunion	952	817

Calculate the following statistics from the table:
a) The overall prevalence of bunions in the population
b) The prevalence separately by regular shoe type
c) The risk ratio for regular wearers of high heels
d) The odds-ratio for regular wearers of high heels

CASE-CONTROL STUDIES

Cross-sectional studies must sample the entire population in order to ascertain the frequency of disease. Where a researcher's purpose is only to identify risk factors, however, a cheaper alternative is provided by the case-control study. Case-control studies sample a group of people who definitely have the disease of interest. For example, they might be recruited from patients receiving treatment. A control group is also recruited who are similar in characteristics to the cases but do not have the disease. The two groups are then compared on potential risk factors to ascertain what differentiates the groups. These studies are much more economical than general population studies in that far fewer participants are required.

Selection of cases and controls requires careful thought. Cases are often recruited from hospital clinics. A potential disadvantage here is that these cases must have been identified by health services (or in some other way) in order to be included in the study. It is possible that identified cases are systematically different from cases that exist undiagnosed in the community. The extent to which this is a problem depends on the nature of the disease. This is a problem for behavioural problems such as ADHD, for example. It is possible that cases that reach clinical services will not be representative of those found in the general population. Children with ADHD who display concurrent antisocial behaviour, for example, may be more likely to be referred to a psychiatrist than those with ADHD alone. In this case findings from case-control studies may not be applicable to cases of ADHD in the general population. Cases need to be selected carefully to be representative of the targeted disease entity in other ways as well. For example, if a disease is linked to mortality then it will be important to sample cases soon after diagnosis. Otherwise the sample will include only those who survive an unusually long time after diagnosis and may only identify the risk factors for this form of the disease.

Controls should be from the same population as the cases, meaning they are at risk of the disease but do not have it. The controls may be formally matched to the cases at an individual or group level. Controls can be selected from the general population or they may be recruited from patients with different diseases. Statistical tests are often more precise when sample sizes are large. This is true in case-control studies as well. While the number of cases available may be limited, the availability of controls may be less restricted. Therefore, studies often increase precision by recruiting more controls than cases, as in the example from the literature below. Clearly, because case-control studies choose how many cases and non-cases are sampled, they are not able to assess the prevalence of disease in a population. They are able to estimate the odd ratios of disease associated with measured risk factors, however.

Example from the Literature: Selective Serotonin Reuptake Inhibitors and Gastrointestinal Bleeding

Selective Serotonin Reuptake Inhibitors (SSRIs) are commonly prescribed for depression. Carvajal et al. (2011) investigated whether this drug is associated with gastrointestinal (GI) bleeding using a case-control design. A total of 581 cases of GI bleeding (as diagnosed by endoscopy) and 1358 controls were identified from four hospitals. The authors describe the selection of controls as follows:

For each case, up to 3 controls >/= 18 year old, matched by sex, age (+/−5 years), date of admission (within 3 months) and hospital were selected; they were recruited from patients who were admitted for elective surgery for non-painful disorders, including inguinal hernia, prostate adenoma and cataracts. Carvajal et al. (2011, p. 2)

The following results were recorded:

	Cases of GI bleeding	Matched controls
Not used SSRIs	558 (96%)	1313 (96.7%)
Used SSRIs	23 (4%)	45 (3.3%)

This provides an odds-ratio of 1.20, allowing for some rounding error. The authors calculated the 95% confidence intervals around this odds-ratio as .72 to 2.01. As the confidence interval includes 1, this shows the relationship between SSRI medication and GI bleeding is non-significant. Often novice researchers are very keen to see significant associations to show their study 'worked'. This is always a mistaken approach to statistical analyses. This study demonstrates the importance of identifying a non-association; this finding increases confidence that SSRIs are not associated with internal bleeding, particularly as the study is well designed with a large sample. However, any one study must be interpreted in the context of other relevant research. Carvajal et al. (2011) review a number of other studies that do report a significant association between SSRI usage and GI bleeding as well as further studies that show no relationship. Their discussion focuses on potential explanations for this body of work as a whole.

COHORT STUDIES

The study designs described so far have been cross-sectional, where data are collected at a single time-point. In contrast, cohort studies involve following a sample across time to examine the development of disease. Often samples will be carefully recruited to be representative of a geographical area as in the prevalence studies discussed above. For example, in the UK there are several national cohort studies that have sampled everyone born in the UK in a particular time period and followed them up regularly across their lifespan. Studies began in 1946, 1958, 1970 and 2000. Typically each contains approximately 17,000 individuals. Much of the data collected is publicly available for analysis (see www.cls.ioe.ac.uk for further details). For example, the 1958 cohort (also known as the National Child Development Study) has been assessed nine times to date, including assessments at birth and ages 7, 11, 16, 23, 33, 42, 46 and 50. At each assessment a range of data is collected addressing medical, social, behavioural and economic circumstances. These studies have made a large contribution to epidemiology. In the UK and internationally there are many other cohort studies of this size.

Smaller cohort studies are often reported in the literature and have also provided much useful information on risk factors for disease. Cohort studies are particularly strong when they begin before the onset of the disease of interest. This offers a greater opportunity to study the factors involved in onset, as risk factors are identified prospectively. Onset is often measured by the *incidence* of the disease. This is the percentage or proportion of participants that develop the disease of interest within a specified period of time.

Cohort studies are usually designed to study risk factors for disease. The longitudinal design provides stronger evidence of causal relationships than can be provided by cross-sectional studies. This is because cause must precede effect. Therefore, if a risk factor is present prior to the onset of disease then the possibility that it is actually a consequence of the disease is ruled out. Let us illustrate this with an extreme example. A cross-sectional study might find smoking is associated with lung cancer. This evidence alone does not rule out the possibility (albeit implausible in this case) that people choose to smoke in an attempt to self-medicate their lung cancer symptoms. In a longitudinal study, smoking at an early time point might be shown to predict later onset of lung cancer. Therefore, this finding is not compatible with the self-medication hypothesis. It is compatible with the hypothesis that smoking causes cancer. However, the longitudinal nature of the relationship does not rule out all alternative explanations. For example, it might be argued that stress causes people to smoke and stress also causes them to have lung cancer, with no direct causal link between smoking and illness.

Example from the Literature: Anxiety and Coronary Heart Disease

An important database has been provided by a cohort of nearly 50,000 young men from Sweden, born between 1949 and 1951. These men were conscripted into military service between 1969 and 1970. They were extensively assessed on psychological and physical health at the beginning of the study and have been followed up via their medical records. Janszky et al. (2010) used this dataset to assess whether depression and anxiety at the initial assessment were risk factors for coronary heart disease over a period of 37 years. Their initial analyses revealed the following results:

	Depressed	Not depressed
No heart disease	616	46811
Heart disease	30	1864
Total	646	48675

	Anxious	Not anxious
No heart disease	148	47279
Heart disease	14	1880
Total	162	49159

Of the men without depression or anxiety at initial assessment, 3.8% developed coronary heart disease during the follow-up period. In those who were depressed and anxious at the initial assessment, 4.6% and 8.6%, respectively, went on to develop heart disease. The statistical analyses showed depression was not a significant risk factor for heart disease. whereas anxiety was significantly associated with later heart disease. The authors consider a number of ways in which anxiety might be associated with later heart disease including the possibilities that anxiety might increase autonomic dysfunction and hypertension.

EXPERIMENTAL DESIGNS

As noted above, cohort studies often offer stronger evidence for causal relationships than do cross-sectional studies. However, they can still be vulnerable to confounding variables. Statistical approaches to confounding are available and are very useful in many instances. However, statistical approaches to confounding can be difficult to interpret, and often not all the important confounding variables will have been identified and measured during a study. Therefore, the evidence for causality is usually weaker in cohort studies than in experimental designs, such as randomised controlled trials (Chapter 15). In these designs the researcher manipulates the treatment the participants receive, allowing much better control over confounding variables. Epidemiologists are sometimes able to conduct randomised trials of the efficacy of interventions such as prevention campaigns, vaccination or drug treatments for disease.

While experimental designs might be the gold standard in identifying causality, the need for non-experimental epidemiological approaches remains. This is for the simple reason that many of the risk factors in which a health scientist might be interested cannot be manipulated in humans because of ethical and practical constraints. For example, a large body of literature has documented social inequalities in health outcomes. Right along the gradient of social class, people of higher status are less likely to suffer a variety of illnesses, such as heart disease, some cancers and depression. These important relationships cannot be studied experimentally, as it is both unethical and impractical to manipulate research volunteers' social background.

Where possible, epidemiologists make use of 'natural experiments' to approach questions of causality. For example, the Great Smoky Mountains Study, mentioned above, included an American Indian reservation in the geographical area studied. During the study a casino was opened on the reservation and the profits were shared amongst all the residents. This led to a substantial boost in their incomes. The, researchers were able to compare the health and wellbeing of the study participants before and after their income improved (Costello et al., 2003). This design is still not as strong as a randomised controlled trial in terms of identifying causal relationships, but experimental manipulation of economic circumstance in a similar way would be impossible. Therefore, this natural experiment has an important place in the body of evidence testing the effect of material circumstance on health outcomes.

Summary

Epidemiology is concerned with studying patterns of health and disease within specified populations. Central aims include specifying the prevalence of disease and identifying factors that increase the risk of disease. Establishing causality is done most effectively in studies that can manipulate the hypothesised variables of interest. Ethical and practical constraints make this difficult in humans, so epidemiologists must use cross-sectional and longitudinal designs carefully to identify the risk factors underlying disease.

In this chapter we touched on a number of important statistics that are routinely used in epidemiological samples, including risk ratios and odds-ratios. In later chapters we will return to these concepts and see how inferential statistics may be used to generalise from the sample to the population as a whole.

MULTIPLE CHOICE QUESTIONS

1. Prevalence studies estimate:
   a) Risk factors for disease in the population studied
   b) The frequency of disease in the population studied
   c) Onset of disease in a particular timeframe
   d) None of the above

2. A study surveys a random sample of 3000 school children from the population of South Yorkshire. On the day of the survey 21 of them report that they have head lice. Therefore the prevalence of head lice is:
   a) $(3000/21)/100 = 1.42\%$
   b) $(21/3000) \times 100 = 0.7\%$
   c) $(3000 + 21)/1000 = 3.0\%$
   d) $(100/3000) + 21 = 21.0\%$

3. Odds-ratios must always be:
   a) between 0 and infinity
   b) between 1 and infinity
   c) between 0 and 1
   d) between −1 and 1

4. The incidence of a disorder refers to:
   a) The proportion of participants who have a disorder onset in a particular time period
   b) The proportion of participants who have a disorder at the start of the study

c) The number of participants who have two or more disorders

d) None of the above

Questions 5–7 refer to a study which finds the risk of having had a cold in the last six months is .17 in those who are unemployed and .09 in those who work full time.

5. In this study the risk ratio for participants exposed to unemployment is:
   a) 1.89
   b) .06
   c) .53
   d) 2.13

6. If the risk of having a cold is .17 then the odds of having a cold are:
   a) .17
   b) .20
   c) .83
   d) .09

7. A researcher calculates an odd ratio of −.08 in this study. This implies:
   a) Employment is protective against colds
   b) People prone to colds are likely to be sacked
   c) The researcher has made a mistake in their calculation
   d) None of the above

8. Odds-ratios are calculated by:
   a) Dividing the odds in one group by the odds in another
   b) Dividing the risk in one group by the risk in another
   c) Multiplying the odds in one group by the odds in another
   d) Squaring the risk ratio

9. Cohort studies involve:
   a) Sampling a group of participants at a single point in time
   b) Studying a military unit
   c) Following a group of participants in a longitudinal study
   d) Randomising groups of participants to receive a particular treatment or not

10. Natural experiments involve:
    a) Conducting experiments in field settings
    b) Manipulating the laws of nature
    c) Manipulating the administration of drugs with natural ingredients
    d) Capitalising on naturally occurring variable manipulation

11. Prevalence estimates may be inaccurate if:
    a) Invited participants with the disorder are likely to refuse to participate
    b) The measurement instrument is inaccurate
    c) The sample size is small
    d) All of the above

12. A study finds that the risk of having a cold in the last three months is similar in smokers and non-smokers. This implies the odds-ratio in this study would be:
    a) Exactly equal to 1
    b) Close to 1
    c) Close to 0
    d) Exactly 0

13. Case-control studies are best suited to:
    a) Identifying risk factors for disease
    b) Estimating the prevalence of disease
    c) Estimating the instance of disease
    d) Identifying a representative sample of the community

14. Odds-ratios and risk ratios will be similar to each other:
    a) Under all circumstances
    b) When the risk of the disease is high
    c) When the risk of disease is low
    d) Under no circumstances

15. A cross-sectional study finds that higher testosterone levels are related to conduct disorder. This finding implies that:
    a) Testosterone causes conduct disorder
    b) Conduct disorder raises testosterone levels
    c) Other factors lead to increases in testosterone levels and conduct disorder
    d) Any of the above may be true

Note

1   Actually, the figures given here refer to hyperkinetic disorder, which is not strictly the same as ADHD, but it is similar.

Introduction to Data Screening and Cleaning

6

Overview

In this chapter we will be looking at how researchers prepare the dataset for their analysis or analyses. Although we will be focussing on a dataset in SPSS, the dataset could be in another statistical program. *Data screening and cleaning* refers to the processes of taking a dataset, looking for errors and missing data, and then dealing with these, so that we have a clean dataset – that is, one which is free from errors and missing data. Data screening and cleaning processes may also involve ensuring that the data meets the assumptions of the various statistics we wish to use – for instance, linear and multiple regressions assume a linear relationship between the variables (see Chapters 11 and 12). This chapter covers the most important issues you need to consider when carrying out your own research, and preparing the dataset. It is also important, however, to understand what data screening and procedures *other* researchers have carried out on the datasets they report in their results sections. Rather than use fictitious data to help you understand this topic, we will be using real data from our own research, and that of our students. You will be able to see the

(Continued)

(Continued)

errors which were in these datasets, and how they were dealt with. We will also be giving you examples from journal articles where researchers from the health sciences have reported the ways in which they screened and cleaned their data.

This chapter can be an introduction only to the topic of data screening and cleaning. There are many available strategies for problems involved in dealing with the very important topic of missing data, for instance. Some of these strategies are too advanced for an introductory textbook. Here we focus on the type of knowledge you will need as an undergraduate in the health sciences.

In this chapter you will learn:

- To minimise possible data entry problems at the design stage
- To test for the accuracy of the data
- To deal with the problem of *outliers*, i.e. scores which are very different from the rest of the dataset
- To identify and deal with missing data, both random and non-random
- How to report data screening and cleaning processes for a laboratory report or a journal article
- The way in which other researchers have reported their data screening and cleaning processes

INTRODUCTION

This chapter refers to inspecting and dealing with the data which has been collected, and typed into a statistical database. When carrying out a study or experiment, there is always going to be at least one error – and probably more. This is especially the case in a very large dataset. What sort of errors could there be? Errors might be attributable to the researchers – perhaps they have given out a questionnaire which has a question missing. Perhaps they have forgotten to ask for the age or sex of the participants. When sending out questionnaire packs to large numbers of people, it's fairly easy to accidentally send two identical questionnaires and omit another. Once the participants receive them, some may overlook questions or simply not answer them.

In a study, experiment or clinical trial where participants need to give data at two or more timepoints, participants might not be contactable, or might simply fail to turn up to a testing session. In studies involving drug or food supplement trials, some may forget to take their tablets for a day, a week, or longer.

Inaccuracies usually occur at the data entry stage. Once the scores have been typed into the statistical database, researchers need to 'screen' the dataset for errors, and then deal with them in some way (this is the 'cleaning' part). This involves checking for inaccurate scores, dealing with missing data and other procedures. Sometimes authors of journal articles say little about the ways in which they prepared their datasets, but it is good practice to inform readers about this. There tend to be strict word count limits for laboratory reports or journal articles. Because of this, it is not necessary to give a very detailed account of the screening and cleaning processes – but it is certainly useful to give basic, concise information, and we will be reproducing some of the results sections in relevant journal articles where authors have provided this information.

MINIMISING PROBLEMS AT THE DESIGN STAGE

There are ways of minimising the effort involved in data screening and cleaning, and that is at the very beginning when the study or experiment is being designed.

In student projects, which are often carried out with limited time and resources, students often use non-copyrighted questionnaires which are available via websites. These usually need to be re-typed by the student in a more user-friendly format – and this is where errors happen. Sometimes two identical questions are typed in by mistake, whilst another is omitted. You'd be surprised how common this is – and yet if someone else had proofread the questionnaire, the problems would have been identified. When hundreds of questionnaire packs are sent out, it is really disappointing to find many of the returned questionnaires can't be used. Some participants react to badly typed or badly presented questionnaires by not answering any of the questions, some answer some questions and leave out others, some write rude comments over the questionnaires.

When questionnaires are printed double-sided there are always some participants who do not turn over and answer the questions on the reverse side. You can reduce the likelihood of this happening by printing in large letters: 'PLEASE TURN OVER – QUESTIONS ON THE OTHER SIDE!' but this won't eliminate the problem entirely.

A common mistake made by novice researchers is to have the response labels printed on page 1 of the questionnaire, but omitted from the reverse side.

Example: A researcher has retyped page 1 of the PSQ-18 questionnaire (Figure 6.1).[1]

The participants can easily rate these questions, although the researcher could have made it easier still by putting SA, A, U, D, and SD instead of the numbers above the five columns.

However, on page 2, the researcher has made an omission, and has forgotten to give the numbers and the labels on this page (Figure 6.2).

This means many participants can't remember what the responses 1, 2, 3, etc. stand for, and they have to keep referring to page 1. Again, some participants will be annoyed by this and decide not to respond to the questions on the reverse side.

Male or Female?

To ensure that you know whether your participants are male or female, write:

'Male/Female/other (please underline)' (rather than 'Sex: ' which leads to the jokers in the study writing things like 'yes please') and gives you additional missing data.

These next questions are about how you feel about the medical care you receive

On the following pages are some things people say about medical care. Please read each one carefully, keeping in mind the medical care you are receiving now. (If you have not received care recently, think about what you would expect if you needed care today). We are interested in your feelings, good and bad, about the medical care you have received.

How strongly do you AGREE or DISAGREE with each of the following statements (tick the appropriate box)

1 = strongly agree
2 = agree
3 = uncertain
4 = disagree
5 = strongly disagree

The researchers could have used the labels instead of numbers

		1	2	3	4	5
1	Doctors are good about explaining the reason for medical tests					
2	I think my doctor's office has everything needed to provide complete medical care					
3	The medical care I have been receiving is just about perfect					
4	Sometimes doctors make me wonder if their diagnosis is correct					
5	I feel confident that I can get the medical care I need without being set back financially					

Figure 6.1   PSQ-18 questionnaire, page 1

No labels here at all!

6	When I go for medical care, they are careful to check everything when treating and examining me				
7	I have to pay for more of my medical care than I can afford				
8	I have easy access to the medical specialists I need				
9	Where I get medical care, people have to wait too long for emergency treatment				
10	Doctors act too businesslike and impersonal towards me				

Figure 6.2   PSQ-18 questionnaire, page 2

ENTERING DATA INTO DATABASES/STATISTICAL PACKAGES

When typing scores into a statistical package, always find someone else to help you, one reading the scores and one entering the data. In small datasets you can easily check scores have been entered correctly, but in a large dataset this is often not possible, so you need to take every precaution against inputting false scores. Good readers can be useful in looking at the dataset and alerting the person entering the data when s/he has made an error. This should be standard practice but it's amazing how many previously sociable students seem to have no friends at the point of data entry.

One word of advice: although SPSS numbers each row (this is what is known as a case number), ensure you create a variable (with an identity or identifier such as 'participant number') because the numbers allotted by SPSS don't change position when you need to 'sort' the datafile (i.e. rather than looking at the dataset as you have typed it in, you might want it sorted by age, sex, or group). You might then be unable to identify which participant is which. What you need is an identity number which moves with the participants data when you re-sort, so ensure you create such a variable.

THE DIRTY DATASET

Let's assume you have a dataset, and that you've done everything right so far – or think you have anyway. You've input the data using a friend to help you. However, you can't assume that everything has been entered accurately. At this stage, the dataset is said to be 'dirty'. The task of the researcher is to ensure the data are screened for problems, and then cleaned.

ACCURACY

Screenshot 6.1 shows some scores from a dataset, from a project carried out by a student of ours. This was a large dataset, but below we show you only ten participants with scores on three different symptoms of illness. The symptoms are rated from 1 (symptom not at all severe) to 7 (extremely severe). You can probably spot the impossible score – because we've only shown you a part of the dataset. So it's quite easy to simply change the 77 to a 7. However, the whole dataset consists of 131 participants and 107 variables, and eyeballing is not a very reliable way of spotting errors.

USING DESCRIPTIVE STATISTICS TO HELP IDENTIFY ERRORS

A simple way of finding mis-entered scores is to perform some descriptive statistics.

Using the *Descriptives*, *Explore* or *Frequencies* options in SPSS (see Chapter 3 page 88) can be very useful in helping you to spot unusual patterns of data. Look to see if the means are as you expect them to be. If they aren't, then either eyeball the dataset itself to find unexpected data values (this is easy for small datasets), or check the output of scores using the *Frequencies* command.

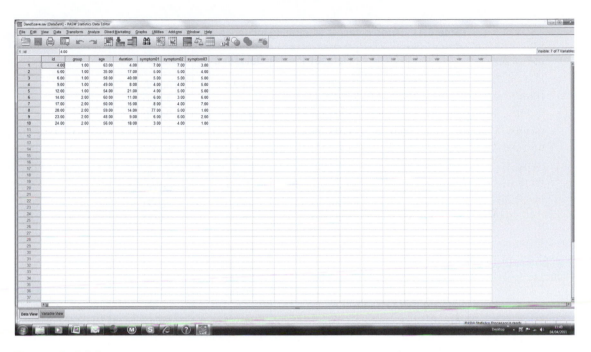

Screenshot 6.1

The range (see Chapter 3 page 83) is also useful in this respect, because if the participants should be responding on a scale of, say, 1 to 7, then seeing a range of 1–77 will alert you to a problem. Again, with a small dataset you can look directly at the SPSS datafile, but with a larger dataset you will need to look through the output from *Frequencies* to see which participant has the error. This then needs to be corrected manually.

Outliers

Outliers are datapoints which are more extreme than the rest of the scores. In quantitative analysis, we are mainly interested in the general pattern of data, and extreme scores could mislead us. For instance, look at the scores in Table 6.1. The mean in the first case is 24.92. Let us change the first score to make it extreme. The mean now is 26.40. Now let us change the first score to 100. The mean is now 29.47.

If we are trying to get an appropriate measure of central tendency – a measure which reflects the general pattern of scores, we might not want the extreme score – 100 – to pull up the mean in this way. Of course we can't simply delete scores just because they are extreme – we need to think about whether this participant differs from the other participants on other measures (not just this one). If the outlier is different in other ways too, then you might want to exclude her from the analysis, since she does not appear to belong to this group, by virtue of being very different from the rest. Outliers are important but relying only on the researchers to spot the outliers is not a reliable method of dealing with these outliers.

Table 6.1   Three datasets illustrating influence of outliers

	Dataset 1	Dataset 2	Dataset 3
	26.00	**54.00**	**100.00**
	23.00	23.00	23.00
	24.00	24.00	24.00
	27.00	27.00	27.00
	25.00	25.00	25.00
	23.00	23.00	23.00
	31.00	31.00	31.00
	30.00	30.00	30.00
	28.00	28.00	28.00
	24.00	24.00	24.00
	22.00	22.00	22.00
	22.00	22.00	22.00
	18.00	18.00	18.00
	25.00	25.00	25.00
	20.00	20.00	20.00
Mean	*24.92*	*26.40*	*29.47*

A fairly easy method is to carry out your statistical analysis using both a parametric test and its equivalent non-parametric test (see Chapter 7). If they give the same overall results then outliers are not a problem. If you get significant results with the parametric but not the non-parametric test then outliers are an issue. This is because outliers reduce the power of parametric tests to a greater extent than non-parametric tests.

If the outlier seems to be similar to the rest of the group (except for the unusual score) then you need to keep her in the analysis, but you can take steps to reduce her influence. So in the example in Table 6.1, in column 3, the outlier has a score of 100 – the highest score of the group. In this case, we can still leave her to have the highest score, but we can reduce her influence by giving her a score of 32 instead of 100. Thus we go back into the dataset and change the score. If there was an outlier who had an extremely low score (imagine some-one had scored 7 in column 3) then we would insert 17 instead of his 7 (since 18 is the next most extreme (lowest) score in the dataset. This isn't 'cheating' (if it's done properly). The outlier still has the highest or lowest score – but their influence on the general pattern of scores is reduced.

Of course it is easy to spot outliers in a small dataset. However, even with a large dataset, the ease with which box-plots and other graphical plots can be produced (see Chapter 3) means that you can easily identify outliers just by looking at the plots for each singe-variable distribution.

Outliers can have a big influence on scores – this is particularly the case in correlational analyses, where we look for relationships between variables. We will be discussing this in Chapter 10.

MISSING DATA

It is very unusual to find a dataset with no missing values at all. Sometimes data goes missing after it's been collected – a computer failure or a memory stick which becomes unreadable can lead to missing data. When this happens, it should be reported in the 'Methods' section of a laboratory report or journal article. As mentioned in the introduction, in an experiment or study which runs over one or more timepoints, there always tend to be drop outs – people who miss one or more testing sessions, or they give up because they don't like the task, they move away from the area, or go missing for a whole host of other reasons. Participants themselves can of course fail to complete questionnaires or assessments given to them. Missing data is increased when researchers use postal questionnaires. If you are able to administer questionnaires in person, and have a fairly small group, then it's possible to check that participants haven't accidentally overlooked some questions. However, since it is not ethical to put pressure onto people to answer questions that they do not want to answer, then you might still find you have missing data. Dealing with missing data is a problem that all of us have to deal with when we analyse data.

How we deal with missing data depends on the reasons why the data are missing. The strategies for dealing with missing data are called *missing data techniques*.

There are three types of 'missingness':

a)   MCAR = missing completely at random
b)   MAR = missing at random
c)   NMAR = not missing at random

MCAR

Missing completely at random is when the missing data has nothing to do with any of the measured or observed variables, or indeed the variable for which there are missing data. The participant might just have overlooked a question, or might have failed to turn up for a testing session because he was ill. This is the best scenario for data screening and cleaning, because we can make a best 'guess' as to what the missing score would be, and replace the missing data with that score. Often, the best 'guess' is the mean of the group.

MAR

Missing completely at random is when missingness is related to another variable in the dataset, but not related to the variable which is missing. Imagine that in a survey relating to drug use, men answered the questions and women did not. The failure to answer questions about drug use depended on whether they were a man or woman, not on their usage of drugs. This means, like MCAR, we can employ one of the missing data techniques which we have at our disposal.

NMAR

Not missing at random is the worse scenario – here we have data which are missing because of systematic influences. Often the missingness is related to the missing variable. Imagine that we ask people how many cigarettes a day they smoke. Some heavy smokers might not like to admit how much they smoke, and so the responses may be greater for non-smokers and light smokers. That is, there will be more missing data for heavy smokers. In this case the missing values (how many cigarettes they smoke) are directly related to how many cigarettes they smoke – and the data for this is missing! In one of our studies, described later (see page 199) around half the participants failed to answer questions relating to their sex lives (or lack of one). Their missing values on this variable probably depended on their sex lives – which we don't know about because the data are missing. Data missing non-randomly is always a problem. It is obviously better to foresee these problems and deal with them at the design stage, for instance piloting some questionnaires on a small group of people to ensure the questions are unambiguous and able to be understood.

NMAR is also a problem in clinical trials, and the longer the trial, the more missing data. Although people often assume data is missing randomly, this may not be the case. Imagine a participant in a clinical trial failed to take her medication for the last two weeks of the trial. This is unlikely to be random. Also, groups might differ in their patterns of missing data, e.g. perhaps the healthy group attended all three testing sessions, but a high percentage of the illness group failed to attend the last two sessions. Here again, the data is not missing randomly. If participants drop out due to problems with the clinical trial, then data is missing non-randomly.

You can tell whether missing values are related to other variables by creating a group for the people who are missing data. For instance, if 'number of cigarettes smoked' had a lot of missing data, you could create a Group 'cigarettesmissing' – everyone who had missing data would be given a value of 1, meaning they are in Group 1. Everyone who had scores for 'number of cigarettes smoked' would be given a value of 2. This is called creating a dummy variable. The easiest way to see whether the group with the missing data differs from the group without missing data is to use a t-test (see Chapter 7). If the groups show a difference then the data is NMAR. If data is NMAR, then advanced techniques are needed to deal with them. As students at an undergraduate level, this level of expertise would not be expected from you if you were carrying out a study or experiment. You could, however, repeat the analysis with and without the missing data when you report your analyses. If the results are similar, then you do not need to do anything else (see how we dealt with a problem like this on page 199 (this chapter). If they are different, however, you need to delve more into the data and find out the reasons for the difference, and then report both sets of results.

Missing Data Techniques

A participant will be deleted from the analysis if s/he has a missing value for the dependent variable being analysed.

Listwise Deletion (Complete Case Analysis)

SPSS gives an option for deleting cases listwise. This means that SPSS will exclude all participants who have a missing value on any of the variables. This means that if a participant has given information on 99 out of 100 variables, the participant will not be included in the analysis. You can see that, using this technique, you might end up with hardly any participants at all.

Pairwise Deletion (Available Case Analysis)

SPSS also gives an option for deleting cases pairwise. A participant will be deleted from the analysis if s/he has a missing value for the variable being analysed. While this might seem to be better than listwise deletion, it is not without its problems – again, sample size can be reduced, and when using correlational techniques (see Chapter 10) problems can occur, as the correlations will be based on different numbers of participants, have different sample sizes and therefore different variances. Sometimes this will lead to correlations above 1 – which is not really possible, and so your statistical program will progress no further!

Inserting a Measure of Central Tendency

In a large dataset, variables tend to be normally distributed and it is acceptable to insert the mean of a group in place of the missing scores. In the absence of any other information, the mean from the rest of the group of participants for that particular variable is the best guesstimate there is, and in general, this should be used. For smaller datasets, the appropriate measure of central tendency may not be the mean – it might be the median (see Chapter 3). Some researchers report which measure(s) of central tendency they used to replace the missing datapoints. The text below is from Castle (2005, p. 121) who was examining the association between the quality of care in nursing homes and the likelihood of closure. Castle had two conditions in this study – 'closed facilities' and 'non-closed facilities'. It was important for Castle to reassure the readers that the two groups were similar in their patterns of outliers and missing values:

> *Following the approach outlined by other researchers using these data, frequency distribution plots were used to identify obvious outliers ... All missing and outlier values for continuous or ordinal variables were replaced by the sample mean ... Duplicate facilities, outlier values, and missing values were found to be evenly distributed in closed and nonclosed facilities.*

Sometimes It Is Not Appropriate to Insert a Measure of Central Tendency

Imagine that there were *five* missing scores in Group 1 (Table 6.2). Here it is not valid to use the other six scores to calculate and insert a measure of central tendency – there is just too much missing data, and putting in a measure of central tendency for 50% of the group may

Table 6.2 Dataset for participants with CFS and healthy participants

Participant	Group 1 – CFS	Participant	Group 2 – healthy people
1	15	12	missing
2	missing	13	13
3	9	14	11
4	missing	15	12
5	missing	16	10
6	14	17	14
7	15	18	12
8	missing	19	10
9	13	20	missing
10	missing	21	13
11	15	22	14
		23	7

be misleading. How much is too much missing data? Newgard et al. (2006) state that it is difficult to determine this. Even 3% missing data may be too much in certain situations. In Table 6.2, we have 27% missing data, so this is definitely too much, especially as the missing data occurs mostly in Group 1.

Here it is best to try to find more participants – although this is not always possible at such a late stage in the research process – especially if participants are selected from rare groups, e.g. people with uncommon illnesses.

LOCF (Last Observation Carry Forward)

This is a technique used in clinical trials and other longitudinal repeated measures research. If, for instance, a person has missed the last five days of a measurement, then the missing data would be replaced with the last recorded value for that participant. Another way of dealing with this would be to take the last five days of the participant's recorded value, and take the mean of that score. However, according to Harris et al. (2009) using this technique may severely bias the estimate of the treatment effect.

However you deal with the missing data, you need to report it. This is what we said for a double-blind placebo trial looking at whether a nutritional supplement helped symptoms of Irritable Bowel Syndrome:

Every participant forgot to take at least one capsule across the duration of the trial, but this was usually one capsule only on any given day. There were two exceptions – one participant took capsules erratically over the last six weeks of the experimental condition and after the first five weeks of the placebo condition. This participant had a change of personal circumstances during this time (she underwent a hysterectomy). The other participant took no capsules for five days in the last week of the experimental condition as she went away and forgot to take the capsules with her ... For symptom recording, three participants had some sequential data missing, i.e. for the first participant this was for seven days in the experimental condition; for the second it was three days in the exper- imental condition, and for the third, three days during baseline. For each missing data point frequency data were obtained for the particular condition in which the missing data occurred, and the most appropriate (representative) measure of central tendency was inserted. Dancey et al. 2006

Activity 6.1

What are the two most important issues to be considered when data screening and cleaning? See page 523.

When writing up the results of a study, researchers should always be honest about these problems, and say how they dealt with them. Here is part of a section on data screening by Booij et al. (2006) describing drop-out rates in their study, which involved seeing how a diet rich in α-lactalbumin could help depressed and non-depressed participants:

Of a total of 49 participants who were included, 43 (23 recovered depressed patients; 20 controls) completed the study. Three recovered depressed patients were included but decided not to participate. Three patients dropped out after the first session; the first case due to nausea (after α-lactalbumin), the second case dropped out because of feeling uncomfortable with venapunction during the first session ...; the third one could not be contacted to schedule the second session on time ... These patients were left out of all analyses. p. 529

They also describe problems they had with technical failures, leading to missing data:

Due to a computer failure, data of the cognitive tasks during the screening session for one control patient were lost. For one patient, data of the Memory Scanning task during the screening session were missing. TOL [Tower of London task] data during the screening session were missing for another patient. Morning assessments of the Left/Right task in the casein condition were unavailable for one patient. Twenty-two of the 172 blood samples

(12.7%) were missing because of difficulties with the venapunction. Cases with missing data were omitted separately by analysis. p. 529.

SPOTTING MISSING DATA

In a large dataset (e.g. perhaps hundreds of variables and/or hundreds of participants) it would be impossible by eyeballing alone to ensure you have spotted all the missing values. Eyeballing here would certainly be the wrong strategy. If you insert measures of central tendency and get as far as analysing the data, you will need to start again if you later realise that you have some values which are still missing. If you have computed totals for any questionnaires when you still have missing data, then you will have to start the whole process again once you realise that you still have missing data.

Missing Values Analysis

SPSS has a Missing Values Analysis (MVA) which can tell you which values are missing. The MVA procedure is complex, and can give us a lot more information than we are going to cover here. Here we are going to discuss a few basic procedures which will help you to identify which cases are missing, and whether they are missing randomly.

The following is output from an MVA carried out on a small dataset on three variables, which are the *total of illness intrusiveness*, the *total of illness uncertainty* and the *total of social support*. The output (Table 6.3) shows that there is one datapoint missing for *illness intrusiveness*, one for *illness uncertainty* and three for *social support*. The output also shows there are no extreme scores outside of the range indicated (see Chapter 3, page 83 for details of the interquartile range).

You could replace the missing data on the variables by the simple mean, and you could of course do this by hand, without performing an MVA. However, in a large dataset where it's difficult to see whether data is missing at random or not, MVA will be very useful. SPSS has different ways of calculating the means which could be inserted instead of missing variables. SPSS can calculate them based on data which is missing pairwise, data which is missing listwise, Expectation-Maximization (EM) estimation and estimation by multiple regression (the latter is covered in Chapter 11). Our example is based on EM.

You can see from Table 6.4 that the EM means are almost identical to the univariate means presented above. The easiest option is to insert the EM means instead of the missing values.

Table 6.5 confirms that three participants have missing values for *social support* (S = missing), and that these cases are number 5, number 8 and number 16 (these are the case numbers allotted by SPSS).

Table 6.3 SPSS Output: Univariate statistics for illness intrusiveness, illness uncertainty, and social support

Means of the variables

For illness intrusiveness, there is one missing score, representing 4.3% of the scores on this variable

Univariate Statistics

	N	Mean	Std. Deviation	Missing Count	Missing Percent	No. of Extremes[a] Low	No. of Extremes[a] High
Illness intrusiveness	22	36.4545	17.29775	1	4.3	0	0
Illness uncertainty	22	58.3636	26.84975	1	4.3	0	0
Social support	20	54.0000	24.90403	3	13.0	0	0

a. Number of cases outside the range (Q1 − 1.5*IQR, Q3 + 1.5*IQR).

Table 6.4 SPSS output: summary of estimated means

Summary of Estimated Means

	Illness intrusiveness	Illness uncertainty	Social support
All Values	36.4545	58.3636	54.0000
EM	36.1608	58.3314	54.0272

Table 6.5   SPSS output: missing patterns analysis

Missing Patterns (cases with missing values)

| Case | # Missing | % Missing | Missing and Extreme Value Patterns[a] | | | Variable Values | | |
			Illness intrusiveness	Illness uncertainty	Social support	Illness intrusiveness	Illness uncertainty	Social support
5	1	33.3			S	55.00	95.00	.
8	1	33.3			S	24.00	97.00	.
16	1	33.3			S	13.00	12.00	.
15	1	33.3		S		35.00	.	55.00
10	1	33.3	S			.	18.00	39.00

'S' represents missing data

- indicates an extreme low value, while + indicates an extreme high value. The range used is (Q1 − 1.5*IQR, Q3 + 1.5*IQR).
a. Cases and variables are sorted on missing patterns.
Note: There are no extreme scores here.

a) Which participant(s) had missing data on illness intrusiveness (give participant number)?

b) Which participant(s) had missing data on illness uncertainty?

If there were any extreme values this would be indicated by a + for a high value and a – for a low value.

Table 6.6   SPSS output: estimated means: Little's MCAR test[a]

EM Means[a]

Illness intrusiveness	Illness uncertainty	Social support
36.1608	58.3314	54.0272

a. Little's MCAR test: Chi-Square = 4.357, df = 6, Sig. = .628

There are several other tables which can be produced, however the important statistic here is the 'Little's MCAR test' (Table 6.6). If the significance level is > .05, then we can conclude that the data is missing at random – luckily for us, because we know that it's a lot easier to deal with missing data if it's missing randomly.

Missing Values Analysis in SPSS

Click on *Analyze, Missing Values Analysis*. A dialogue box appears (Screenshot 6.2).

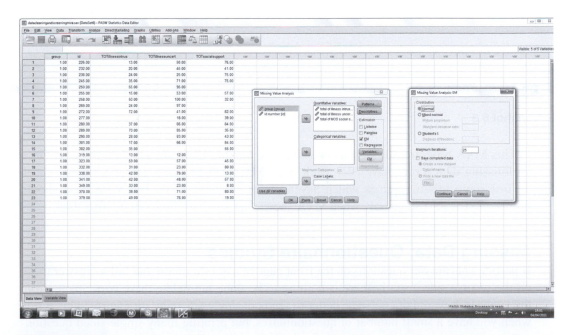

Screenshot 6.2

Check *EM* (expectation-maximization), then *Continue*, then *Patterns*.

Click on the *Cases with missing values, sorted by missing value patterns* and *Sort variables by missing value pattern* and then move the variables (illness intrusiveness, illness uncertainty and social support)from the left-hand side to *Additional information for:* on the righthand side (Screenshot 6.3). Then *Continue*, then *OK*.

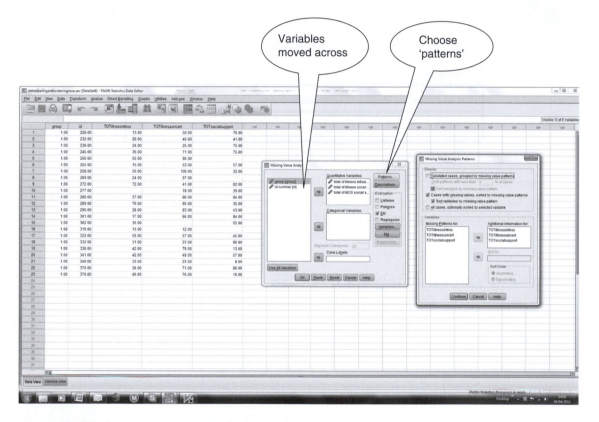

Screenshot 6.3

This MVA program allows someone to check whether there are any data missing. Once the missing data scores have been dealt with, MVA can be run again as a further check against some missing values which haven't been spotted. If you run MVA, you should proceed to the next stage only when MVA shows that you have no more missing data.

Missing Data: Questionnaire Studies

If participants answer questions on the front page of a questionnaire but fail to answer those on the reverse side, usually there is nothing to be done but delete these participants from the analysis. It would of course be better to send out single-sided questionnaires. This is fine when you have a small number of questionnaires, but printing many single-sided question-naires, raises costs considerably, and also looks more daunting for the participants.

Participants who fail to answer one or more questions on one or more of the questionnaires probably need to be excluded from the analyses. Many questionnaires have sub-scales embedded within them. For instance, a Quality of Life (QOL) questionnaire may have sections relating to health, work, social life, personal life and so on. Questions relating to health would be summed, giving a total 'health sub-scale' score. Questions relating to other scales would also be summed. Then all the sub-scale scores would be added to give a total QOL score. Unless you design your own questionnaires, you will be using extant questionnaires which have been already tested, and for which their reliability and validity are known. If, because of missing data, it is not possible to calculate a sub-scale, then this sub-scale cannot contribute to the total QOL score. Although you could calculate a total QOL score without the missing sub-scale, you would not then know whether it was reliable or valid (because it has been altered, and the known reliability and validity measures are based on the QOL with all sub-scales included). This is what happened in a study conducted by one of our students. A proportion of the men and a larger proportion of the women failed to answer questions which made up a 'sexual relations sub-scale' in a QOL questionnaire. With such a large amount of missing data, we did not feel we could simply insert a measure of central tendency. We thought about leaving this scale out entirely, but we didn't know how this would affect the validity of the questionnaire. On the other hand, including it meant that the sexual relations sub-scale would be based on only a small number of participants – participants who might be very different from the ones who did not answer. Our solution was to perform our analyses twice – both with the sub-scale included, and without it. Luckily the analyses were almost identical, so we decided to use the QOL scale without the sexual relations sub-scale.

With most problems, there are always ways to deal with them.

Below we report how we dealt with this situation:

> *The QOL comprises nine life domains, one of which is sexual relations. Unfortunately, a large number of participants – 18 men (33%) and 26 women (41%) – either wrote 'not applicable' in this section, or did not answer the questions relating to sex. The total QOL score was computed both with and without this scale: results were almost identical in all analyses. The results in this paper refer to the total QOL scale with the sex sub-scale excluded.* Dancey et al. (2002, p. 393)

A More Advanced Way to Deal with Missing Data

For non-randomly missing data, there are more advanced ways of dealing with missing data. One of these involves predicting what the individuals *would* have scored if they were not missing, based on the data they have given. This technique is included in MVA and involves the use of regression analysis – and therefore we cover this technique in Chapter 11.

NORMALITY

Generally we make a reasonable assumption – that all variables are drawn from a population which is normally distributed (see Chapter 4, page 140). If a variable, or variables, are not normally distributed then the distribution will either have a positive or a negative skew (see Chapter 4, page 141). To check skewness, it is usual to look at histograms (see Chapter 4, page 141) or to look at the skewness statistics, produced under the *Analyze, Descriptives, Frequencies*, command. Below is the mean and skewness statistics for a variable called 'biological causes' produced with these commands (Table 6.7).

As you know, the larger the sample size, the more the distribution approaches normality (see Chapter 4, page 140). If scores were perfectly normally distributed the skew would be 0.00 – but as we are unlikely to have such a perfect normal distribution in our studies, a skewness figure which is near zero is acceptable. The skewness statistic here is .024, which is near zero. A histogram confirms that in this case, we have a fairly normal distribution (Figure 6.3).

For multivariate statistics (see Chapter 12) we assume that all combinations of the variables are normally distributed.

The skewness statistic should be read in conjunction with the standard deviation of the skew. If the SD is 1.98 or above (this equates to $p = .05$) then we can say that it is skewed enough for us to decide to:

a)   use non-parametric statistics or
b)   transform the scores so that they are less skewed.[2]

Sometimes, however, transforming the data does not lead to an improvement in skewness. People have different views about whether data should be transformed, and whether it is useful to do so. Also, many people find it difficult to both transform the data, and to understand the meaning of the statistics once they've been transformed. For students using statistics at the undergraduate level, it is probably better to stay away from transformations. However, you need to know that researchers do sometimes transform their data in this way. For example, researchers Gunstad et al. (2006) reported that one of their variables was

Table 6.7   SPSS output: descriptive statistics for biological causes

Statistics

biological causes

N	Valid	116
	Missing	2
Mean		18.3966
Median		19.0000
Mode		19.00
Skewness		.024
Std. Error of Skewness		.225

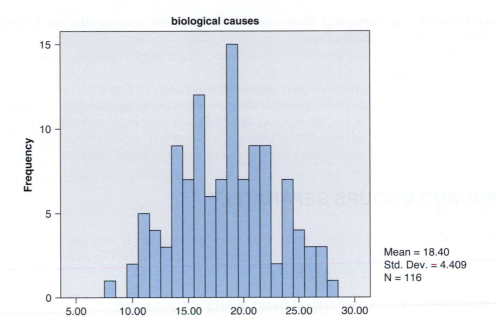

Figure 6.3   SPSS output: histogram for biological causes

skewed, and showed readers that they had considered transforming it. They then gave the reason why they didn't do this. Their description of their data screening process is both concise and informative:

Data Screening
Before analysis, the performances of all 364 individuals were examined for missing values and fit between distributions and assumptions. No participant had missing data. Assumptions of normality and possible extreme scores were then determined separately for each age group and variable. A slightly positive skew was detected for the executive function measure (Switching of Attention–II) in each age group. However, this minor violation is consistent with theoretical models of executive function and was not transformed. p. 60

Booij et al. (2006) gave a brief description of the ways in which they screened and cleaned their data. Notice they do not go into detail about which participants had missing data, or how they dealt with it. Journal editors work using very strict word-counts, and authors do not need to go into great detail in respect of data cleaning. In the following example, readers know that the authors are aware of data cleaning and screening procedures, and that they have dealt with the important issues of accuracy and missing data, and that they met the assumptions of their statistical analyses . You will see that one of their measures – reaction times on a task called the Tower of London – were transformed by a log10 transformation,[3] and that they have informed readers that they used non-parametric statistics on the POM scores because transformations were unsuccessful, i.e. transformations did not lead to a normal distribution of these scores.

Statistical analysis
Prior to analysis, all variables were examined for accuracy of data entry, missing values and fit between their distributions and the assumptions of the statistical analyses …. Reaction Times of the Tower of London task and Left/Right task were log10 transformed prior to analysis. The Profile of Mood State (POM) scores were analysed with nonparametric statistics because transformations were unsuccessful, as shown by visual inspection … p. 530

SCREENING GROUPS SEPARATELY

If there are sub-groups within a dataset, e.g. men and women, illness and heatlhy, etc., then it is good practice to screen and clean the groups separately. Gunstad et al. (2006) see above – reported that they had done this.

REPORTING DATA SCREENING AND CLEANING PROCEDURES

We believe that describing the data cleaning and screening processes which arise from quantitative analyses should be included in reports and journal articles. In practice, many authors do not include information about the ways in which they cleaned and screened their data, and of those who do, there is a great deal of variability in both the type and amount of information they include. Of course, part of this variability could be due to the space constraints of the journal concerned. At the minimum, there should be a brief paragraph which details the ways in which missing data and outliers have been dealt with. If there are no missing data, or outliers (see below) it is an good idea to say so.

Example from the Literature

Byford and Fiander (2007) worked out a prospective method of collecting information on professional input into the care of people with severe mental health problems.

A two-sided A5 sheet was used to record information on all contact between professionals and their patients. The full description of the study can be accessed online (see Byford and Fiander, 2007). For the purposes of this chapter, we report the section which relates to data screening and cleaning:

The data were entered into SPSS Data Entry II, usually within a month of collection, and omissions and obvious errors investigated in writing at this time. The completeness of the event record data was verified by audits of the clinical and social work notes of all study participants. Audits took place at approximately yearly intervals to identify direct and attempted face-to-face patient contacts not recorded on event records. Staff were sent lists of missing data and asked to complete an event record for each missing event. Data cleaning was thorough, with each variable being subjected to frequency tests and any incorrect, missing or unusual entries investigated, first with reference to the paper event record and where necessary by referring to the staff member who had completed the record. Once data cleaning had been completed, any remaining missing data for the variables based on continuous data (i.e. time) were imputed from the average for that type of event performed with a particular patient or, where this was impossible (e.g. because the patient received no other care activity of that type), from the average for that type of event performed with all patients in the patient's treatment group. The time was rounded to the nearest five minutes according to the data-recording protocol. Although missing categorical data could not be imputed its incidence was low.

Here is an example of a rather brief statement regarding data cleaning and screening, which is perhaps a bit ambiguous?

Data cleaning occurred before the breaking of the randomisation code and the statistician was blinded during the statistical analysis. Silveira et al. (2002)

Activity 6.3

Look at the dataset in Screenshot 6.4. Type the data into your statistical package, and decide on the best way to deal with the missing data. For example, which figure should be inserted into the missing cells for 'age', which for symptoms, and so on?

Compare your findings to ours. Data cleaning and screening is not an exact science – so in some cases, we may have made different decisions to you.

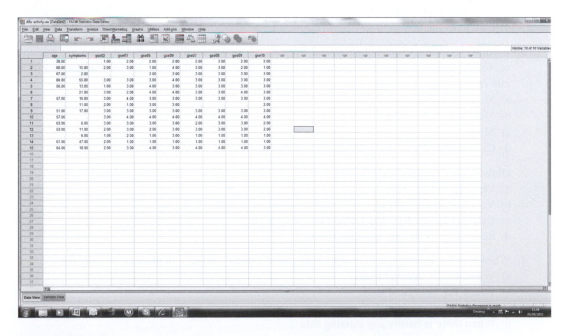

Screenshot 6.4

Summary

Data screening and cleaning techniques involve inspecting the data and ensuring it is 'clean', i.e. that there are no errors, that missing data have been dealt with, and that the data meet the assumptions of the analyses which the researchers intend to use (e.g. that scores are normally distributed and have equal variances). Techniques for screening and cleaning are generally available through statistical packages such as SPSS. The problem of missing data is perhaps the hardest to deal with, and depends on whether the data are missing at random, or whether there is a pattern to missingness. This chapter has discussed various methods that researchers use in order to deal with problems surrounding accuracy and missing data. Good researchers will always report their screening and cleaning techniques in their write-ups.

MULTIPLE CHOICE QUESTIONS

1. A dirty dataset is one that:
   a) Hasn't been screened
   b) Hasn't been cleaned
   c) May have incorrect scores
   d) Has all of the above

2. Assume you have a small dataset and the data are not normally distributed. Data are missing randomly. Which measure of central tendency is likely to be the most appropriate for insertion into empty cells?
   a) Mean
   b) Median
   c) Mode
   d) Can't tell

3. Outliers are datapoints which are:
   a) Very high scores only
   b) Very low scores only
   c) Extreme data scores which could be low or high
   d) Something to do with a cricket match

4. When is it *not* appropriate to insert a measure of central tendency in place of missing data?
   a) When data is interval level
   b) When data is ordinal level
   c) When there is too much missing data
   d) When there is hardly any missing data

5. SPSS is able to carry out an analysis of missing data. This gives information on:
   a) How many participants have missing data for selected variables
   b) How many participants have extreme scores
   c) Which cases have missing data
   d) All of the above

6. When data is drawn from a normal population and is not skewed, the most appropriate measure of central tendency to use in replacing missing values is likely to be the:
   a) Mean
   b) Median
   c) Mode
   d) Standard deviation

7. The biggest practical problem in a dataset is:
   a) Inaccurate data
   b) Missing data
   c) Multicolinearity
   d) Non-normal data

8. Deleting data listwise means a participant who has missing values:
   a) On any of the variables will be excluded
   b) On over 3% of the cells will be deleted
   c) On the dependent variable being analysed will be deleted
   d) On all of the above will be deleted

9. Assume you have a large dataset – there are some randomly missing data in variables such as *age*, *IQ*, *height* and *weight*. Which is the most likely appropriate measure of central tendency?
   a) Mean
   b) Median
   c) Mode
   d) Can't tell

10. When the missing data has nothing to do with any of the measured or observed variables, or indeed the variable for which there is missing data, we say that the data is:
    a) Missing completely at random
    b) Missing at random
    c) Not missing at random
    d) Last observation carried forward

11. Deleting data pairwise means:
    a) In a repeated measures analysis, pairs of participants will be deleted if either has missing values on the variables
    b) Excluding all participants who have a missing value on any of the variables
    c) A participant will be deleted from the analysis if s/he has a missing value for the variable being analysed
    d) All of the above

12. If data are not normally distributed, it is possible to force them into normality by:
    a) Deleting outliers
    b) Performing arithmetical transformations
    c) Using parametric statistics
    d) All of the above

13. If, in a clinical trial, a person has missed the last five days of a measurement, then the missing data could be replaced with the last recorded value for that participant. This technique is known by the following acronym:
    a) MCAR
    b) MAR
    c) NMAR
    d) LOCF

14. The worse case scenario for dealing with missing data is:
    a) MCAR
    b) MAR
    c) NMAR
    d) LOCF

15. If participants in a clinical trial drops out due to problems with the clinical trial itself, then data are:
    a) MCAR
    b) MAR
    c) NMAR
    d) Can't tell

Notes

1   Only five questions are shown on each of the two pages of the PSQ-18 shown here
2   To transform scores a mathematical calculation is carried out, e.g. the simplest transformation is to add a constant to all participants' scores on a variable (e.g. adding 50 to everyone's score). Calculations such as using a square root or a logarithmic transformation are more common in this situation.
3   A logarithm is the power a number must be raised to in order to get the original number. Here the researchers have used logarithms with the base of 10. So 1 is 10^0 because 10 to the power of $0 = 1$. 100 is 10^2 because 10 to the power of $2 = 100$.

Differences Between Two Groups

7

Overview

This chapter will be looking at statistics which tell us whether two conditions or groups differ from each other on one or more variables. The two conditions can either be:

a) The same group of people tested in two conditions (traditionally called A and B), or

b) Two different groups of people, who perform in either condition A or condition B[1]

This chapter will illustrate the ways in which researchers test their hypotheses, based on the research questions that they have. The tests covered in this chapter are parametric ones (see Chapter 4, page 142 for an explanation): the t-tests and the z-test, and their non-parametric equivalents: the Mann–Whitney U test and the Wilcoxon signed rank test. We will give you a basic conceptual understanding of the tests, show how researchers report their results, how to perform the tests in SPSS, and how to interpret the output. We will cover confidence intervals and effect sizes (see Chapter 4, pages 155–161) specifically relating to two groups.

From this chapter you will:

- Gain a conceptual understanding of two-group tests of difference
- Be able to decide when to use a two-group test of difference
- Be able to identify whether you should use a parametric or a non-parametric test, and whether the test should be repeated-measures or independent
- Learn to interpret effect sizes, and confidence intervals around the mean for two-group tests
- Be able to interpret the results of researchers who have used these techniques and reported them in their results sections
- Be able to understand and use these techniques in your own work

INTRODUCTION

In comparing two groups or conditions researchers hypothesise that there will be a statistically significant difference between them. The null hypothesis is that any differences in the scores between the conditions are due to sampling error (often called chance) (see Chapter 4, page 129).

Sometimes the researchers predict the direction of the difference. In this case, the hypothesis is directional, e.g. that Group A is predicted to score, on average, higher than Group B, in which case a one-tailed test can be used.[2] Sometimes researchers predict that there will be a significant difference between conditions, but they cannot specify the direction of the difference, in which case a two-tailed test will need to be used (see Chapter 4, page 147).

The parametric test comparing two groups is called the t-test. Parametric tests were designed for datasets which were normally distributed, and so for many years students were told that before carrying out parametric tests such as the t-test, they had to ensure that their samples had to be drawn from a population which was normally distributed, and that the variances in each condition had to be similar (the homogeneity of variance assumption).

It was (and still is) difficult to know whether the scores were drawn from a population which is normally distributed. So students were told to look at their sample distributions, and if they were skewed, they could infer that the population scores were skewed. They therefore had to conclude that a parametric test was not the right test to use. You can see that this was/is an inexact science!

However, recent advances in statistical theory and practice indicate that the violation of these assumptions does not make much difference to the results (i.e. they are 'robust' in respect of violations of the assumptions). With the advent of computerised statistical programs, it is easy to compare parametric and non-parametric tests for the same dataset, and for many datasets, you will see that there is very little difference in the results.

Statistical programmes such as SPSS can adjust the t-test formula when the homogeneity of variance assumption is violated. Where researchers believe that their distribution is too skewed to be normal, an alternative method of calculating the t-test has become available, called bootstrapping. This approach makes no assumptions about the distribution of the dependent variable. Bootstrapping is not common at the moment, but is likely to become so (see the companion website).

Even though bootstrapping is now available, it is not available for all statistical procedures, and many people still don't use them. Many researchers still use non-parametric equivalents of the t-test. These tests are still available in modern statistical packages and are often used in research papers relating to the health sciences.

Non-parametric statistics make no assumptions about normal distribution, type of data or equivalence of variances, and because of this, their power to detect a statistically significant difference between the conditions is lower than those of parametric tests.

So how should you decide on whether to use a parametric test or not?

If your data are normally distributed, then use the t-test. However, in the health sciences in particular, researchers often have small samples with skewed data. If you are carrying out your own research, we recommend that you look to see if your data are significantly skewed (see Chapter 4, pages 140–141). If they are, you can use the bootstrapping approach to t-test calculation or the traditional non-parametric tests. The non-parametric equivalents of the t-test are the Mann–Whitney for independent groups, and the Wilcoxon for repeated measures.

All of the tests in this chapter are 'inferential tests' because they go beyond descriptive statistics – you can actually infer something from them, i.e. whether any differences between groups are real (or due to chance), and furthermore, the direction of the difference.

Here are some aims/hypotheses which show clearly that the researchers are looking for differences between conditions. As you read them, think about whether the design is independent groups, or repeated measures.

1) Yu et al. (2007) were looking at the effectiveness of a breast cancer screening training programme. The group they tested were trainees (who were training as lay health advisors for promoting breast cancer screening). The potential trainees were given a pre-intervention questionnaire measuring knowledge and self-efficacy. The group were then engaged in a three-month self-study of training materials. At the end of the programme they were again given the questionnaires to measure knowledge and self-efficacy.

2) Skumlien et al. (2007) investigated the benefits of intensive rehabilitation in patients with Chronic Obstructive Pulmonary Disease (COPD). They looked at changes in functioning disability and health in relation to pulmonary rehabilitation (PR). Forty people with COPD attended an in-patient multidisciplinary PR. This consisted of endurance training, resistance training, education sessions and individual counselling sessions. They compared this group to a patient group who were on a waiting list. This is called a *waiting list control group*.

3) Shearer et al. (2009) compared glucose point-of-care values with laboratory values in critically ill patients. Sixty-three critically ill patients had their blood glucose levels measured by a glucose meter at a bedside point-of-care (POC). This method is often used on its own, rather than sending the blood specimens to a laboratory. In this study, the blood was also sent to the laboratory. Shearer et al. then compared the glucose values obtained in the 63 patients by both methods.

4) Giovannelli et al. (2007) wanted to see whether physiotherapy increases botulinum toxin type A effects in reducing spasticity in patients with Multiple Sclerosis (MS). There were 38 patients in this study, which was a randomised controlled trial, consisting of an intervention group (given botulinum toxin A injection plus additional physiotherapy) and a control group (botulinum injection).

In 1), the design is 'repeated measures' as there is one group of people who are tested as both timepoints – before and after a training programme.

In 2), the design is 'independent groups', i.e. an intervention group and a control group.

In 3), the design is 'repeated measures', as the blood given by patients was measured both in the laboratory and by a glucose meter.

In 4), the design is 'independent measures' as a treatment group was compared to a control group.

You need to identify whether you have independent groups or repeated measures. The formula to calculate t differs according to the two different designs.

CONCEPTUAL DESCRIPTION OF THE t-TESTS

Let us say there are two groups of people. Group 1 are patients with MS who are being given a new treatment, Group 2 are patients on the waiting list (control group). The independent variable is 'Treatment' and the dependent variable is a measure of memory.

You can see (Table 7.1) that the treatment scores vary from 10 to 18. Although all ten patients in the treatment condition have MS, their memory scores show variability within the group (or within the column). The waiting list control patients also vary. Their scores vary from 4 to 14. So we have two measures of within-participants variation, one for the treatment group, and one for the control group.

There is also variation in scores across the groups (or between the groups). This is called between-groups variation (between the columns).

There are different measures of variation. You have learned these in Chapter 3, pages 82–87.

If we want to know whether the two groups differ, we can't simply look at the group means. We have to know whether the between groups variance (what we are really interested in) differs from the within groups variance (which, if we want to find statistically significant results, is just a nuisance to us!).

The test statistic t is calculated by calculating the difference between the two means and then dividing the result by a measure representing the variation in scores for the groups. This measure of variance is the 'Standard Error of the Difference'.

Table 7.1 Dataset for treatment and control groups

Patient number	Treatment	Patient number	Control
1	14	11	9
2	18	12	7
3	10	13	12
4	13	14	11
5	15	15	14
6	15	16	5
7	12	17	4
8	12	18	10
9	10	19	9
10	12	20	9
Mean	*13.1*	*Mean*	*9*

The *t*-test formulae can be thought of as:

difference between the means (signal) ÷ unwanted variability (noise)

The 'noise' is the variability for each group.

The more noise there is, the lower the signal–noise ratio will be (*t*-value will be lower); the less noise there is, the greater the signal–noise ratio (*t*-value will be higher). Look at Figure 7.1.

Figure 7.1 shows that group 1 has a higher mean (13.10) than group 2 (9). The mean difference is 4.1. However, the variability is similar (but not identical) in each. There is not too much overlap between the groups – this gives a clear signal, as 'noise' is reduced. The *t*-value is going to be large and the *p*-value is going to be statistically significant. Although the distributions overlap, the results of the *t*-test are statistically significant: $t = 3.3$, $p = .002$ (you will need to take our word for this, at this stage).

Look at Figure 7.2, the means differ by four, the same as in Figure 7.1. However, in this case the within-participant variability for both groups is wide, so there is more overlap in this case. The noise' obscures the signal – the *t* will be smaller than in the case of groups 1 and 2, because the noise is large.

A '*t*-value' can be negative or positive; this depends on which group is coded as 1 and which group is coded as 2. For example, using the earlier example of groups 1 and 2, we coded the treatment group 1, and the control group 2. Our hypothesis is that the treatment group will score significantly higher than the control group. We find that the means of the group are as follows:

- Group 1 treatment group: mean 13.10
- Group 2 control group: mean 9.00

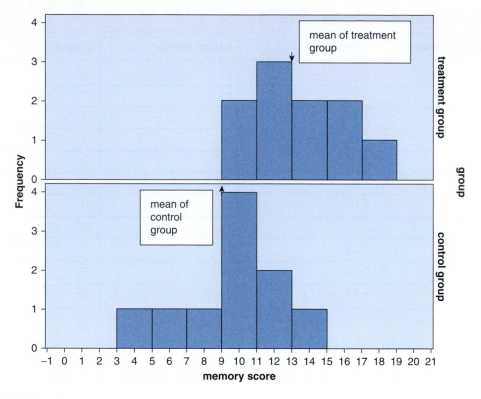

Figure 7.1 Frequency histograms for two groups on memory measure (small overlap)

The mean difference is positive, and the *t*-value is therefore positive.

What happens if we code the control group as Group 1 and the treatment group as Group 2?

- Group 1 control group: mean 9.00
- Group 2 treatment group: mean 13.10

The mean difference (−4.1) is negative, and the *t*-value is therefore negative.

This leads to a value of $t = -3.3$, $p = .002$.

So it doesn't matter which way we code the groups, a negative *t*-value is just as important/ significant as a positive value.

The paired *t*-test, used for repeated measures designs, is more sensitive than the independent groups *t*-test, i.e. you are more likely to find a statistically significant result. This is because variability is reduced, as each participant acts as his or her own control. The formula for the repeated measures *t*-test takes this into consideration.

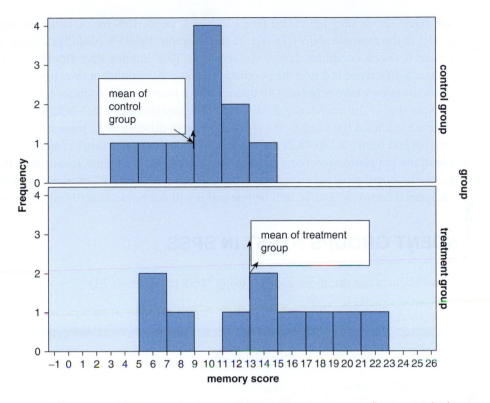

Figure 7.2 Frequency histograms for two groups on memory measure (larger overlap)

GENERALISING TO THE POPULATION

Anyone who carries out research involving looking at differences between two groups or conditions tries to ensure their sample group or groups are representative of the population from which they are drawn. Researchers want to be able to generalise to the population (see Chapter 4, page 155). Although we might find that our two conditions differ significantly, we want to be able to generalise to the wider population. This is achieved by confidence intervals, explained in Chapter 4, pages 155–161, and below.

Extending the example above, if we have a *t*-value of 3.3, *p* = .002, we can conclude that our two samples were significantly different, and that our hypothesis is confirmed: the treatment group scored significantly higher than the control group. However, the means of both groups are 'point estimates'. If we had carried out this experiment on a different day, with a new sample, or even the same sample, the means would most likely have been slightly different. If we carried out the experiment yet again, the means might have been different again. So there is always a certain amount of error when we carry out our experiments, or studies. There is a way of calculating the likely error, and obtaining a range within which we can be confident that the population means will fall. With the *t*-test, we are able to find these 'confidence intervals' as they are called (see Chapter 4, pages 155–161) around the mean difference (4.1 in the example above). In fact, in this example, the 95% confidence limits for the difference between condition means is 1.49–6.71. This implies that although in the sample the mean difference is 4.1, in the population we are 95% confident that the mean difference would be somewhere between 1.49 and 6.71. The narrower the confidence intervals, the better. Note that if the confidence limits had been something like 3.9–4.2, the sample mean difference is almost the same as the population mean difference. If, however, the confidence interval had been –4.1 to +8.2, the range is so wide that we couldn't even be certain that people in the population receiving the treatment would have a higher mean score than the people in the population who were not receiving the treatment. When the confidence interval includes 0 (zero) the t-value will be low and it will not be statistically significant.

INDEPENDENT GROUPS t-TEST IN SPSS

Let's see how to carry out the above analysis using SPSS (Screenshot 7.1).

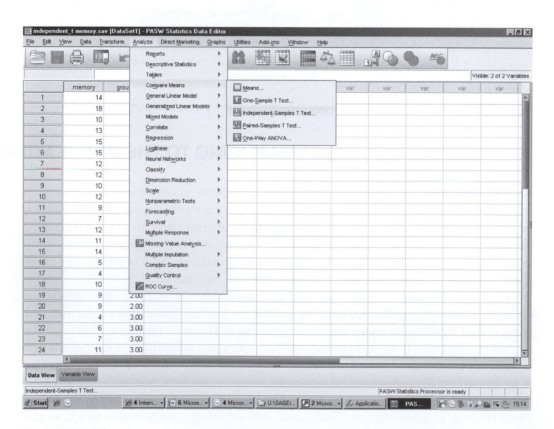

Screenshot 7.1

1) Select *Analyze*, *Compare means*, *Independent_Samples T Test*. This obtains Screenshot 7.2.

2) Move the variable of interest (*memory measure*) to the *Test Variable(s)* on the right.

3) Move the grouping variable (*group*) to the *Grouping Variable* box on the right. This obtains Screenshot 7.3.

4) Click the *Define Groups* button. This obtains the *Define Groups* dialogue box (Screenshot 7.4).

5) As we have called our groups 1 and 2, enter these values as shown above, then press *Continue*. You will now see Screenshot 7.5.

6) Press *Options*. This gives you the *Options* dialogue box (Screenshot 7.6).
   You could change the confidence interval – to 99% or 90% for instance. But it is usual to have 95% confidence intervals.

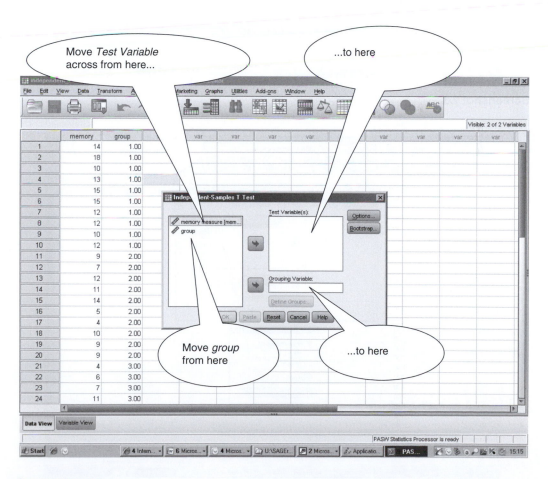

Screenshot 7.2

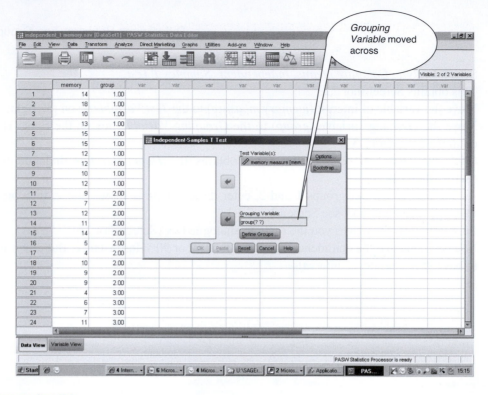

Screenshot 7.3

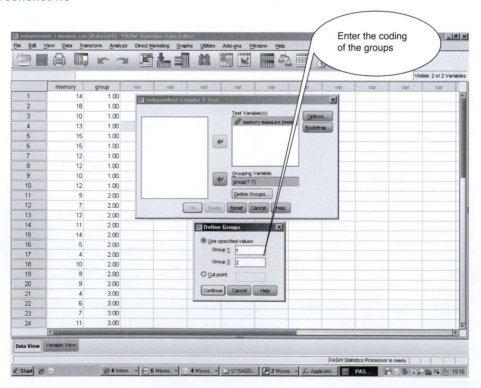

Screenshot 7.4

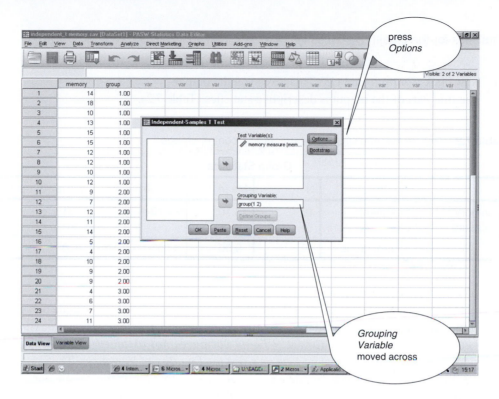

Screenshot 7.5

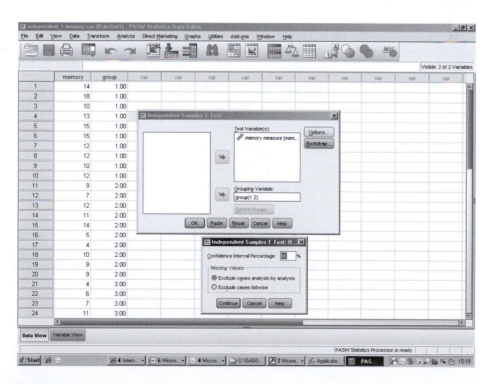

Screenshot 7.6

7) Now click *Continue* and *OK*. This gives you the output.
The first part of the output is descriptive statistics (Table 7.2).

Table 7.2 Descriptive statistics for treatment and control groups

			Group Statistics		
	Group	N	Mean	Std. deviation	Std. error mean
memory measure	treatment group	10	13.10	2.470	.781
	control group	10	9.00	3.055	.966

The second part is the inferential statistics (Table 7.3).

The first thing you need to know is that SPSS uses a slightly different formula according to whether the variances are similar for the two groups (row 1 = *Equal variances assumed*) or whether they are dissimilar (row 2 = *Equal variances not assumed*). In order to find which row we should use we look at *Levene's Test for Equality of Variances*. The important figure is the *p*-value. If it is non-significant, we can assume that our variances are equal, and we can report the figures in the first row. This is the case for our example.

A detailed report of this result might say:

> *Results showed that the treatment group scored higher on memory (x = 13.10, SD = 2.47) than the control group (x = 9.00, SD = 3.06). The mean difference (4.1) between the two groups was statistically significant (t = 3.3 (18); p = .002). The 95% confidence interval showed that the population mean difference is likely to fall within 1.49 and 6.71.*

Note that:

a)   the degrees of freedom (*df*) are reported in parentheses;
b)   we have halved the *p*-value – this is because the *t*-test results give a *p*-value which is relevant to a two-tailed test, so in order to find the *p*-value for a one-tailed test, we have to halve it.

If Levene's test were found to be statistically significant, this would mean our group variances were significantly different from each other, and we would have to report statistics from row 2. Differences in the figures, as you can see, are slight. In respect of the *df*, which looks a little strange, don't worry, we simply report this correct to two decimal places, i.e. *df* = 17.24.

Table 7.3 Independent t-test for differences between groups on memory measure

Independent Samples Test

| | | Levene's test for equality of variances | | t-test for equality of means | | | | | 95% confidence interval of the difference | |
		F	Sig.	t	df	Sig. (2-tailed)	Mean difference	Std. error difference	Lower	Upper
memory score	Equal variances assumed	.132	.721	3.300	18	.004	4.100	1.242	1.490	6.710
	Equal variances not assumed			3.300	17.243	.004	4.100	1.242	1.482	6.718

Levene's test is not significant so we can use the 'equal variances assumed' row

There is a significant difference between the groups

We are 95% confident that the population mean difference is between 1.5 and 6.7 (correct to one decimal place)

COHEN'S *d*

Cohen's *d* is a measure of effect. Once you have found a significant difference in the means between groups, you really want to be able to say something about the *size* of the difference. Simply knowing that the means differ by 4.1 isn't good enough, especially if we want to compare the effect size from this study with an effect size from another study where the dependent variable might have been scored on a different metric. What we need to do is convert the 4.1 into a standardised score. The standardised score is the *z*-score (see Chapter 4, page 143). SPSS doesn't calculate this for us. However, there are online programs which do calculate them, e.g.http://www.uccs.edu/~faculty/lbecker/.

However, it's very easy to calculate by hand. You take mean 2 and subtract it from mean 1. Then you divide this figure by the mean of the standard deviations for the two groups. You get these descriptive statistics from the *Group Statistics* output (Table 7.4).

1) Mean 1 – mean 2 = 4.1 (subtract mean 2 from mean 1)
2) 2.470 + 3.055 = 5.525 (add up the two standard deviations)
3) 5.525 ÷ 2 = 2.7625 (find the mean standard deviation by dividing by two)
4) 4.1 ÷ 2.7625 = 1.48 (divide the mean difference from step 1 by the mean standard deviation

Therefore, z^3 is 1.48. This means that the means differ by 1.48 standard deviations. As you know, the standardised normal distribution is like Figure 7.3.

Table 7.4 Means and standard deviations for treatment and control group

Group	Mean	Standard deviation
Treatment group	13.10	2.470
Control group	9.00	3.055

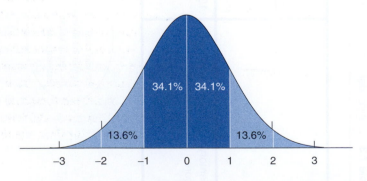

Figure 7.3 Normal distribution curve

When you see Cohen's *d* reported, you should immediately be able to visualise where the figure is on the curve, even if you haven't got it in front of you. Cohen's *d* is often reported with the *t*- and *p*-values, but sometimes it is reported without the *t*-test values.

Cohen has produced guidelines on what constitutes a small, medium or large effect. A *d* of 0.2 for instance, is small; this represents an overlap of the two distributions of 85%. A medium effect (0.5) equates to 67% overlap and a large effect (0.8) represents an overlap of 53%. A very large effect (1.5+) represents 25% of the overlap.

Example from the Literature

Oman et al. (2008) in a randomised control trial found that meditation lowers stress and supports forgiveness among college students. There were two groups: students who were 'treated' by being taught meditation techniques, and students who were waiting to be treated (waiting list controls). The authors say:

> *Compared with controls, treated participants (N=29) demonstrated significant benefits for stress* (p < .05, *Cohen's* d = −.45) *and forgiveness* (p < .05, d = .34)... p. 56

Although they have not given the *t*-value here, they have given the effect size, *d*. So for stress, the difference between the means of the two groups equated to a difference of nearly half of a standard deviation. For forgiveness, the effect size was a third of a standard deviation. The authors tell us that the difference was in favour of the treated group, i.e. they showed less stress and more forgiveness. From this study therefore, there is evidence that meditation works in relation to stress and forgiveness.

Example from the Literature

Jaiswal et al. (2010) looked at the effect of antihypertensive therapy on the cognitive function of patients with hypertension. They compared patients who were being treated for hypertension for three months with a group who had blood pressure within the normal range.

First, they used the independent *t*-test to compare the two groups at baseline. There were 50 participants in each group. The means, standard deviations and *p*-values of (some of) the cognitive function measures for the two groups are given in Table 7.5.

Table 7.5 Means and standard deviations for patients and control groups

	Patients		Control group	
	Mean	SD	Mean	SD
Remote memory	5.82	0.44	5.81	0.44
Recent memory	5.00	0.00	4.95	0.20
Immediate recall	**8.80**	**1.28**	**9.77**	**1.50*****

Table 7.5   Cont'd

	Patients		Control group	
	Mean	SD	Mean	SD
Mental balance	6.13	0.96	6.63	1.12*
Backward digit span	3.28	0.66	3.43	0.69
Word list memory	**4.88**	**0.95**	**5.36**	**0.83*****

*p-value < .05; **p–value < .01; ***p-value < .001; unpaired t-test

Of the above tests, 'Immediate recall' and 'Word list memory' show statistically significant differences between the groups at the beginning of the study.

Here are the other six results which we omitted in Table 7.5.

Table 7.6   Means and standard deviations for patients and control groups

	Patients		Control group	
	Mean	SD	Mean	SD
Paired associate test	3.13	0.99	3.47	1.32
Ray's figure test	5.82	2.08	6.31	1.73
Recognition	10.73	1.07	11.34	0.88**
Six-letter cancellation test	14.11	3.9	17.31	3.48***
Line test	8.48	0.75	8.34	0.91
Delayed recall test	3.48	1.16	3.84	1.41

*p-value < .05; **p-value< .01; ***p-value < .001; unpaired t-test

Write a brief paragraph interpreting these results. Compare it with our interpretation at the end of the book.

Activity 7.1

PAIRED t-TEST IN SPSS

The paired, or related t-test is used when the same participants perform in both conditions, that is, it is a within-participants design. The paired t-test compares each participant with him- or her-self, and so you would expect that the two scores would be correlated. This reduces the error variance, and leads to a more sensitive test. If you have 60 participants in an independent groups design, you only need 30 for a paired t-test to achieve the same power level (see Chapter 4, page 151).

To illustrate the paired *t*-test, we are going to use part of a dataset from our own research which had three independent groups (people with Inflammatory Bowel Disease, people with Irritable Bowel Syndrome, and healthy controls). Participants were measured on a number of variables, including their Performance IQ (PIQ), and their Verbal IQ (VIQ). In this study, there were 99 participants, and the design was a mixed one (not covered in this introductory text, but see Dancey and Reidy (2011) if you want to know more about more complex ANOVAs).

However, in order to illustrate the way in which paired t tests are carried out, we will focus on just 20 participants with chronic illness and two variables, PIQ and VIQ. All participants were measured on both PIQ and VIQ and so this is a repeated measures design with two conditions. For this example, we are going to predict that there will be a significant difference in the scores of people with chronic illness on PIQ and VIQ, such that people will score significantly lower on their VIQ than their PIQ. The hypothesis was derived from the literature, which shows that contrary to healthy people, those with some chronic illnesses have a lower VIQ score than their PIQ (Attree et al., 2003).

1) Choose *Analyze*, *Compare Means*, *Paired-Samples T Test* (Screenshot 7.7).

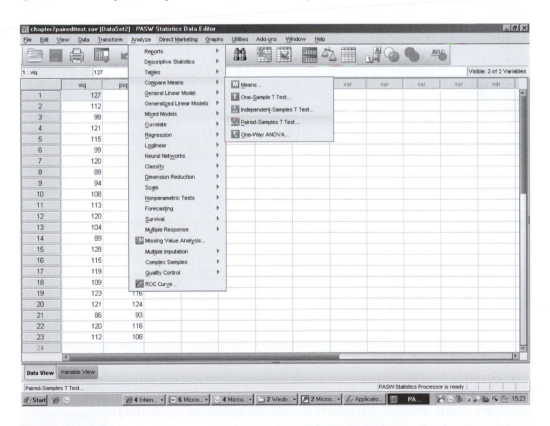

Screenshot 7.7

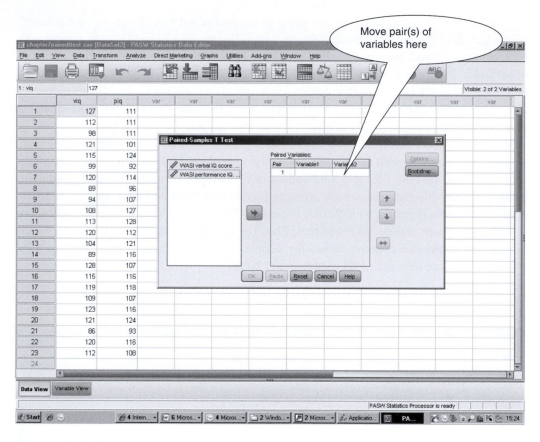

Screenshot 7.8

This gives the dialogue box shown in Screenshot 7.8.

2) Highlight the pair of scores (the VIQ and the PIQ) and move them to the *Paired Variables* box on the right.

Press *OK*. This gives Screenshot 7.9.

3) Press *Options* and you will see the *Paired Samples T-Test Options* box. Press *Continue*, then *OK*.

The relevant output is given in Table 7.7.

This shows the means, number of participants in the study, the standard deviation and the standard error of the mean.

There are some circumstances in which one should not use the paired *t*-test, and that is when the scores are not correlated. It can be seen in Table 7.8 that the correlation between the scores is only moderate (.41) and is statistically significant at $p = .05$. This shows we are correct to use the paired *t*-test (Table 7.9).

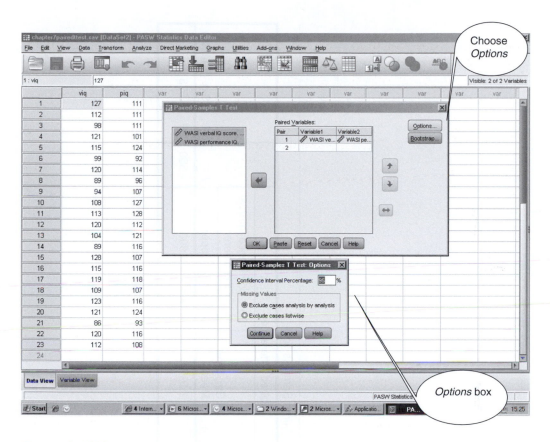

Screenshot 7.9

Table 7.7 Paired samples statistics for chronic illness participants

		Mean	N	Std. deviation	Std. error mean
			Paired Samples Statistics		
Pair 1	WASI verbal IQ score.	110.52	23	12.587	2.625
	WASI performance IQ.	112.00	23	9.968	2.078

Table 7.8 Paired samples correlations for chronic illness participants

		N	Correlation	Sig.
		Paired Samples Correlations		
Pair 1	WASI verbal IQ score. & WASI performance IQ.	23	.409	.053

Table 7.9 Paired samples *t*-test for chronic illness participants

		Paired Samples Test							
		Paired differences							
					95% confidence interval of the difference				
		Mean	Std. deviation	Std. Error Mean	Lower	Upper	*t*	*df*	Sig. (2-tailed)
Pair 1	WASI verbal IQ score. – WASI performance IQ.	–1.478	12.457	2.597	–6.865	3.908	–.569	22	.575

mean difference

not statistically significant

Levene's Test of Equal Variances is not relevant here, as we only have one group of participants. Here we can see that the mean difference is −1.478, and the *t*-value is −.569. The minus occurs simply because the VIQ scores have been coded as variable 1 and the PIQ scores have been coded as variable 2. The significance level is *p* = .575, i.e not statistically significant. Here the hypothesis has not been confirmed. Even though the group did have a higher PIQ than their scores on VIQ, we cannot reject the null hypothesis, that this difference has arisen just by sampling error, or chance. We might say:

> *Although the difference between the groups was in the expected direction, results showed that this was not statistically significant:* t = .569 (22), p = .575.

There is not enough evidence therefore, to conclude that the participants differed on their VIQ and PIQ measures.

Example from the Literature

Anzalone (2008) wanted to determine whether there were significant differences in blood glucose sampled at the earlobe relative to fingertip sites. Fifty participants provided samples from both the fingertip and earlobe sites. This is what is said:

> *The results indicated that the mean finger stick glucose result (M = 180.14, SD = 64.16) was significantly statistically greater than the mean earlobe glucose result (M = 174.38, SD = 63.18),* t(49) = 2.81, p = .007) *.[4] The standardized effect size (d) was .40 (small effect). The 95% confidence interval of the mean difference between the two results was 1.64 to 9.89.*

This gives us a lot of information – not only the means, the direction of the difference and the test statistics – but also effect sizes and confidence intervals. Everything we need to properly interpret the analysis. Based on their results section, it seems that there is enough evidence to conclude that there are significant differences in blood glucose sampled at the earlobe and fingertip sites.

Activity 7.2

Jaiswal et al. (2010), discussed on page 221 also carried out a paired *t*-test, to compare the way in which the patients changed from the beginning of the study, and at the three-month follow-up. Table 7.10 gives the results.

(Continued)

Activity 7.2 Cont'd

Table 7.10   Means and standard deviations for patients at baseline and three months

	Patients' initial score (n = 50)		Patients' score at 3 months (n = 45)	
	Mean	SD	Mean	SD
Remote memory	5.82	0.44	5.75	0.48
Recent memory	5.00	0.00	4.97	0.14
Immediate recall	8.80	1.28	9.42	1.28***
Mental balance	6.13	0.96	6.28	0.96
Forward digit span	4.77	0.79	4.88	0.48
Backward digit span	3.28	0.66	3.31	0.55
Word list memory	4.88	0.95	5.17	0.77*
Paired associate test	3.13	0.99	3.13	0.97
Ray's figure test	5.82	2.08	6.13	1.70
Recognition	10.73	1.07	11.42	0.72***
Six-letter cancellation test	14.22	3.90	16.77	3.57***
Line test	8.48	0.75	8.44	0.69
Delayed recall test	3.48	1.16	4.06	1.13***

*p–value < .05; **p–value < .010; ***p-value < .001; paired t-test

Write a paragraph interpreting the results. Compare it with ours at the end of the book.

TWO-SAMPLE z-TEST

This test is sometimes used instead of a t-test. It has traditionally been used when the sample size is over 30, and when the data are normally distributed. It tended to be used because it had no requirement for the variances of the groups to be equal. With the advent of computerised statistical programs such as SPSS, where SPSS can correct for unequal variances, this test has become somewhat redundant, as most people prefer to use the more popular t-test. Occasionally, however, the two-sample z-test can be found in the research literature.

If you want to use the two-sample z-test, then refer to the companion website. However, you need to know how to interpret articles which have used the z-test.

Example from the Literature

It was quite difficult to find an article which used the *z*-test. One which did was the Morbidity and Mortality Weekly Report for 1 May 2009 which discussed the prevalence and most common causes of disability among adults in the United States in 2005. It presented the estimated number and percentage of adults with self-reported disabilities by age group. The report says:

> *Differences in the prevalence of disability by sex across age groups and other comparisons were assessed by z-test and considered statistically signficant if the 95% confidence interval (CI) of the difference excluded zero (p < .05).* p. 422

The analyses were based on a total estimated population of 47,501 people. They presented the Figure 7.4.

They then performed *z*-tests to compare men and women, for the different age groups, hence three *z*-tests. They say:

> *Disability prevalence is significantly higher among women than men for all age groups (z-test for women–men differences by age group: 18–44 years, p = .006; 45–64 years, p < .0001; ≥65 years, p < .0001).* p. 426

The computed values of the *z*-scores were not reported, although we would recommend including statistics of this sort in your own write-ups.

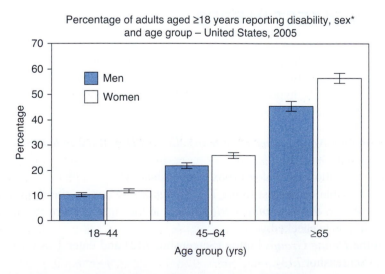

Figure 7.4 Disability by sex and age group († 95% confidence interval)

NON-PARAMETRIC TESTS

The following non-parametric tests transform scores into ranked data. Thus the tests are resistant to outliers and skewness, making them ideal for small, skewed samples.

MANN–WHITNEY: FOR INDEPENDENT GROUPS

The Mann–Whitney test uses the ranking of scores in a formula which calculates the test statistic 'U'. In fact, if you took data you had used for an independent *t*-test, and ranked the conditions, then performed a Mann–Whitney test, the probability value would be almost identical to that of the *t*-test. Before computerised statistical programs, in order to carry out a Mann–Whitney test, students would rank the scores by hand (see Chapter 3, page 80). Scores are given ranks from both groups together. From this a mean rank for each group was found. If there are no significant differences between conditions A and B, then the ranks should be equally distributed throughout both conditions. Mann–Whitney U was calculated on the bases of the ranks and the sample size.

Ranking by hand used to cause students a lot of problems, especially when there were a large number of cases and/or a large number of ties, e.g. perhaps ten people scored 3.00. It was then necessary to find the mean rank of the ten cases (3/10 = .3)! Statistical programs are of course far more reliable. SPSS calculates the number of times that a rank score from condition A precedes a score from condition B, and the number of times that a rank score from Group B precedes a score from condition A. The appropriate measure of central tendency could be the mean or the median (see Chapter 3, page 80).

MANN–WHITNEY TEST IN SPSS

Imagine we have a small sample of patients; eight have had treatment to improve fatigue and seven are on the waiting list. Fatigue is rated on a scale of 1 = 'hardly any fatigue' through to 7 = 'severe fatigue'. The hypothesis is that the treated sample will have lower fatigue. This is a directional hypothesis so that we can use a one-tailed test.

1) Choose *Analyze*, *Nonparametric Statistics*, *Legacy Dialogs*, *2 Independent Samples*, as shown in Screenshot 7.10.
   This gives the following dialogue box (Screenshot 7.11).
2) Move the variable of interest to the *Test Variable List* box on the right, and move the group variable to the *Grouping Variable* box on the right. Ensure the *Mann–Whitney U Test Type* box is checked.
3) Click on the *Define Groups* button (Screenshot 7.12) and enter 1 as *Group 1* and 2 as *Group 2* (Screenshot 7.13).
4) Then press *Continue*, followed by *Options*. This gives another dialogue box (Screenshot 7.14).

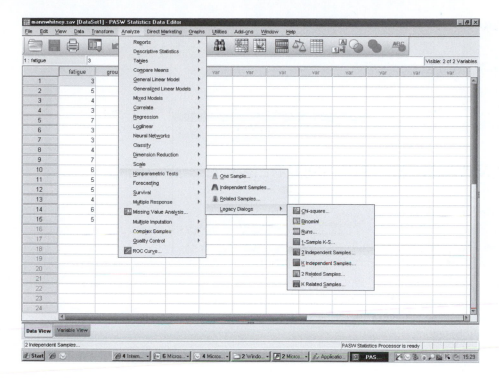

Screenshot 7.10

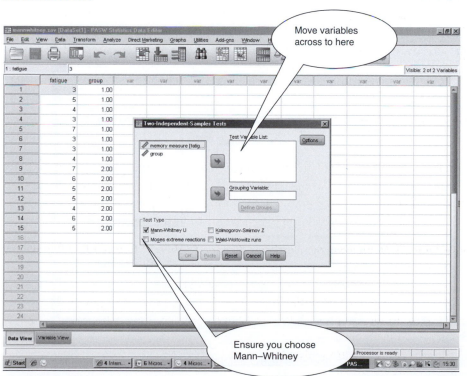

Screenshot 7.11

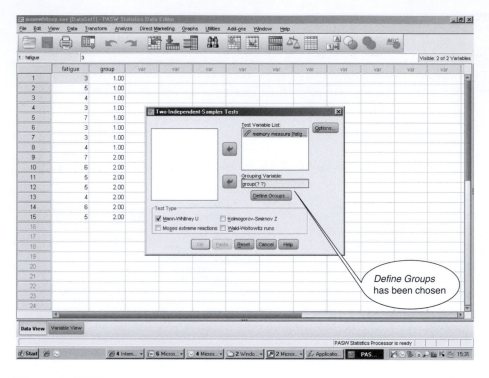

Screenshot 7.12

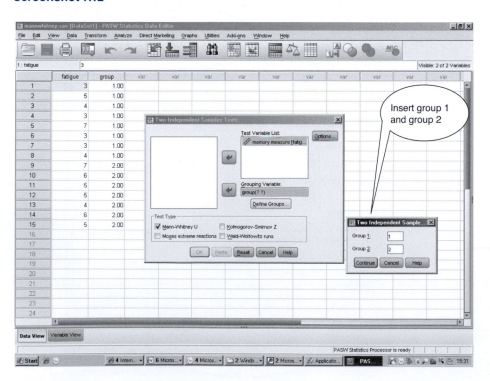

Screenshot 7.13a

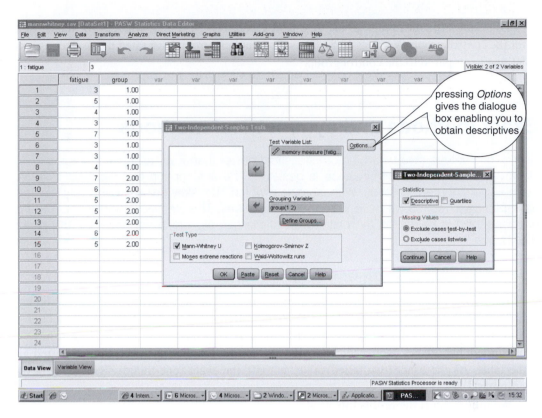

Screenshot 7.13b

5) Check *Descriptives* if you want to, then *Continue*, then *OK*.
   Table 7.11 gives the relevant part of the output.

Table 7.11 Mean rank and sum of ranks for treatment and control groups on measure of memory

		Ranks			
	Group	N	Mean rank	Sum of ranks
memory measure	treatment group	8	5.75	46.00
	control group	7	10.57	74.00
	Total	15		

This shows the mean rank of the treatment group ($N = 8$) is 5.75, whereas the mean rank for the control group ($N = 7$) is 10.57. Thus the treatment group have rated themselves as less fatigued compared to the control group.

Exact methods and symmetrical methods

Asymptotic values give us a bit more statistical power than if we had used exact values. However, the statistical significance is based on the assumption that we have a large, normally distributed dataset. With samples which are skewed *we can't* rely on the asymptotic values, so we have to report exact values. The statistical significance of the exact method is based on the distribution of the sample which we have, i.e. the exact distribution.

Table 7.12 gives more information than we need. The test statistic is Mann–Whitney U (commonly just referred to as U) and you will often see this reported in results sections. You may also see z reported. In this case then, $U = 10$ and $z = -2.133$. If you have a one-tailed hypothesis, you need to halve the two-tailed significance value reported in the table. As the exact (two-tailed)value is .040, the exact (one-tailed) significance level becomes .020.

We might report the results this way:

A Mann–Whitney test showed that the treated group rated themselves as less fatigued than the control group (U = 10, z = 2.133, p = .020).

Table 7.12   Test statistics for memory measure

Test Statistics[b]

	Memory measure
Mann-Whitney U	10.000
Wilcoxon W	46.000
Z	−2.133
Asymp. Sig. (2-tailed)	.033
Exact Sig. [2*(1-tailed Sig.)]	.040[a]

a. Not corrected for ties
b. Grouping Variable: group

However, results sections in many of the journals related to health sciences do not report either the U or the z-value, but simply report that Mann–Whitney was used to compare two groups and give the p-value associated with the statistical test.

Example from the Literature

Blake and Batson (2008) had the following research question:

> *Does participation in a Qigong exercise intervention improve mood, self-esteem, perceived flexibility, coordination, physical activity and social support in people with traumatic brain injury?* p. 590

In order to answer this question, Blake and Batson carried out a Tai Chi Qigong exercise intervention for an hour weekly for eight weeks, on 20 people with brain injury. Twenty other people participated in an eight-week non-exercise-based activity, acting as a control. The authors checked that groups were similar on the dependent variables before the intervention.

The authors presented results as in Table 7.13.

You can see that the authors have given the median scores for both groups at baseline and follow-up, and have also given the median change score. For each of the measured variables, they have carried out a Mann–Whitney test between the exercise and control groups at follow-up. They have given the U-value, and associated exact probability value, flagging up the one significant difference.

They also give the interpretation of these results as text:

> *Mann–Whitney U-tests conducted on outcome measures at eight weeks follow-up showed a significant difference between exercise and control groups in mood on the General Health Questionnaire-12. There were no significant differences between exercise and control group on measures of Social Support for Exercise Habits from family or friends, Physical Self Description Questionnaire coordination, self-esteem, flexibility and physical activity.* p. 593

Activity 7.3

We asked the authors of this paper if we could have the SPSS data file so that we could use it as an exercise in this book, and they agreed. For the purposes of this exercise, we are going to ask you to carry out a Mann–Whitney test on their GHQ-12 data (see Table 7.13). Look at the data shown in Screenshot 7.14. The dependent variable is the score on GHQ-12 and the groups are control (coded 0) and exercise (coded 1). Carry out the Mann–Whitney test, obtaining the output and check your results against those of Blake and Batson. The correct output is shown in the Answers section at the end of the book.

Table 7.13 Comparison between control and exercise groups

	Control group (n = 10)			Exercise group (n=10)			Eight-week comparison Mann-Whitney U-test*	
	Baseline median (IQR)	Followup median (IQR)	Change median (IQR)	Baseline median (IQR)	Followup median (IQR)	Change median (IQR)	U	p-value (2-tailed)
SSEH family support	20.5 (10)	14 (13.25)	−6.5 (3.25)	23.5 (14)	16 (12.25)	−7.5 (−1.75)	42.5	0.567
SSEH friend support	18 (10.75)	12.5(4.75)	−5.5 (−6)	21 (14)	14 (13.5)	−7 (−0.5)	35.5	0.266
GHQ-12	3.5 (4.75)	2.5 (2.75)	−1 (−2)	1.5 (3.75)	0 (1)	−1.5 (−2.75)	22	0.026*
PSDQ coordination	3.75 (2.55)	4.25 (2.67)	0.5 (0.12)	3.42 (2.67)	3.42 (2.66)	0 (−0.01)	45.5	0.733
PSDQ self-esteem	2.55 (1.12)	2.88 (1.16)	0.33 (0.04)	2.83 (0.96)	3.44 (1.12)	0.61 (0.16)	37.5	0.344
PSDQ flexibility	3.58 (2.59)	4.17 (3.09)	0.59 (0.5)	3.33 (1.96)	2.92 (1.62) −	−0.41 (−0.34)	41	0.496
PSDQ physical activity	1.5 (3.12)	1.67 (3.41)	0.17 (0.29)	3.17 (1.71)	3.50 (2.04)	0.33 (0.33)	34.5	0.240

SSEH, Social Support for Exercise Habits Scale; GHQ-12, General Health Questionnaire-12; PSDQ, Physical Self-Description Questionnaire; IQR, interquartile range, U, Mann-Whitney U statistic.
*Significant at P<0.05.
*Mann-Whitney U-tests were conducted to compare control group with exercise group on each outcome measure at follow-up.

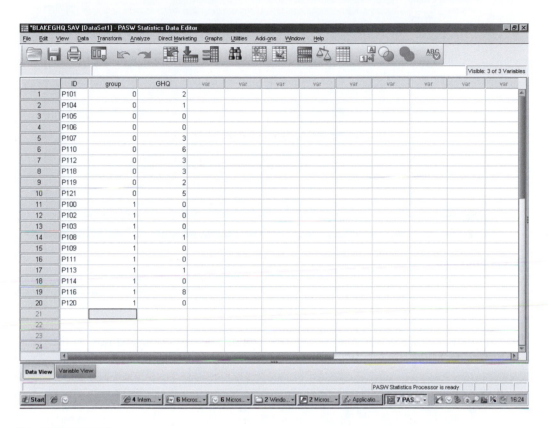

Screenshot 7.14

WILCOXON SIGNED RANK TEST: FOR REPEATED MEASURES

The Wilcoxon test is similar, but, like the paired t-test, makes use of the knowledge that participants perform in both conditions. Instead of ranking the scores in the combined dataset, as in the Mann–Whitney test, for each case one score is taken from the other (these are called 'difference scores') and then the differences of the group are ranked. The sum of the positive ranks and negative ranks are calculated separately. When calculating a Wilcoxon signed rank test by hand, the sum of the ranks of the least occurring sign gives the test statistic which is called T. When carrying out the test by using a statistical program such as SPSS, the test statistic given is z.

WILCOXON SIGNED RANK TEST IN SPSS

We are going to use the following dataset to illustrate the Wilcoxon signed ranks test. Twenty patients were measured on a depression scale before and after an intervention.

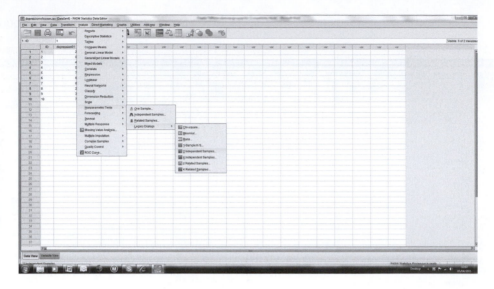

Screenshot 7.15

1) Choose *Analyze*, *Nonparametric Statistics*, *Legacy Dialogs*, *2-related samples* (Screenshot 7.15).

   This gives a dialogue box (Screenshot 7.16).
2) Highlight the pair of variables on the left, and move them to the text box on the right-hand side. Make sure the *Wilcoxon* test is checked.

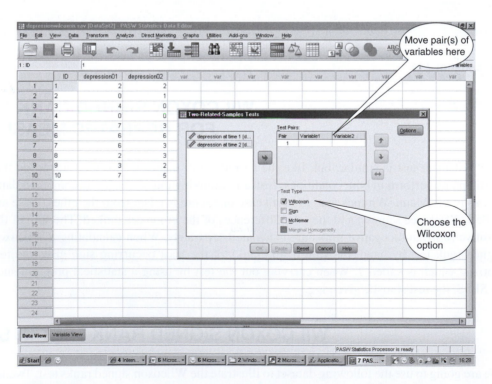

Screenshot 7.16

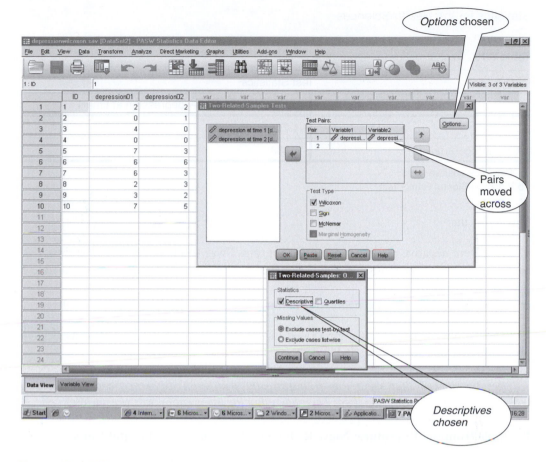

Screenshot 7.17

1) Click on *Options*
2) Pairs moved across
3) Check *Descriptives* if you want them (Screenshot 7.17), then *Continue*, then *OK*.

Table 7.14 gives the relevant output.

Table 7.14 Ranks for depression at time 1 and time 2

		N	Mean Rank	Sum of Ranks
depression at time 2 – depression at time 1	Negative Ranks	5[a]	4.80	24.00
	Positive Ranks	2[b]	2.00	4.00
	Ties	3[c]		
	Total	10		

a. depression at time 2 < depression at time 1
b. depression at time 2 > depression at time 1
c. depression at time 2 = depression at time 1

Table 7.15   Test statistics for depression

Test Statistics[b]	
	depression at time 2 – depression at time 1
Z	−1.706[a]
Asymp. Sig. (2-tailed)	.088

a. Based on positive ranks.
b. Wilcoxon Signed Ranks Test

This shows that

a)   Five were negative ranks, i.e. depression at time 2 was less than depression at time 1
b)   Two were positive ranks, i.e. depression at time 2 was more than depression at time 1 and
c)   There were three ties, i.e. depression at time 2 was equal to depression at time 1

The value of the Wilcoxon test uses z (Table 7.15). In this case $z = -1.706$, with an associated probability of .044 for a one-tailed hypothesis. In this case, we might say:

> *Results showed that there was a statistically significant difference between the two conditions ($z = 1.71$),[5] p = .044. This shows that the intervention was worthwhile.*

Example from the Literature: Noise Reduction Programme in Hospital Units

Taylor-Ford et al. (2008) wanted to determine whether a noise reduction programme reduced sound levels and disturbance due to sound as perceived by patients on two different hospital units. Patients who had completed the Topf Adapted Sound Disturbance Survey for Patients during a pre-intervention and post-intervention phase provided data. The researchers selected Wilcoxon as their test of choice, and say the following:

> *The possible scores ranged between 30, indicating no sound disturbance, and 150, indicating severe sound disturbances. The difference in Wilcoxon Rank Sum means and medians on the sound disturbance scores between the two units was not significant (p = .16), and the difference between the pre and post scores on the treatment unit was not significant (p = .67) p. 81*

Activity 7.4

What conclusions can you draw from the above results section, in terms of evidence-based practice? Check your answer with ours at the end of the book.

ADJUSTING FOR MULTIPLE TESTS

As you have seen, many researchers carry out two-condition comparisons on more than one variable. Carrying out multiple tests in this way makes it more likely that one or more of the t-tests were significant just by sampling error, or chance. It is then advisable to 'adjust' the significance level to make it stricter. For instance, if we have carried out three t-tests, say, then we adjust by dividing our usual significance level (.05) by the number of comparisons made (3): .05/3 = .017 (correct to two decimal places). This means that only the t-tests with $p < .017$ will be declared statistically significant, although we report this as $p < .05$. This alteration of the significance level is known as the Bonferroni correction, and you will learn more about this in the following chapters (in particular 8 and 9).

Summary

If you are carrying out your own research, we recommend that you look to see if your data are significantly skewed (see Chapter 4, pages 140–141). If they are, you can use the bootstrapping approach to t-test calculation or the traditional non-parametric tests. The appropriate descriptive statistics for t-tests are the means and standard deviations. Confidence intervals around the differences between the means allow you to generalise to the population – you can state that the population mean difference is likely to fall within a certain range. An effect size, Cohen's d, allows you to state the strength of the difference between conditions, in standardized units (z-score).

When using the MannWhitney for independent groups and the Wilcoxon signed rank tests for repeated measures, choose an appropriate measure of central tendency (see Chapter 3, page 82). Confidence intervals based on the mean are not appropriate for these non-parametric statistics.

MULTIPLE CHOICE QUESTIONS

1. If Cohen's $d = -.33$ then:
   a) Groups differ by 3.3 SD
   b) Groups differ by a third of a SD
   c) Groups differ by less than 30% of a SD
   d) They do not differ

The following relates to questions 2 and 3 below.

A researcher predicts that an exercise intervention with patients who have respiratory problems will improve physical function, measured by muscle force and oxygen uptake. There was an intervention ($N = 20$) and a control ($N = 20$) group.

2. This is a:
   a) Two-group independent design
   b) Two-group repeated measures design
   c) Correlational design
   d) One-sample z-test

3. From those listed below, an appropriate statistical test to analyse these data is:
   a) One-sample z-test
   b) Paired t-test
   c) Mann–Whitney test
   d) Wilcoxon

4. If Cohen's $d = 2.5$, this is considered:
   a) A small effect
   b) A medium effect
   c) A large effect
   d) An impossible result

5. Levene's test shows whether:
   a) Scores from two independent groups have roughly equal variances
   b) Scores from one group of people performing in two conditions have equal variances
   c) Scores are normally distributed
   d) All the of above

6. A researcher carries out a t-test to analyse the differences between two conditions. She wishes to use a one-tailed hypothesis. The output from SPSS gives a two-tailed probability of 07. Which value should she use to report the one-tailed associated probability?
   a) .070
   b) .035
   c) .05
   d) .14

The following relates to questions 7 and 8 below.

Ten people with Chronic Fatigue Syndrome rated their fatigue on a scale of 1–5 at two time points, before and after lunch. Data is skewed.

7. This is a:
   a) Two-group independent design
   b) Two-group repeated measures design
   c) Correlational design
   d) One sample z-test

8. The appropriate statistical test to analyse these data is:
   a) Independent *t*-test
   b) Wilcoxon signed ranks test
   c) Mann–Whitney test
   d) Paired *t*-test

9. Which one of the following was traditionally *not* an assumption underlying the independent samples *t*-test:
   a) Scores must be drawn from a normally distributed population
   b) Variances should be roughly equal in both groups
   c) There should be a linear relationship between scores in condition 1 and condition 2
   d) The data should be interval level

The following relates to questions 10–12 below.

   Look at the following output, which compares the amount of movement measured in patients with Multiple Sclerosis after treatment (0 = no movement, 5 = much movement) with those patients waiting for treatment (control group)

Group Statistics

	Group	N	Mean	Std. deviation	Std. error mean
movement	treatment group	12	4.00	.853	.246
	control group	12	1.67	1.435	.414

Independent Samples Test

		Levene's Test for equality of variances		t-test for equality of means					95% Confidence interval of the difference	
		F	Sig.	t	df	Sig. (2-tailed)	Mean difference	Std. error difference	Lower	Upper
movement	Equal variances assumed	3.667	.069	4.841	22	.000	2.333	.482	1.334	3.333
	Equal variances not assumed			4.841	17.905	.000	2.333	.482	1.320	3.346

10. Which is the most appropriate conclusion?
    a) The treatment group shows more movement than the control group, and this difference is statistically significant $p < .001$
    b) The control group shows more movement than the control group, and this difference is statistically significant $p < .001$
    c) The treatment group shows more movement than the control group, and this difference is statistically significant $p = .069$
    d) The control group shows more movement than the control group, and this difference is statistically significant $p = .069$

11. Which is the most appropriate conclusion? We are 95% confident that the population mean difference:
    a) Is 2.33
    b) Lies somewhere between 1.33 and 3.33
    c) Lies somewhere between 1.32 and 3.35
    d) Is 4.84

12. Which is the most appropriate conclusion?
    a) Scores in the treatment group are more variable than the control group
    b) Scores in the control group are more variable than the treatment group
    c) The groups have identical variances
    d) It is not possible to determine which group has the most variance

13. A researcher tests two groups of participants ($N = 300$) on a measure of stress (units: 1–20). If Cohen's d is found to be 1.5 then the groups differ by:
    a) 1.5 standard deviations
    b) 1.5 units of stress
    c) 150
    d) 15 SD

The following relates to questions 14 and 15.

   This is a repeated measures analysis with movement in nine people with Multiple Sclerosis at two timepoints (an intervention was given between pre-test and post-test). The hypothesis was that movement would be greater after the intervention. Look at the output:

Ranks

		N	Mean rank	Sum of ranks
movement at posttest – movement at pretest	Negative Ranks	1[a]	2.00	2.00
	Positive Ranks	6[b]	4.33	26.00
	Ties	2[c]		
	Total	9		

a. movement at posttest < movement at pretest
b. movement at posttest > movement at pretest
c. movement at posttest = movement at pretest

Test Statistics[b]

	Movement at posttest – movement at pretest
Z	−2.058[a]
Asymp. Sig. (2-tailed)	.040
Exact Sig. (2-tailed)	.063
Exact Sig. (1-tailed)	.031
Point Probability	.023

a. Based on negative ranks
b. Wilcoxon Signed Ranks Test

14. Which is the most appropriate conclusion:
    a) There were six ranks where post-test movement was greater than pre-test movement
    b) There were six ranks where pre-test movement was greater than post-test movement
    c) There was one rank where post-test movement was greater than pre-test movement
    d) There was one tie

15. Which is the appropriate probability value to report?
    a) .040
    b) .063
    c) .031
    d) .023

Notes

1 When writing up the results of your own studies, however, *you should always give the variables meaningful names*, such as sex, illness group, etc.
2 Although we call the conditions A and B to illustrate the method, when writing up reports you should always ensure that your conditions have meaningful names.
3 Note that this is identical to Cohen's *d*.
4 Note that the calculation of degrees of freedom for paired *t*-tests is $N − 1$.
5 Remember that it does not matter whether *z* is positive or negative, it is just the way we have coded the variables; we have also rounded the figures to two decimal places.

Differences Between Three or More Conditions

8

Overview

This chapter will be looking at statistics which tell us whether three or more conditions or groups differ from each other on one or more variables. This follows on from the two-condition tests in the last chapter. The conditions can be either:

a) The same group of people tested in all the conditions, or
b) Different groups of people, who perform in one condition only

This chapter will illustrate the ways in which researchers test their hypotheses, based on the research questions which they have. The tests covered in this chapter are parametric ones, the Analysis of Variance (ANOVA), and their non-parametric equivalents, the Kruskal–Wallis test and Friedman's ANOVA. We will give you a basic conceptual understanding of the tests, show how researchers report their results, how to perform the tests in SPSS, and how to interpret the output. We will also cover confidence intervals and effect sizes.

(Continued)

(Continued)

From this chapter you will:

- Gain a conceptual understanding of Analyses of Variance
- Be able to decide when to use the ANOVA, which is a parametric test, and when to use bootstrapping or the non-parametric equivalents to parametric ANOVAs: Kruskal–Wallis or Friedman's ANOVA
- Learn to distinguish between planned comparisons and post-hoc tests
- Learn how carry out Analyses of Variance in SPSS
- Learn how to report effect sizes and confidence intervals for ANOVA
- Learn how to interpret the findings of researchers who have used parametric and non-parametric ANOVAs in their published articles

INTRODUCTION

When researchers manipulate a single variable with three or more conditions and hypothesise that there will be a significant difference between them, they use one of the tests covered in this chapter. The experimental hypothesis would be that there will be a significant difference between some or all of the conditions. The null hypothesis is that any differences in the scores between the conditions are due to sampling error (chance).

The parametric test for three or more conditions is simply called the Analysis of Variance (ANOVA). There are two types of ANOVAs, one for independent groups, and one for a repeated measures design.

Students have traditionally been told to ensure that such parametric tests meet certain assumptions before they can use them (see Chapter 7, page 208).

In practice, similar to the *t*-test, ANOVA is said to be 'robust' with respect to these assumptions. So we recommend that unless your sample scores are skewed (see Chapter 4, pages 140–141) then you should go ahead and use ANOVAs. Where you have skewed data, the non-parametric equivalents can be used. These are the Kruskal–Wallis ANOVA for independent groups, and Friedman's ANOVA for repeated measures. These, however, are much more restricted in scope than ANOVA.

Activity 8.1

Here are some studies which show clearly the researchers are looking for differences between some or all of the three or more conditions. As you read them, think about whether the design is independent groups, or repeated measures. Check your answers at the back of the book.

(Continued)

(Continued)

Activity 8.1

- Scarpellini et al. (2008) state that antibodies directed against citrullinated peptides are the most specific serological markers for the diagnosis of rheumatoid arthritis (RA). The authors wanted to determine whether there were significant differences in cyclic citrullinated peptide (CCP) between people with RA, people with osteoarthritis, those with psoriatic arthritis and those with other arthritic conditions. They found that the CCP was significantly higher in RA than in the other conditions.
- Button (2008) investigated the possible differences in stressors and health levels between different grades of nurses, i.e. auxiliary nurses, staff nurses, ward sisters, senior nurses and midwives. She found that there was a significant difference in 'time stress levels', with ward sisters reporting higher time stress than auxiliary nurses, staff nurses and midwives.
- Paterson et al. (2009) wanted to discover whether caffeine would disrupt sleep and also whether two sleep-promoting drugs would reverse the potential disruption. Twelve healthy men participated in a double-blind study where they all received placebo, caffeine, caffeine plus zolpidem and caffeine plus Trazodone.
- Gariballa and Forster (2009) carried out a study on the effects of smoking on nutrition status and response to dietary supplements during acute illness. As part of that study, nutrition status was compared between current smokers, ex-smokers and those who never smoked.

ANOVA is an extension of the *t*-test. In fact, if an ANOVA on two groups is carried out instead of using the *t*-test, results will be the same, although for the ANOVA, the test statistic is called *F*. There is a direct relationship between the *t*-test and the *F*-test ($t^2 = F$). Therefore, ANOVA can actually be used in place of the *t*-test with identical outcomes in terms of significance levels.

ANOVA shows whether there are any significant differences between the conditions. So for a three-condition design, a statistically significant ANOVA will usually mean that either :

a) condition 1 could be significantly different from condition 2, and/or
b) condition 1 could be significantly different from condition 3, and/or
c) condition 2 could be significantly different from condition 3

Further tests can be applied to explore these possibilities as discussed on pages 251–252.

For a true experimental design, the researchers would assign participants randomly to the different conditions (see Chapter 3), but in the health sciences it is more likely that participants in the group would be pre-existing groups, e.g. men and women, or different illness groups. This design is called quasi-experimental, and the conclusions that can be drawn about cause and effect cannot be as strong as the true experimental design. The statistical analysis is the same in true and quasi-experiments, however; ANOVA is applicable to both.

CONCEPTUAL DESCRIPTION OF THE (PARAMETRIC) ANOVA

The *analysis of variance* investigates the different sources from which variation in the scores arise.

Look at Table 8.1, which gives fictitious data to help explain our point. The data are scores on a test.

Table 8.1

Group A	Group B	Group C
3	10	20
3	9	18
3	10	28
3	11	22
3	10	24
3	11	20
3	10	16
3	9	20
3	10	12

Activity 8.2

Which group shows the most variability?[1] Which group shows the least? See the end of the book for answers.

The variation *within* each group is called *within-groups variance*. There is almost always variability within a group of people, simply because they are different people and they don't always react in the same way to treatments. The within-groups variance can also be a function of the measures used. Unfortunately, there is always some error due to problems in the methods or running of our studies and experiments – participants are not well during the experiment, equipment fails and so on. In particular, 'measurement error' will also contribute to within-groups variance. To take an extreme example, if the experimental equipment went wrong and messed up the score recorded for one participant, then this score would probably vary a lot from all of the others in the group. Error variance will be represented in both the within-group and between-group variance estimates. Everything we measure has some measurement error, no matter how sophisticated the measuring instrument. What we hope for is that our within-groups variance and the variance due to experimental errors is small.

Looking at the Table 8.1, can you see that there will also be a difference in the *means* of each group – even without calculating the means, you can probably easily tell which group has the highest mean. This variation between the groups is, unsurprisingly, called the *between-groups variance*. When we carry out an experiment or study, we hope that the reason the groups differ is because of our intervention, or because the groups are really different (and not just because of measurement error or sampling error – or something the researchers did wrong!)

When conducting a between-groups ANOVA we split all the variance in the dataset into within-groups variance and between-groups variance:

a) between groups variance (BG variance) – due to our treatment effects, individual differences and experimental error

b) within groups variance (WG variance) – due to individual differences and experimental error

ONE-WAY ANOVA

A one-way ANOVA means that there is only one independent variable. We call the independent variables 'factors'. In our example below, the factor is 'illness group'.

A one-way ANOVA could have three or more *levels* of the factor.

For example, if we were testing three different illness groups, then the factor could be called 'illness group' and the three levels could be 'Multiple Sclerosis'; 'Irritable Bowel Syndrome' and 'Chronic Fatigue Syndrome'. Alternatively, if we were testing five different drug doses on people with Multiple Sclerosis, then the factor would be 'drug levels' and there would be five levels of 'drug levels', e.g. placebo, 5 mg, 10 mg, 15 mg, 20 mg.

> **Activity 8.3**
>
> A researcher wanted to determine whether there were significant differences in cortisol level between people with Chronic Fatigue Syndrome, those with Irritable Bowel Syndrome, those with Inflammatory Bowel Disease and those with Rheumatoid Arthritis.
>
> Identify both the independent variable and the dependent variable. State how many levels the independent variable/factor has. Check your answers at the end of the book.

In any dataset the total variance measures the spread of each observation around the grand mean of all the observations, ignoring any different groups or conditions that have been specified in the design. The formula for a one-way ANOVA partitions the total variance into BG variance and WG variance. The WG variance estimate includes individual differences and measurement error, whereas the BG variance additionally includes the treatment effects. Therefore if the effect of the independent variable is larger, then the BG estimate will be a lot larger than the WG.

As in the t-test, if the BG variance is relatively larger than the WG variance, the F-value will be larger; if the WG variance is larger, then the F-value will be smaller. The relative size of the BG and WG variance is expressed as a ratio. This is called the F-ratio (usually abbreviated to F) and it is at the heart of significance testing in ANOVA.

$$F\text{-ratio}^2 = \text{estimate of between groups variance} \div \text{estimate of within groups variance}$$

Each one-way ANOVA calculates only one F-ratio. This is called the 'omnibus F-ratio'. In the past, students were told to look at the omnibus ratio, and, if it was significant, they could then look to see where those differences were. However, there may be differences somewhere between the conditions, whether the omnibus F-ratio is statistically significant or not. When you are carrying out your own research we suggest that you consider the use of pairwise comparisons to look for where any differences might lie. Note, however, that you might find instances where authors of papers, noting a non-significant omnibus F, decide to go no further. See Howell (2009) for a more in-depth discussion of these points.

Sometimes researchers decide which pairwise comparisons they wish to carry out before the main analysis. These are called *planned comparisons* (sometimes called *a priori*). Often researchers use t-tests for this. In other instances, comparisons are not planned in advance, but it becomes clear during the study that they would be useful.

These are called post-hoc tests, and SPSS has options for a variety of these tests. Further details of these tests are provided in the Box describing multiple comparison tests.

Multiple comparison tests

As you have learned, the omnibus F-value does not tell you where any significant differences lie. You might ask why the researchers don't perform every possible comparison. The reason why this isn't desirable is because with every pairwise comparison, the Type I error increases (i.e. it increases the probability that you will falsely reject the null hypothesis: you will call a finding statistically significant when really there is no difference in the population – see Chapter 4, page 148). When making planned comparisons, researchers choose the pairwise comparisons carefully, according to theory and hypotheses, without looking at the data beforehand. In this way fewer pairwise comparisons are made and the chances of a Type I error are reduced. If you don't have any theoretical grounds for choosing particular comparisons to make, then a post-hoc test is the multiple comparison procedure of choice. Post-hoc tests make all possible pairwise

(Continued)

(Continued)

comparisons amongst a set of means. For instance, if we have one factor with three conditions (e.g. group 1, people with IBD; group 2, people with IBS; and group 3, healthy people) then the comparisons would be: 1 versus 2; 1 versus 3 and 2 versus 3). The probability of making a Type I error is controlled across the set of comparisons. A range of different methods of controlling the error rates are available, and they differ in how stringently they control the probability of Type I error. When making a large number of comparisons, you should use a test which is conservative, that is, that errs on the side of caution in deciding whether a pairwise comparison is statistically significant. A description of the tests offered by SPSS can be found by pressing the *Help* button and searching for post-hoc tests. A detailed discussion of these tests is beyond an introductory statistics book, but can be found in Howell (2009).

ONE-WAY ANOVA IN SPSS

The following is a real dataset from a study which we carried out in 2009 (Attree et al.). For this example, we wish to find out whether the groups (Inflammatory Bowel Disease – IBD, Irritable Bowel Syndrome – IBS and healthy controls – HC) differ from each other. We predicted that people with IBD and IBS would have lower Verbal IQ scores (VIQ) than the healthy controls. This is because previous literature showed that other illness groups showed lower VIQs than healthy controls.

1) Choose *Analyze*, *Compare Means*, *One-Way ANOVA*.

   This gives a dialogue box (Screenshot 8.1).

2) Move the variable of interest (VIQ) to the *Dependent List* on the right, and move the grouping variable (group) to the *Factor* box on the right (Screenshot 8.2). Then press the *Post Hoc* button. This will enable you to see where the differences lie, if indeed there are any significant differences between groups. Pressing the *Post Hoc* button gives the another dialogue box (Screenshot 8.3).

   For the purposes of this example, we have chosen the Bonferroni as our post-hoc test.

3) Then click *Continue*. Then *Options* to obtain descriptive statistics (Screenshot 8.4).

   Then *Continue*, and *OK*. The output is obtained is given in Table 8.2.

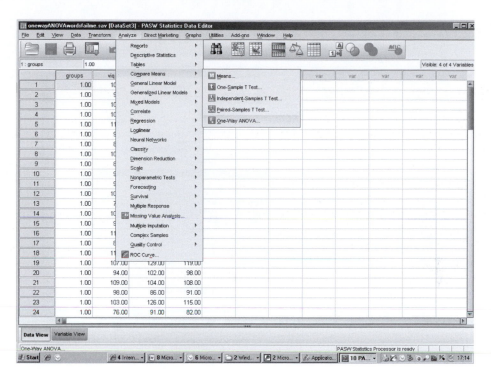

Screenshot 8.1

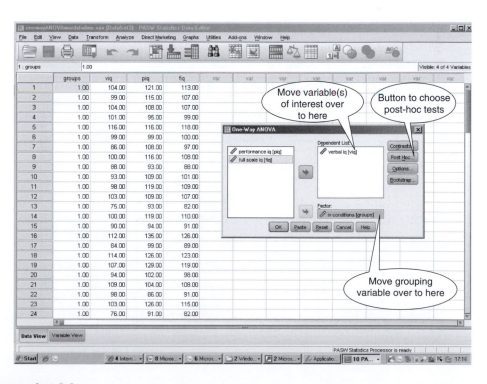

Screenshot 8.2

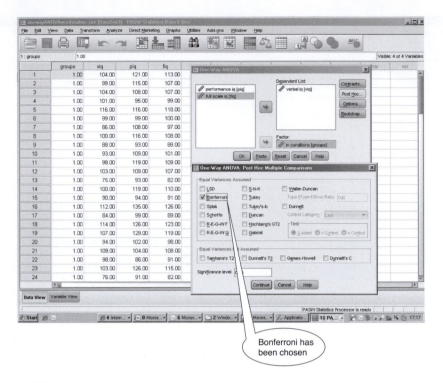

Bonferroni has been chosen

Screenshot 8.3

Options button leads to the dialogue box below

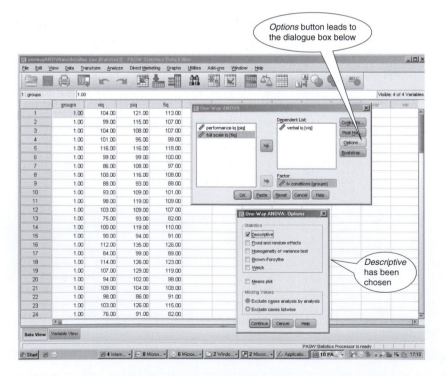

Descriptive has been chosen

Screenshot 8.4

Table 8.2 Descriptive statistics for IBD, IBS and healthy controls

Descriptives

verbal iq

| | N | Mean | Std. deviation | Std. error | 95% confidence interval for mean | | Minimum | Maximum |
					Lower bound	Upper bound		
ibs	29	97.4828	11.26188	2.09128	93.1990	101.7666	75.00	116.00
ibd	29	93.2069	13.42008	2.49205	88.1022	98.3116	67.00	119.00
controls	30	107.8667	11.66998	2.13064	103.5090	112.2243	80.00	129.00
Total	88	99.6136	13.52259	1.44151	96.7485	102.4788	67.00	129.00

The table shows the number of people in each group – you can see there was one more person in the control group than in the other two groups. The control group has a higher VIQ than the other two groups. Whether or not this is a statistically significant difference cannot be seen from the descriptives. The groups are fairly equal in variance, as shown by the standard deviation for each group, and the standard error. The 95% confidence interval allows us to generalise to the population. So for the IBS group, the mean is 97.48, and we can be 95% certain that the true population mean for people with IBS is somewhere between 93.20 and 101.77 (rounded up).

The ANOVA output (Table 8.3) tells us whether there is a statistically significant difference between some or all of the groups. This is what is known as the overall (or omnibus) F. F-ratios always come with two separate figures for degrees of freedom; one related to the BG variance and one relating to the WG variance. They are 2 and 85 in this case and it is conventional to quote these when reporting the F-ratio. The significance level is also given as .000 which should be reported as $p < .001$. In this case the full report should be $F_{2,85} = 11.40$, $p < .001$. So there is a significant difference between some or all of the groups.

Table 8.3 ANOVA table for IBD, IBS and healthy controls

ANOVA

verbal iq

	Sum of squares	df	Mean square	F	Sig.
Between Groups	3365.397	2	1682.698	11.403	.000
Within Groups	12543.467	85	147.570		
Total	15908.864	87			

Table 8.4 Multiple comparisons for IBS, IBD and control groups

Verbal IQ
Bonferroni

Multiple Comparisons

(I) iv conditions		(J) iv conditions		Mean difference (I-J)	Std. error	Sig.	95% confidence interval	
							Lower bound	Upper bound
	IBS	dimension3	IBD	4.27586	3.19018	.551	−3.5155	12.0672
			controls	−10.38391*	3.16348	.004	−18.1100	−2.6578
Dimension 2	IBD	dimension3	IBS	−4.27586	3.19018	.551	−12.0672	3.5155
			controls	−14.65977*	3.16348	.000	−22.3859	−6.9337
	controls	dimension3	IBS	10.38391*	3.16348	.004	2.6578	18.1100
			IBD	14.65977*	3.16348	.000	6.9337	22.3859

* The mean difference is significant at the 0.05 level.

Now we wish to conduct a multiple comparison test to identify which groups are significantly different from which. Table 8.4 gives pairwise comparisons for significant differences once the Bonferroni correction has been applied. The asterisk signifies a statistically significant difference between the pairs. The first row shows IBS was not significantly different from IBD. The mean difference is only 4.28 and the associated probability is .551. IBS can be seen to be different from the controls – the mean difference is 10.39, and the associated probability value is $p = .004$. In the second row, the IBD group can be seen to be significantly different from the controls – a bigger difference here (14.66). This is significant at $< .001$. The 95% confidence intervals are confidence limits around the mean difference (as in the t-test).

We could report this in a results section as follows:

> A one-way between-participants ANOVA showed that there were significant differences between the illness groups in terms of IQ scores ($F_{2,85} = 11.40$, p $< .001$). A post-hoc test (Bonferroni correction) showed that controls had significantly higher IQ than both the IBS and IBD groups (p $= .004$ and p $< .001$ respectively). The difference between IBS and IBD groups was not statistically significant (p $= .551$).

Notice how the report above gives the direction of effect when a significant difference is reported. We do not simply say control and IBS groups differed. We say the control group had a significantly *higher* IQ than the IBD group. It is crucial to give direction of effect in this way whenever significant statistical tests are reported. It is often useful to be able to calculate the effect size *d* by hand, when reading the results sections of journal article. Eventually you may become familiar enough with the formula to do a rough calculation in your head. The formula is given in Chapter 7, page 220.

Activity 8.4

Using information from the descriptive statistics (above) calculate Cohen's *d* for the significant comparisons above (correct to two decimal places) and state whether the effect is weak, moderate, or strong.

Rewrite the reported results section above, this time incorporating the effect sizes. Check what you've written with our revised section at the end of the book.

Example from the Literature

Button (2008), as mentioned at the beginning of this chapter, wanted to investigate possible differences in stressors and health levels between different grades of nurses, i.e. auxiliary nurses, staff nurses, ward sisters, senior nurses and midwives. It can be seen that this is a quasi-experimental design, because of the lack of random allocation to the conditions, i.e. the groups are pre-existing ones. There were 212 nurses in the study. As part of this study, they looked at 'time stress', a composite variable composed of items such as hours contracted per week and actual hours worked per week. Higher scores indicate a greater level of stress. They carried out a one-way ANOVA to determine the differences in time stress between job grades. Table 8.5 relates to the analysis.

Table 8.5   Time stress levels depending on job grade

	Auxiliary nurses	Staff nurses	Ward sisters	Senior nurses	Midwives
Mean	−0.56[a,b]	0.01[c]	0.99	0.50	−0.33[d]
SD	0.86	0.91	0.26	0.54	1.05
N	8	160	13	20	11

a Ward sister versus auxiliary nurse $p < 0.001$
b Auxiliary nurse versus senior nurse $p < 0.05$
c Ward sister versus staff nurse $p < 0.001$
d Ward sister versus midwife $p < 0.005$

The authors report

> *There was a significant difference in time stress levels, with ward sisters reporting higher time stress than auxiliary nurses, staff nurses and midwives [F(4,207) = 6.72, p < 0.005]. In addition to ward sisters, auxiliary nurses also reported lower time stress than senior nurses.*

This relates to the overall, omnibus F-test – i.e. there was a significant difference between some or all of the groups. To provide definitive statistical evidence of which groups differ from which, a multi-comparison test is required to follow-up on the significant omnibus F-ratio.

ANOVA MODELS FOR REPEATED-MEASURES DESIGNS

We saw in the between-participants ANOVA that the total variation in scores was broken into between-group variation and within-group variation. As noted on page 210, these sources of variation represent:

a) Between-groups variation (BG variation) – due to our treatment effects, individual differences and experimental error
b) Within-groups variation (WG variation) – due to individual differences and experimental error

The defining feature of a repeated-measures design is that everyone takes part in all conditions. Therefore participants act as their own controls. This means the between-conditions variance cannot include individual differences. For example, in an experiment on reaction time you might have one participant with lightning fast reactions. In a between-participants experiment this might seriously reduce the mean of one group relative to the others. In a repeated measures design, however, this person appears in all conditions and will affect all of their means in the same way. So an extreme individual will not make any one condition look different from another.

The formula for the repeated-measures ANOVA takes this into account. The variance due to individual differences in the dataset can be estimated and removed from the equation:

$$F = \text{between-groups variance} \div \text{within-groups variance (with individual differences removed)}^3$$

Repeated-measures ANOVAs are based on the same assumptions as those which were traditionally required for the independent-groups ANOVAs. One difference, however, is that it is assumed that the variances of the differences between each individual's scores in a pair of conditions is approximately equal across all pairs of conditions. This is called 'sphericity', and although it sounds complicated you probably don't need to understand it fully. If you really want to understand it fully, then Andy Field gives a readable account in his textbook (Field, 2009). What you do need to understand is that the assumption is frequently violated in repeated-measures experiments.

Given that violation of sphericity is such a problem, the good news is that SPSS produces all the information to deal with a violation by default when you ask for a repeated-measures ANOVA. First of all it gives you a test that tells you whether your data violate the assumption of sphericity: Mauchly's test of sphericity. If this test is significant then it indicates a violation of the assumption. Therefore, you are now in the somewhat new territory of hoping that a test result is non-significant ($p > .05$). If Mauchly's test is significant you know you have a problem and you must correct your significance testing to avoid a Type I error. SPSS also produces ANOVA results corrected for violation of sphericity by default. Actually, it produces a number of approaches to correction including the widely used Greenhouse–Geiser correction.

REPEATED-MEASURES ANOVA IN SPSS

The following example is based on a dataset consisting of patients with Irritable Bowel Syndrome. The dataset looked at the way in which duration of illness, rumination and depression related to cognitive measures. Here, we are simply looking at the differences between four cognitive tests, taken by all the participants. Thus the four related conditions are analysed by a repeated-measures ANOVA. Repeated-measures ANOVAs produce an F-ratio, degrees of freedom and p-value similar in format to between-participants ANOVAs. The interpretation of effects and the need for multiple comparison tests is also the same. The way the test is conducted in SPSS is a little different, however.

1) Choose *Analyze*, *General Linear Model*, *Repeated Measures* (Screenshot 8.5).

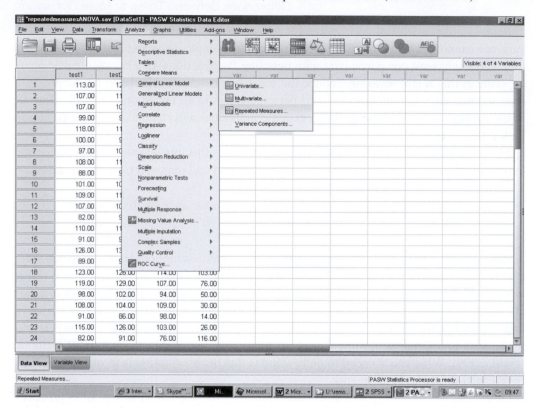

Screenshot 8.5

This gives a dialogue box (Screenshot 8.6).

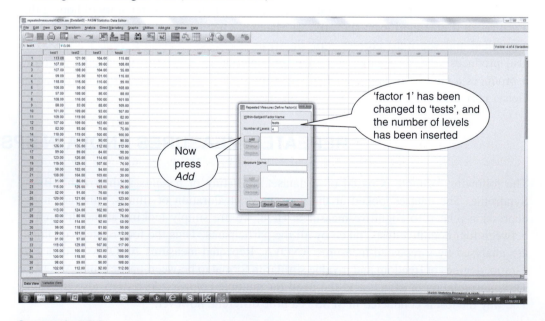

Screenshot 8.6

2) Change the word 'factor' to a sensible name – here we have changed it to 'tests' and then insert the number of levels – here we have four. Then press *Add*.

3) Then press *Define* (Screenshot 8.7).

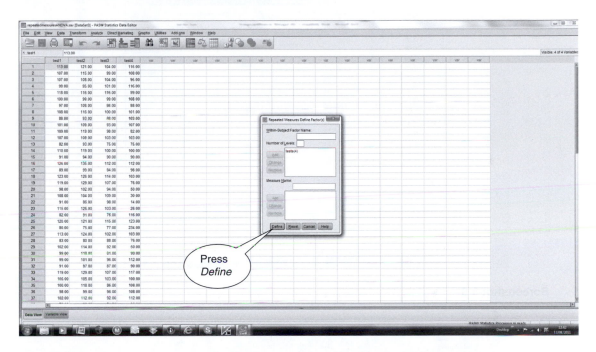

Screenshot 8.7

4) Highlight the within-participants variables and move them to the *Within-subjects variables (tests)* on the right (Screenshot 8.8). Note you need to move these over in the order in which you want them to appear.

5) Press *Options* (Screenshot 8.9):

6) Move the variables from the left to *Display means for* on the right; check the *Compare main effects* box. By default, the Bonferroni post-hoc test is given. Check *Descriptive statistics* and *Estimates of effect size* (Screenshot 8.10).

7) Then *Continue*, and *OK*.

The output is as in Table 8.6.

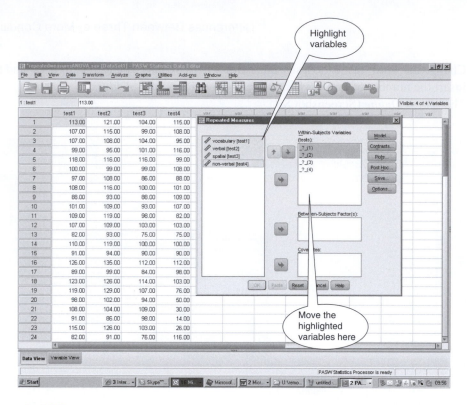

Screenshot 8.8

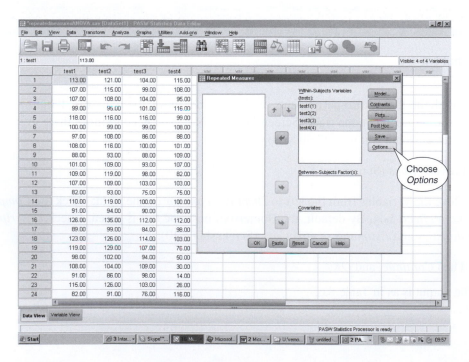

Screenshot 8.9

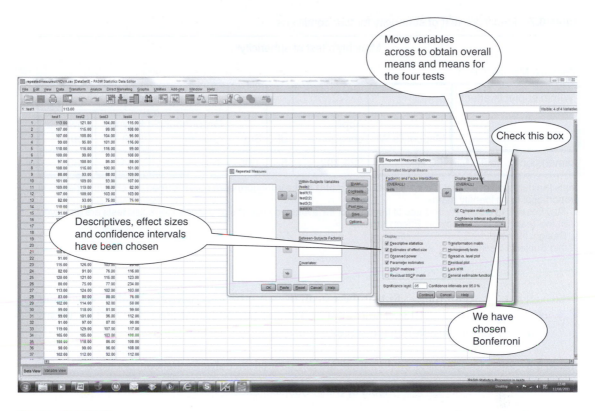

Screenshot 8.10

Table 8.6 Descriptive statistics for four conditions

Descriptive Statistics

	Mean	Std. deviation	N
vocabulary	102.7667	13.29759	60
verbal	108.9167	14.15566	60
spatial	96.1333	12.99213	60
non-verbal	98.8000	29.67725	60

This shows the means, SDs and Ns of our four conditions.

Mauchly's test of sphericity shows that we cannot assume sphericity (Table 8.7) (see page 259), so we correct for this by using the Greenhouse–Geisser part of the main ANOVA output. If Mauchly's test was non-significant you would report the figures from the sphericity assumed line.

Table 8.7   Mauchly's test of sphericity for four conditions

Mauchly's test of sphericity[b]

Measure:MEASURE_1

Within subjects effect		Mauchly's W	Approx. chi-square	df	Sig.	Epsilon[a]		
						Greenhouse-geisser	Huynh-feldt	Lower-bound
dimension1 tests		.004	324.792	5	.000	.391	.394	.333

Tests the null hypothesis that the error covariance matrix of the orthonormalized transformed dependent variables is proportional to an identity matrix.
a. May be used to adjust the degrees of freedom for the averaged tests of significance. Corrected tests are displayed in the Tests of Within-Subjects Effects table.
b. Design: Intercept
Within Subjects Design: tests

It can be seen (Table 8.8) that there is an overall difference between the four conditions ($F_{1.17, 69.26}{}^4 = 6.01$, $p = .013$). The overall measure of effect (partial eta^2) is .092. This means that 9.2% of the variation in the scores is due to the different conditions.

Table 8.8   Tests to determine whether there are any differences between the four conditions

Tests of Within-Subjects Effects

Measure:MEASURE_1

Source		Type III sum of squares	df	Mean square	F	Sig.	Partial eta squared
tests	Sphericity Assumed	5556.446	3	1852.149	6.005	.001	.092
	Greenhouse-Geisser	5556.446	1.174	4733.525	6.005	.013	.092
	Huynh-Feldt	5556.446	1.183	4695.358	6.005	.013	.092
	Lower-bound	5556.446	1.000	5556.446	6.005	.017	.092
Error(tests)	Sphericity Assumed	54590.804	177	308.423			
	Greenhouse-Geisser	54590.804	69.257	788.234			
	Huynh-Feldt	54590.804	69.820	781.878			
	Lower-bound	54590.804	59.000	925.268			

The part of the output shown in Table 8.9 shows the means of the four conditions, with 95% confidence intervals around the means.

And Table 8.10 shows the significance of the pairwise conditions using the Bonferroni corrections.

Table 8.9   Mean, standard error and 95% confidence intervals for the four conditions

Estimates

Measure:MEASURE_1

tests	Mean	Std. error	95% confidence interval	
			Lower bound	Upper bound
1	102.767	1.717	99.332	106.202
2	108.917	1.827	105.260	112.573
3	96.133	1.677	92.777	99.490
4	98.800	3.831	91.134	106.466

Table 8.10   Pairwise comparisons for the four conditions (Bonferroni)

Pairwise Comparisons

Measure:MEASURE_1

(I) tests		(J) tests		Mean difference (I-J)	Std. error	Sig.[a]	95% confidence interval for difference[a]	
							Lower bound	Upper bound
dimension1	1	dimension2	2	−6.150*	.857	.000	−8.489	−3.811
			3	6.633*	.758	.000	4.565	8.702
			4	3.967	4.349	1.000	−7.906	15.840
	2	dimension2	1	6.150*	.857	.000	3.811	8.489
			3	12.783*	1.560	.000	8.524	17.043
			4	10.117	4.479	.166	−2.113	22.346
	3	dimension2	1	−6.633*	.758	.000	−8.702	−4.565
			2	−12.783*	1.560	.000	−17.043	−8.524
			4	−2.667	4.355	1.000	−14.556	9.223
	4	dimension2	1	−3.967	4.349	1.000	−15.840	7.906
			2	−10.117	4.479	.166	−22.346	2.113
			3	2.667	4.355	1.000	−9.223	14.556

Based on estimated marginal means
* The mean difference is significant at the .05 level
a. Adjustment for multiple comparisons: Bonferroni

Activity 8.5

Which conditions are significantly different from each other? See the answers at the end of the book.

NON-PARAMETRIC EQUIVALENTS

In the health sciences it is often the case that samples are small and distributions skewed. If you are carrying out your own research, we recommend that you look to see if your data are significantly skewed (see Chapter 4, page 140). If they are, then use the equivalent non-parametric tests. As you know, non-parametric tests make no assumptions in relation to normal distribution.

The Kruskal–Wallis one-way ANOVA is the non-parametric equivalent to the parametric between-participants ANOVA. It is an extension of the Mann–Whitney test, which is the non-parametric test used for two groups. The Kruskal–Wallis test is used for three or more groups. This test is based on the ranks of the scores, and the test looks for a significant difference between the mean ranks of the groups. The descriptive statistic appropriate for this test is sometimes the median rather than the mean.

THE KRUSKAL–WALLIS TEST

The formula for this test works by taking the scores for all the conditions and ranking them. The ranks for each group are then added together, and a mean rank obtained for each group. These are then compared using chi-square (see Chapter 9, page 287). The null hypothesis would be that the groups would have similar ranks, since if there really are no differences, ranks should be randomly distributed in the different groups. The experimental hypothesis is that there will be a difference in the ranks of the groups. The researchers are not likely to formulate the experimental hypothesis in these terms, however; they are more likely to say they are looking for differences between groups, and to specify the direction of the difference.

When tests were hand calculated, a test statistic called H was obtained, and so you might find that sometimes this test is referred to as Kruskal–Wallis H. However, statistical packages such as SPSS convert H into a chi-square value. The output gives the mean ranks of the groups, the chi-square value and the associated probability value.

The median test is also used to find whether three or more conditions are drawn from populations with the same median. However, this test relates only to the number of cases that are greater than and less than or equal to the median in each category, and is therefore less powerful than the Kruskal–Wallis test.

The difference in power can be seen by comparing the results of the Kruskal–Wallis test to the median test using the same dataset; this is shown in the next section.

KRUSKAL–WALLIS AND THE MEDIAN TEST IN SPSS

1) Choose *Analyze, Nonparametric tests, Legacy Dialogs, K Independent Samples*.

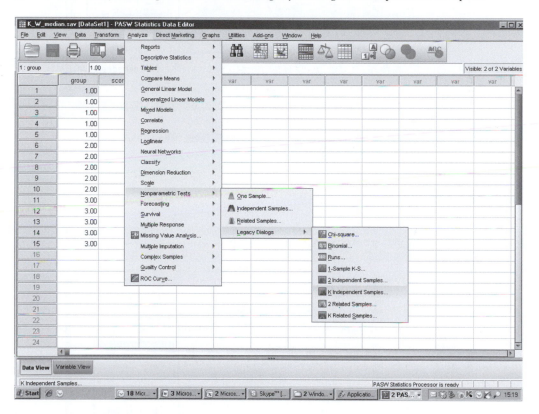

Screenshot 8.11

This gives a dialogue box (Screenshot 8.11).

2) Move the test variable *score* from the left-hand side to the *Test Variable List*, and move the grouping variable *group* to the *Grouping Variable* box on the right. Click *Define Range*. This gives another dialogue box (Screenshot 8.12).

3) Enter the range for the *Grouping Variable*, in this case the minimum is 1 and the maximum 3. Press *Continue*, then *Options* (to choose descriptives). If you want the *Median* test, then check the relevant box.

Then *Continue*, then *OK* (Screenshot 8.13).

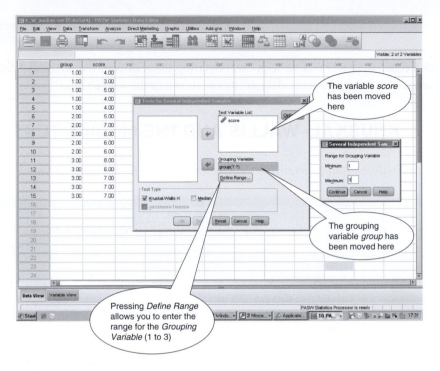

Screenshot 8.12

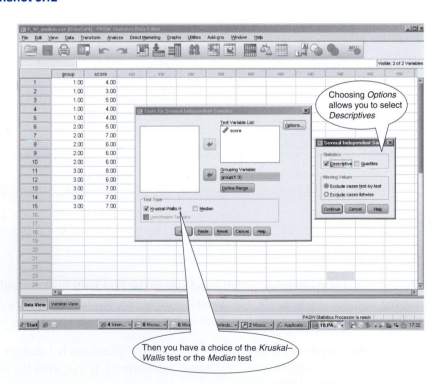

Screenshot 8.13

Table 8.11 gives the relevant part of the output.

Table 8.11   Mean ranks of the three groups

	Ranks		
	Group	N	Mean rank
score	1.00	5	3.10
	2.00	5	8.70
	3.00	5	12.20
	Total	15	

This output shows that group 1 had the lowest mean rank, group 3 the highest, and group 2 was intermediary.

Table 8.12   Test statistics for the three groups

Test Statistics[a,b]	
	Score
Chi-square	11.027
df	2
Asymp. Sig.	.004

a. Kruskal Wallis Test
b. Grouping Variable: group

The test statistic for Kruskal–Wallis is given as chi-square (Table 8.12). We might report findings in this way:

A Kruskal–Wallis test showed that there was a significant difference between groups (chi-square = 11.03, df = 2, p = .004). Group 3 > group 2 > group 1.

If pairwise comparisons are needed, then it would be appropriate to compare groups using the Mann–Whitney test, with significance levels corrected for multiple testing.

Example from the Literature: Kruskal–Wallis

Doest et al. (2007) used the Theory of Planned Behaviour (TPB) to determine the explanatory power of planned behaviour constructs in relation to smoking and not smoking in 248 Dutch secondary students. The authors explain that there are

four ways to conceptualise and operationalise the determinants of the TPB in relation to smoking. These are: a) the not smoking model; b) the smoking model; c)
the dual assessment model; and d) the mixed assessment model. If you wish to
know more about this article, it is available on the companion website This study
evaluated and compared the ability of these four assessment models to account for
adolescents' intentions to smoke or not to smoke. The authors say 'because of differences in sample size and variance between the four categories of self-reported
smoking behavior, a nonparametric test (Kruskal–Wallis) was used to evaluate group
differences' (p. 664).

Table 8.13   TPB Constructs and Current Smoking Behavior

	Current smokers (n = 22)		Ex-smokers (n = 181)		Experimenters (n = 62)		Never smokers (n = 143)		Kruskal–Wallis χ^2(3 df)	Pairwise comparisons
	M	SD	M	SD	M	SD	M	SD		
ATT-S	3.47	0.73	2.36	0.88	1.51	0.55	1.31	0.55	84.47***	Cur >*** Ex >*** Exp >** Nev
ATT-NS	5.45	0.93	5.63	0.82	5.99	1.45	6.26	1.47	42.63***	Cur = Ex <* Exp <** Nev
SN	3.50	0.87	2.78	1.24	1.91	1.15	1.65	0.97	49.19***	Cur >* Ex >** Exp = Nev
PBC-S	6.27	1.52	6.33	1.28	4.90	2.15	4.17	2.38	27.43***	Cur = Ex > *Exp >* Nev
PBC-NS	4.41	2.36	6.11	1.53	6.34	1.44	6.19	1.68	18.77***'	Cur <* Ex = Exp = Nev
INT-S	5.07	1.58	2.22	1.61	1.40	0.99	1.17	0.73	109.61***	Cur >*** Ex >* Exp >** Nev
INT-NS	2.63	1.63	5.50	1.75	6.34	1.37	6.72	0.80	99.45***	Cur <*** Ex <* Exp <** Nev

NOTE: TPB = theory of planned behavior; ATT = attitude; SN = subjective norm; PBC = perceived behavioral control;
INT = intention; –S = construct assessed for smoking; –NS = construct assessed for not smoking; Cur = current
smokers; Ex = ex-smokers; Exp = experimenters; Nev = never smokers.
*p <.05. **p<.01. ***p<.001.

One of the tables of results, reproduced here (Table 8.13) shows the means and
standard deviations for the four independent groups on seven constructs. The
Kruskal–Wallis test statistic, here chi-square, is given, along with the df.[5] Each value
is asterisked, showing that p < .001. The authors have also given the results of

the pairwise comparisons they have carried out, showing the direction of differences in the means of the various groups on the seven constructs. The researchers considered that the mean was the best measure of central tendency to report in their study.

The researchers concluded on the basis of these results (and others not reported here) that 'attitudes towards smoking, perceived subjective norm and perceived behavioural control over both smoking and not smoking – best explained the adolescents' smoking intentions and smoking behaviour'. (p. 660)

THE MEDIAN TEST

As mentioned above, the median test shows only the number of cases that are greater than and less than or equal to the median in each category; it does not take into account the distance from the median.

Table 8.14   Frequencies of scores for three groups

Frequencies

		Group		
		1.00	2.00	3.00
score	> Median	0	1	4
	<= Median	5	4	1

In group 1, there were no scores that were higher than the median, but five scores which were equal or lower than the median. In group 3, there were four scores which were higher than the median, and one lower than the median (Table 8.14).

The test statistic (also chi-square) = 7.8; $df = 2$, $p = .02$ (Table 8.15). Notice how, using the same dataset, the chi-square-value is lower and the p-value higher, when using the median test .

The median test is rarely used, as it is hard to see the advantages when compared to the Kruskal–Wallis test.

Table 8.15 Tests statistics for three groups

Test Statistics[b]

	Score
N	15
Median	6.0000
Chi-square	7.800[a]
df	2
Asymp. Sig.	.020

a. 6 cells (100.0%) have expected frequencies less than 5. The minimum expected cell frequency is 1.7.
b. Grouping Variable: group

Example from the Literature

Al-Faris (2000) compared students' evaluations of a traditional and an innovative undergraduate family medicine course in Saudi Arabia. The traditional approach was very much teacher-centred, and mostly was taught by traditional lectures. The assessment focussed on the knowledge gained by students. The innovative approach consisted of a mixture of group discussions and interactive lectures and the assessment focussed on the appraisal of students' performance in health clinics.

Table 8.16 Comparison of old and new course students' evaluation of different aspects of their curricular as measured by the median test

Items	Old course students No. (%) above median score	New course students No. (%) above median score	p-value
Teaching in form of lectures	6 (26.1)	5 (18.5)	0.76
Teaching in form of group discussion	10 (41.7)	15 (55.6)	0.48
Accessibility and availability of references	8 (33.3)	14 (51.9)	0.29
Curriculum content	7 (29.2)	7 (26.9)	0.89
Competence of health center's tutors	0	2 (7.7)	0.49
Interest of health center's tutors	0	7 (25.9)	0.01*
Assessment in general	2 (8.3)	4 (14.8)	0.78

*p-value < 0.05 using the median test

Al-Faris randomly divided students into two groups. Twenty six were taught according to the old course, and 27 students followed the new course. The author states that 'The Median Test (a non-parametric test) … was used to estimate significance' (p. 233). Al-Faris provides the results given in Table 8.16.

You can see that there is only one result which is statistically significant. The author says 'both groups of students were relatively dissatisfied with the competence of the health clinic tutors. Students in the new course were significantly more satisfied with the tutors' interest' (p. 234).

FRIEDMAN'S ANOVA FOR REPEATED MEASURES

Friedman's test is the non-parametric equivalent of the repeated-measures ANOVA and is an extension of the Wilcoxon test for two conditions. Friedman's ANOVA is therefore used for three or more conditions. For each of the participants, the variables are ranked and the sum of ranks over the participants is calculated. For example, if there were three conditions and participants scored highest in the second condition, next highest in the third condition and lowest in the first condition, the following would be the ranks for each condition for this person (Condition 1 = 3, Condition 2 = 1, Condition 3 = 2). It is rather like the parametric repeated-measures ANOVA, but using ranks of the participants' scores instead of the scores themselves. The null hypothesis is that the ranks of the different conditions will be similar (since if there are really no differences between them, then the ranks will be more or less the same in each group). The experimental hypothesis is that there will be differences in the ranks between each group. Researchers do not usually express the experimental hypothesis in this form however, they are more likely to specify the hypothesis in terms of differences between the conditions, and to specify the direction of the differences. The test statistic is chi-square.

FRIEDMAN'S ANOVA IN SPSS

Six participants with Chronic Fatigue Syndrome reported how fatigued they felt by answering a 20-item fatigue questionnaire. The total scores they could have obtained ranged from 0 to 100. They then were given an intervention which showed them how to reduce their fatigue. This included showing them how to pace themselves (daily, weekly and monthly) and giving advice on how to relax and practice various meditation techniques. They were then given the questionnaire again immediately after the intervention and then again at 6- and 12-month follow-ups. Small participant numbers meant a non-parametric analysis was relevant.

1) Click on *Analyze*, *Nonparametric Tests*, *Legacy Dialogs* and *K Related Samples* (Screenshot 8.14).

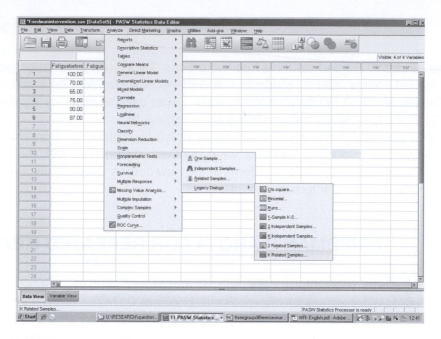

Screenshot 8.14

This gives the Screenshot 8.15.

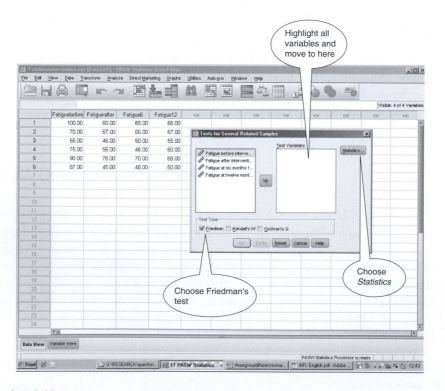

Screenshot 8.15

2) Move all the fatigue scores from the left to the *Test Variables* box on the right, then press *Statistics*. This gives Screenshot 8.16.

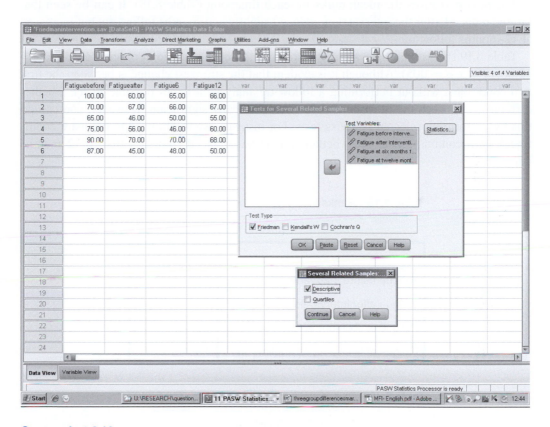

Screenshot 8.16

Check *Descriptives* if you want, then press *Continue*, then *OK*, this gives the output in Table 8.17:

Table 8.17   Descriptive statistics for fatigue at four timepoints

Descriptive Statistics					
	N	Mean	Std. deviation	Minimum	Maximum
Fatigue before intervention	6	81.1667	13.34791	65.00	100.00
Fatigue after intervention	6	58.6667	12.64384	45.00	78.00
Fatigue at six months follow up	6	57.5000	10.61603	46.00	70.00
Fatigue at twelve months follow up	6	61.0000	7.32120	50.00	68.00

The table shows the number of participants, the mean fatigue scores and standard deviations for fatigue at each timepoint, and the minimum and maximum scores.

The next part gives the mean ranks for each timepoint (Table 8.18). It can be seen that fatigue reduced after the intervention, reduced slightly at 6-months follow-up, but increased at 12-months follow-up.

Table 8.19 shows that there was a statistically significant change in fatigue (chi-square = 12.86, $df = 3$, $p = .005$). Although it is evident that the strongest change is between the first two conditions, without performing a follow-up analysis, it is not possible to see whether differences between the other conditions are statistically significant. However, you can do this by performing selected pairwise tests. For instance, we might want to compare condition 1 with condition 4, to see whether fatigue has reduced from baseline to 12 months later.

Table 8.18   Ranks for fatigue at four timepoints

Ranks

	Mean rank
Fatigue before intervention	4.00
Fatigue after intervention	1.75
Fatigue at six months follow up	1.67
Fatigue at twelve months follow up	2.58

Table 8.19   Test statistics for fatigue at four timepoints

Test Statistics[a]

N	6
Chi-square	12.864
df	3
Asymp. Sig.	.005

a. Friedman Test

Activity 8.6

Carry out an appropriate pairwise test between fatigue at baseline and fatigue 12 months later. Report the appropriate statistics, and give an interpretation of the results. You may need to refer to Chapter 7. Compare this to our results in the answers section.

Example from the Literature

Chiou and Kuo (2008) wanted to assess the effect of betel-quid chewing on autonomic nervous modulation by using a spectral heart-rate variability analysis. Betel quid is a psychoactive substance, widely used around the world. Twenty participants were measured using Heart Rate Variability (HRV) analysis after 5 minutes chewing, 30 minutes chewing and 60 minutes chewing. The researchers measured the participants using normal chewing gum, as well as after chewing betel-quid. Both the data from the normal chewing gum and the betel-quid gum were analysed by (separate) Friedman ANOVAs. Part of their table of results is reproduced in Table 8.20.

Table 8.20   Sequential changes in HRV measures before and after chewing betel quid

HRV measures	Before	5 minutes	30 minutes	60 minutes
Mn_{RRI} (ms)	885 +/– 119	772 +/– 113*	896 +/– 116	939 +/– 137*
HR (bpm)	69.0 +/– 9.3	79.3 +/– 11.6*	68.1 +/– 9.4	65.2 +/– 9.7*
SD_{RR} (ms)	61.2 +/– 25.7	53.5 +/– 17.8	67.3 +/– 31.6	66.5 +/– 22.8
CV_{RR} (%)	6.82 +/– 2.38	6.80 +/– 1.58	7.40 +/– 2.82	7.10 +/– 1.99

Data was presented as the mean +/–SD. *$p < .05$ compared with the before chewing betel-quid (Friedman repeated measures ANOVA on ranks)
Mn_{RR}, mean RR interval; HR, heart rate; SD_{RR} standard deviation of RR intervalse; CV_{RR} coefficient of variation of RR intervals; ms, millisecond; bpm, beats per minute

The table shows that there is a significant difference between the first two measures before chewing started, and after chewing for 5 minutes, and also between before chewing and after 60 minutes. The authors present means and standard deviations, but no test statistic. However, we do know that these comparisons are significant at the $p < .05$ level.

The researchers concluded, on the basis of these results and other significant findings (not reported here) that 'the short-term effect of chewing betel-quid was an initial increase in the sympathetic modulation and reduced vagal modulation, followed by gradual increase in the sympathetic and vagal modulations of the subject'.

Summary

In order to test for differences between three or more groups or conditions, you need to choose an ANOVA model.

We suggest that unless you have skewed data, you choose the one-way ANOVA for independent groups or the repeated-measures ANOVA for within groups. The appropriate descriptive statistics are the means and standard deviations. Confidence intervals around the means, and measures of effect, are appropriate for these statistics. Partial eta^2 (an effect size) can be obtained as part of the SPSS output. When carrying out ANOVA, the descriptive statistics might lead you to believe, for instance, that there is a significant difference between groups 1 and 2, rather than 2 or 3. Follow-up tests can confirm whether the differences lie. The equivalent non-parametric test for an independent-groups ANOVA is the Kruskal–Wallis test, and for the repeated measures ANOVA it is Friedman's.

MULTIPLE CHOICE QUESTIONS

1. A test which looks for a significant difference between the mean ranks of three or more independent groups is called the:
   a) Mann-Whitney test
   b) Wilcoxon test
   c) Friedman's ANOVA
   d) Kruskal–Wallis test

2. In order to determine the strength of the difference between pairs of conditions using a parametric test, which is the most suitable?
   a) Cohen's d
   b) Eta^2
   c) t-test
   d) Mann–Whitney

3. A researcher carries out five pairwise comparisons, and decides to adjust the criterion significance level to control for a Type I error. The most sensible probability level at which the findings should be declared statistically significant is:
   a) $< .05$
   b) .04
   c) .50
   d) .10

4. A researcher has four different groups of participants, measured on a scale which is interval level. The scores are normally distributed and the groups have similar variances. Which is the most appropriate test of difference?
   a) Kruskal–Wallis test
   b) Friedman's ANOVA
   c) One-way independent-groups ANOVA
   d) Repeated-measures ANOVA

5. A research group investigates three groups of patients; each group suffers from a rare disease and so participant numbers are small and the scores are not normally distributed. In addition, data are at the ordinal level. Which is the most appropriate test of difference?
   a) Kruskal–Wallis test
   b) Friedman's ANOVA
   c) One-way independent-groups ANOVA
   d) Repeated-measures ANOVA

6. After performing an ANOVA and finding an overall significant difference, researchers need to find where the significant differences lie. They achieve this by performing a:
   a) *t*-test
   b) Least Significant Difference (LSD) test
   c) Tukey's test
   d) Any of the above

Questions 7 to 9 relate to the output for a one-way ANOVA, below.

Descriptives

Anxiety

	N	Mean	Std. deviation	Std. error	95% confidence interval for mean		Minimum	Maximum
					Lower bound	Upper bound		
IBS	29	15.1034	4.26233	.79150	13.4821	16.7248	7.00	27.00
IBD	29	14.6552	3.83849	.71279	13.1951	16.1153	8.00	23.00
Controls	30	12.5000	3.60794	.65872	11.1528	13.8472	7.00	21.00
Total	88	14.0682	4.03090	.42970	13.2141	14.9222	7.00	27.00

ANOVA

Anxiety

	Sum of squares	df	Mean square	F	Sig.
Between Groups	114.850	2	57.425	3.758	.027
Within Groups	1298.741	85	15.279		
Total	1413.591	87			

Multiple Comparisons

Anxiety
LSD

(I) iv conditions	(J) iv conditions	Mean difference (I-J)	Std. error	Sig.	95% Confidence interval Lower bound	Upper bound
IBS	IBD	.44828	1.02652	.663	−1.5927	2.4893
	Controls	2.60345*	1.01793	.012	.5795	4.6274
IBD	IBS	−.44828	1.02652	.663	−2.4893	1.5927
	Controls	2.15517*	1.01793	.037	.1313	4.1791
controls	IBS	−2.60345*	1.01793	.012	−4.6274	−.5795
	IBD	−2.15517*	1.01793	.037	−4.1791	−.1313

* The mean difference is significant at the 0.05 level.

7. Rounding to the nearest integer, we are 95% confident that the mean anxiety level in the IBS population will fall between:
   a) 13.48 and 16.72
   b) 13.20 and 16.12
   c) 11.15 and 13.85
   d) 13.21 and 14.92

8. Which is the most appropriate statement?
   a) There is a statistically significant effect of group on anxiety ($F_{2,85} = 3.76$; $p = .027$)
   b) There is a statistically significant effect of group on anxiety ($F_{2,87} = 3.76$; $p = .027$)
   c) There is no statistically significant effect of group on anxiety ($F_{2,85} = 3.76$; $p = .027$)
   d) There is no statistically significant effect of group on anxiety ($F_{2,87} = 3.76$; $p = .027$)

9. Which groups are not statistically significantly different from each other?
   a) IBD and controls
   b) IBS and IBD
   c) IBS and controls
   d) All of the above

Questions 10 to 12 relate to the following repeated-measures ANOVA output.

Descriptive Statistics

	Mean	Std. deviation	N
Motivation	8.4659	4.61619	88
Distraction	11.1364	4.08581	88
Emotion	12.4091	4.36716	88

Mauchly's test of sphericity[b]

Measure:MEASURE_1

Within subjects effect	Mauchly's W	Approx. chi-square	df	Sig.	Epsilon[a]		
					Greenhouse-Geisser	Huynh-Feldt	Lower-bound
Rumination	.994	.518	2	.772	.994	1.000	.500

Tests the null hypothesis that the error covariance matrix of the orthonormalized transformed dependent variables is proportional to an identity matrix.
a. May be used to adjust the degrees of freedom for the averaged tests of significance. Corrected tests are displayed in the Tests of Within-Subjects Effects table.
b. Design: Intercept
Within Subjects Design: rumination

Tests of Within-Subjects Effects

Measure: MEASURE_1

Source		Type III sum of squares	df	Mean square	F	Sig.	Partial Eta squared
Rumination	Sphericity Assumed	712.795	2	356.398	18.597	.000	.176
	Greenhouse-Geisser	712.795	1.988	358.540	18.597	.000	.176
	Huynh-Feldt	712.795	2.000	356.398	18.597	.000	.176
	Lower-bound	712.795	1.000	712.795	18.597	.000	.176
Error(rumination)	Sphericity Assumed	3334.538	174	19.164			
	Greenhouse-Geisser	3334.538	172.960	19.279			
	Huynh-Feldt	3334.538	174.000	19.164			
	Lower-bound	3334.538	87.000	38.328			

Pairwise Comparisons

Measure:MEASURE_1

(I) rumination	(J) rumination	Mean difference (I-J)	Std. error	Sig.ª	95% Confidence interval for differenceª	
					Lower bound	Upper bound
1	2	−2.670*	.668	.000	−3.998	−1.343
	3	−3.943*	.677	.000	−5.288	−2.598
2	1	2.670*	.668	.000	1.343	3.998
	3	−1.273*	.634	.048	−2.534	−.012
3	1	3.943*	.677	.000	2.598	5.288
	2	1.273*	.634	.048	.012	2.534

Based on estimated marginal means
* The mean difference is significant at the .05 level.
a. Adjustment for multiple comparisons: Least Significant Difference (equivalent to no adjustments).

10. Has the assumption of sphericity been met?
    a) Yes
    b) No

11. The overall repeated measures analysis shows that:
    a) There is/are significant difference(s) between some or all of the rumination conditions ($F_{2,174} = 18.60, p < .001$)
    b) There is/are significant difference(s) between some or all of the rumination conditions ($F_{2,173} = 18.60, p < .001$)

12. Which pairwise comparison shows the strongest effect?
    a) Conditions 1 and 2
    b) Conditions 2 and 3
    c) Conditions 1 and 3
    d) We cannot tell

13. In the one-way ANOVA procedure, the Bonferroni test is:
    a) A type of fast car
    b) A post-hoc test
    c) A planned comparison
    d) None of the above

14. A research group has four categories of self-reported smoking behaviour. There are differences in sample size and variance between the categories. The appropriate test to determine whether there are differences in the four independent groups is:
    a) One-way ANOVA
    b) Repeated-measures ANOVA

    c) Kruskal–Wallis test

    d) Friedman's ANOVA

15. In a repeated-measures ANOVA, an appropriate overall measure of effect obtained by SPSS is:

    a) Partial eta^2

    b) Cohen's d

    c) Chi-square

    d) None of the above

Notes

1 Note that this table is for illustrative purposes only. As ANOVA analyses the sources of the different variances, it is not appropriate when all scores in one or more conditions are identical.

2 These estimates are represented in ANOVA by the mean square values in the ANOVA table.

3 This is usually called residual error.

4 Rounded to two decimal places.

5 For Kruskal–Wallis, df = number of groups −1.

Testing Associations Between Categorical Variables

9

Overview

This chapter focusses on tests of association between two categorical, or nominal, variables. Categorical variables can take on a limited number of values and no natural ordering of categories is assumed. We will discuss the tabulation of pairs of categorical variables (in contingency tables) and consider the descriptive statistics that are most useful when summarising the results. The significance of association is assessed using the chi-square statistic. We will consider the conceptual basis of the test and its implementation in SPSS. We will also address the interpretation of SPSS output, and how the results should be written up.

The chi-square test of association does not require the assumptions of parametric tests but it does have assumptions of its own. We will discuss these and consider

(Continued)

(Continued)

what you can do if these assumptions are not met, including coverage of Fisher's Exact test. Finally, we will also cover application of the chi-square statistic to the analysis of a single categorical variable; the chi-square goodness-of-fit test.

  After reading this chapter you will:

- Understand where a contingency table analysis is appropriate
- Appreciate the conceptual basis of the chi-square test
- Be able to choose between a straightforward chi-square analysis and Fisher's Exact test
- Know how to conduct the relevant analyses using SPSS and interpret the results
- Be able to draw contingency tables and write up the results
- Understand the use of contingency table analysis in the published literature

INTRODUCTION

As the name suggests, categorical variables group participants into a limited number of categories. We can count the frequency with which participants fall into each category. For example, gender is one categorical variable with two possible values: people may be categorised as 'male' or 'female'. Categorical variables may have more than two values. For example, people may be categorised according to their occupation. This could produce lots of values (e.g. nurse, radiologist, doctor, teacher, university lecturer, investment banker, thief, gangster). You can only include each person in one category, however. So if someone was a doctor by day and a gangster by night you would have to choose which single category was most representative for them. Depending upon your research question, you may want to combine some categories together (often called collapsing categories). This is perfectly permissible so long as the collapsed categories are meaningful. For example, you could form larger categories such as health workers (collapsing doctors and nurses), educators (collapsing teachers and lecturers) and criminals (including the investment bankers at your discretion).

  Many research hypotheses boil down to predicting that one variable is associated with another. In many cases these variables are categorical. Here are some example studies that have studied associations of this type.

- Rowe et al. (2004) tested the hypothesis that low reading ability in children (defined as being in the worst 10% on a reading test) would be associated with suffering an unintentional poisoning.
- Merline et al. (2004) investigated whether level of college education (defined as none, some, or a college degree) was associated with substance use (present or absent) at age 35.

Table 9.1

	No crash	Crash	Total
Women	**51**	**5**	56
Men	**29**	**15**	44
Total	80	20	100

• Green et al. (2005) tested the hypothesis that the presence of child mental disorder would be associated with family socioeconomic classification (e.g. higher profession, routine occupation, etc.)

The association between two categorical variables can be summarised in a contingency table. The categories of one variable are listed across the top row of the table and the categories of the second variable are listed down the first column. For example, we might hypothesise that male drivers are at more risk of car crash than females. To test this hypothesis we might recruit 100 car drivers and ask them whether they have ever been involved in a crash. We could count the number of crashes they have been involved in, but there will probably be very few participants who have had multiple crashes. Therefore, we will create a simple categorical variable with two possible values. One value is for people who have never had a crash. The other value is for people who have had one or more crashes.

So of our 100 participants, imagine 56 of the participants are women (so 44 are men). Twenty participants have had a car crash (so 80 have not). The observed frequencies are shown in Table 9.1. We have listed crash involvement on the first row and gender in the first column. It would make no difference if you drew the table the other way around, with gender on top and crash involvement in the first column. The highlighted cells show the frequency count for each combination of the values. For example, 51 of the observations were *both* female and had not been involved in a crash.

The inferential test of the association between these variables is not based on percentages, but it can be helpful to summarise the data as percentages as described in Chapter 5. We think the most helpful ones are the percentages of men and women who have had a crash. To calculate the percentage of women who have crashed we simply divide the number of female crashers (5) by the total number of women (56), which gives us the proportion of women who have crashed (.09). We multiply this by 100 to get the percentage: 9% of women reported they had been involved in a car crash.

Activity 9.1

Calculate the percentage of men who report a crash history. The answer is in the paragraph below (but no peeking).

We hope you calculated that 34% of the men had been involved in a crash. The figure of 34% sounds a lot more than the 9% for women. Therefore, you might think there is an association between gender and crash involvement, such that men are more likely to have crashed than women. We only have a sample, however, so the apparent differences could be the product of sampling error. We need an inferential statistic to test the probability that this association could have been observed by chance. The chi-square statistic (χ^2, pronounced kai-square) is appropriate here. As with the other inferential statistics you have encountered, we calculate the probability that the observed data could be generated if the null hypothesis is true (i.e. that crashes are not associated with gender). All other things being equal, the larger the χ^2 statistic, the smaller the probability of the null hypothesis being true. If the probability is $< .05$ then we reject the null hypothesis and accept that an association exists in the population.

RATIONALE OF CONTINGENCY TABLE ANALYSIS

The calculation of the χ^2 statistic is based on the frequencies in the cells of the contingency table. As we'll see below, SPSS will do the calculation for you. First of all it calculates the frequencies you would expect in each cell if the null hypothesis was true. These are known as the *expected frequencies*. In our example the null hypothesis is that there is no association between gender and car crash. You might think that under this null hypothesis we would expect our observations to fall equally into the four cells with 25 in each. This is not the case, however. We know that only 20 of our sample overall have had a car crash, so it does not make sense to predict there will be 25 in each of the crash cells. We also recruited uneven numbers of women (56) and men (44), possibly because women are more likely to volunteer to take part in research studies. These row and column totals must be taken into account when calculating the expected frequencies in each cell. To find the expected frequency for each cell we simply multiply the observed row total by the observed column total and divide by the number of participants in the whole table. For example, as we have 56 women and 20 crash-victims in the study of 100 people, we would expect to observe 11.2 females with a crash history ($(56 \times 20)/100$) under the null hypothesis. The expected frequencies in all four cells are shown in Table 9.2.

Table 9.2

	No crash	Crash	Total
Women	44.8	11.2	56
Men	35.2	8.8	44
Total	80	20	100

Table 9.3

	No crash	Crash
Women	$(51-44.8)^2/44.8 = 0.86$	$(5-11.2)^2/11.2 = 3.43$
Men	$(29-35.2)^2/35.2 = 1.09$	$(15-8.8)^2/8.8 = 4.37$

$\chi^2 = 0.86+3.43+1.09+4.37 = 9.75$

The χ^2 statistic is based on the difference between the observed frequencies and expected frequencies. For each cell the expected frequency is subtracted from the observed frequency. This number is then squared, so that we can deal with the mixture of positive and negative numbers that will inevitably be calculated. This works because both positive and negative numbers become positive when squared. Next we divide by the expected frequency. Then we simply add up the figures calculated in each cell and this gives us the χ^2 statistic. The larger the statistic the greater the difference between the observed and expected values across the cells. The calculation is illustrated in Table 9.3.

Next we need to test the significance of this χ^2 statistic. We will look at this as we see how to run the calculation using SPSS.

RUNNING THE ANALYSIS IN SPSS

Entering the Data

Usually in the SPSS data viewer, you have to enter data for each participant on a separate line and you can run a contingency table analysis on data in this form. There is also a data entry short cut you can take if you have already constructed your contingency table, where each line in the data sheet represents a cell in the contingency table. We will focus on this approach. You require three variables to do this; the first two tell SPSS which category of each variable the cell refers to, the third contains the number of observations that fall into that cell. This variable is often called frequency, or 'freq' for short. For example, in our analysis above the data sheet would look as shown in Screenshot 9.1.

We have coded gender as 1 for male and 0 for female, crash involvement is coded 1 for those with a history of involvement and 0 for those who do not have a crash history. We have provided labels for those values and SPSS is displaying the value labels in the data sheet to make it more informative.

	gender	crashhist	freq
1	women	no crash	51.00
2	women	crash	5.00
3	men	no crash	29.00
4	men	crash	15.00
5			
6			

Screenshot 9.1

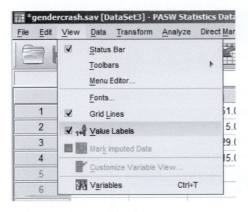

You can toggle this view feature on and off using the *Value Labels* tick box on the *View* menu, as shown in Screenshot 9.2.

Currently SPSS does not know that you have entered a contingency table, it thinks you have a dataset with four observations. In order to set it straight, you need to select *Weight Cases* from the bottom of the *Data* menu (Screenshot 9.3).

In the *Weight Cases* dialogue box you should click the radio button to select the *Weight cases by* option. Then identify *freq* as the frequency variable to weight the cases by moving it from the list on the left to the *Frequency Variable* box

Screenshot 9.2

on the right, as shown in Screenshot 9.4. Next press *OK*. Now SPSS knows that each line on the dataset represents the number of cases specified in the *freq* variable.

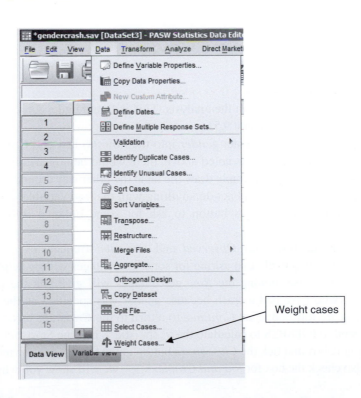

Screenshot 9.3

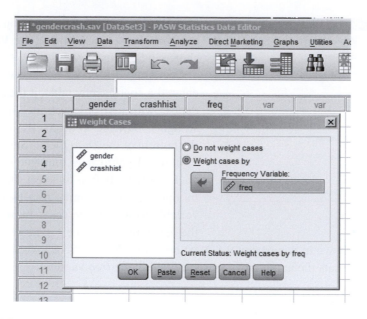

Screenshot 9.4

Running the Analysis

Now the data are set up we can run the analysis. This is found under *Analyze*, *Descriptive Statistics* and *Crosstabs* (Screenshot 9.5).

In the crosstabs dialogue box, enter *gender* into the *Rows(s)* box and *Crashhist* into the *Column(s)* box. (Screenshot 9.6) As noted above, there would be no harm in entering them the other way round – this would simply draw the table the other way around. The χ^2 statistic would remain the same. You should not do anything with the *freq* variable.

Next you should click the *Cells* button to ask for some optional information to be displayed.

You should tick the boxes for *Observed* and *Expected* frequencies to be displayed (Screenshot 9.7). It is also likely that asking for some percentages will be helpful in writing up the result. In this case, ticking the *Row* percentages will give you the percentage of women and men who have had a crash because gender was specified as the row variable above. When you are finished, click *Continue* to return to the *Crosstabs* box.

Finally we need to tell SPSS to calculate the χ^2 statistic. Click the *Statistics* button in the *Crosstabs* dialogue box and tick the *Chi-square* button at the top left as shown in Screenshot 9.8. You can also check the box for *Phi and Cramer's V* – we will show you why this is helpful below.

Once you have done this click *Continue* and then *OK* to run the analysis.

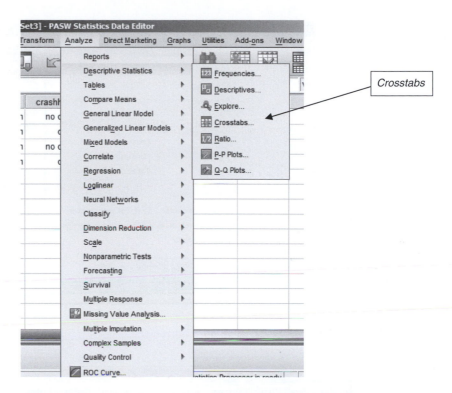

Screenshot 9.5

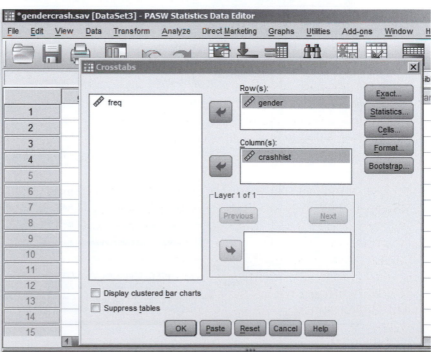

Screenshot 9.6

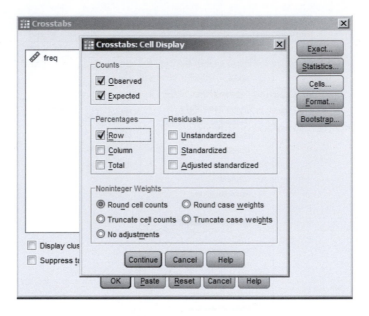

Screenshot 9.7

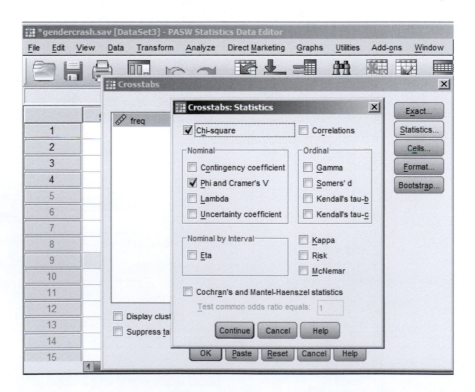

Screenshot 9.8

Interpreting the Output

As often happens with SPSS, more output is printed than you require. The main results table to focus on is the *gender * crashhist Crosstabulation* (i.e. the contingency table) and the box of *Chi-Square Tests* below this. The crosstabulation (Screenshot 9.9) shows the observed frequencies in each cell (labelled *Count*) and the expected frequencies.

SPSS prints a range of test results in the *Chi-Square Tests* box (Screenshot 9.10), only some of which need concern you at this stage.

We described the calculation of the Pearson χ^2 statistic above, and this is the line you should look at first. This shows a χ^2 value of 9.750. The degrees of freedom for a χ^2 analysis

gender * crashhist Crosstabulation

			crashhist		
			no crash	crash	Total
gender	women	Count	51	5	56
		Expected Count	44.8	11.2	56.0
		% within gender	91.1%	8.9%	100.0%
	men	Count	29	15	44
		Expected Count	35.2	8.8	44.0
		% within gender	65.9%	34.1%	100.0%
Total		Count	80	20	100
		Expected Count	80.0	20.0	100.0
		% within gender	80.0%	20.0%	100.0%

Screenshot 9.9

Chi-Square Tests

	Value	df	Asymp. Sig. (2-sided)	Exact Sig. (2-sided)	Exact Sig. (1-sided)
Pearson Chi-Square	9.750[a]	1	.002		
Continuity Correction[b]	8.241	1	.004		
Likelihood Ratio	9.918	1	.002		
Fisher's Exact Test				.002	.002
Linear-by-Linear Association	9.653	1	.002		
N of Valid Cases	100				

a. 0 cells (.0%) have expected count less than 5. The minimum expected count is 8.80.

b. Computed only for a 2x2 table

Screenshot 9.10

are calculated as the number of rows (in the contingency table) minus 1, multiplied by the number of columns minus 1. Hence we have one degree of freedom in this analysis. SPSS tells us that the probability of observing a χ^2 value of 9.750 with one degree of freedom is .002 if the null hypothesis is true. This is very unlikely and below the .05 critical cut off. Therefore we can reject the null hypothesis. The results show men are more likely to have had a crash than women. SPSS reports a two-tailed test of significance (see Chapter 4).

MEASURING EFFECT SIZE IN CONTINGENCY TABLE ANALYSIS

As noted in Chapter 4, there are different measures of effect size available. For this analysis, SPSS produces Cramer's *V*. This provides an intuitive measure of effect size in analyses where both variables have two categories; its interpretation is similar to a Pearson correlation coefficient (*r*). As shown in Screenshot 9.11, the Cramer's *V* is .31.

Writing Up the Result

A good report of a contingency table analysis would name the variables involved, indicate the value of the χ^2 statistic, the degrees of freedom, the number of observations, and the *p*-value. You should also provide the effect size, some descriptive statistics and give the direction of the effect when the result is significant. In our example we could say:

There was a significant association between gender and crash involvement ($\chi^2(1, N = 100)$ = 9.75, p = .002). Men were significantly more likely to have had a crash (34.1%) than women (8.9%). The Cramer's V measure of effect size was .31.

It is the degrees of freedom that is written in the brackets first, then the number of observations is given as the *N*. Instead of the percentages it would also be possible to give the odds-ratio (see Chapter 5).

Symmetric Measures

		Value	Approx. Sig.
Nominal by Nominal	Phi	.312	.002
	Cramer's V	.312	.002
N of Valid Cases		100	

Screenshot 9.11

Example from the Literature

Chris Armitage (2006) studied the role of implementation intentions in dietary change. Implementation intentions involve participants forming explicit plans of how they will behave in critical situations to avoid unwanted behaviours (e.g. eating high fat food). In this study participants were randomly allocated to either an implementation intention or a control condition. The main outcome measures of the study were continuous and showed the implementation intention approach improved dietary behaviour. The continuous nature of these measures made them unsuitable for contingency table analysis. An important initial step in the analysis, however, was to ensure that the implementation intention and control groups did not differ in terms of their composition. Contingency table analysis was used to check allocation was equal in respect of categorical variables including gender. Regarding gender, a contingency table (Screenshot 9.12) can be reconstructed from the details given in the paper.

The χ^2 was not significant ($\chi^2(1, N = 554)=2.2$, $p = .138$). Therefore, as expected, there was no evidence of an unequal gender distribution between experimental and control groups.

LARGER CONTINGENCY TABLES

So far we have only looked at contingency tables in which each variable can have two values. This is often referred to as a 2×2 table as you require two rows and two columns to display the data. We may easily extend the analysis to variables with more categories (e.g. a 3×2 table or a 4×3 or a whatever you like × whatever you like table). For example, imagine our original crash data only included people who had been involved in crashes where they were not at fault. We could easily add some data from people who had been involved in crashes

condition * gender Crosstabulation

			gender female	gender male	Total
condition	control	Count	178	80	258
		Expected Count	185.8	72.2	258.0
	experimental	Count	221	75	296
		Expected Count	213.2	82.8	296.0
Total		Count	399	155	554
		Expected Count	399.0	155.0	554.0

Screenshot 9.12

Table 9.4

	No crash	No-blame crashes	Blame-worthy crashes
Women	51	5	3
Men	29	15	16

where the police blamed them for the crash. Now the crash history variable has three categories: no crashes, no-blame crashes and blame-worthy crashes. It would be possible for the same person to have had (separate) blame-worthy and no-blame crashes. We would need to decide how to categorise these people, as they cannot be counted in both categories. One approach would be to include anyone with a blame-worthy crash in that category, irrespective of whether they had had no-blame crashes as well. The resulting 3×2 table might be as shown in Table 9.4.

Activity 9.2

What would the SPSS datasheet look like if you were setting up this analysis?

In this analysis we still have a significant result ($\chi^2(2, N = 119)=19.9$, $p < .001$). Note that the degrees of freedom are now two as we have a 3×2 table. The significant result still implies that crash history and gender are associated, but in the larger table interpretation is no longer so straightforward. The significance of the χ^2 does not tell us whether the distribution of men and women differs between all categories of the crash variable or only between some of them. One way to solve the problem is to collapse categories until you have a 2×2 table. For example, you could collapse the blame and no-blame categories into a single crash category if all crashes was really your theoretical interest, irrespective of blame.

Contingency table analysis of the form discussed in this chapter is limited to two categorical variables. If you wish to include more variables then loglinear analysis may be appropriate and this is beyond the scope of our book. However, logistic regression (Chapter 13) may be helpful for some analyses of this sort, and also has the advantage that both continuous and categorical variables may be included as predictors.

CONTINGENCY TABLE ANALYSIS ASSUMPTIONS

As we have seen already, the categories of each variable must be mutually exclusive. Each participant may only be placed in one category of each variable. This means contingency table analysis is not suitable for within-participants designs.

Table 9.5   Chi-square tests

	Value	df	Asymp. Sig. (2-sided)	Exact Sig. (2-sided)	Exact Sig. (1-sided)
Pearson Chi-Square	9.750[a]	1	.002		
Continuity Correction[b]	8.241	1	.004		
Likelihood Ratio	9.918	1	.002		
Fisher's Exact Test				**.002**	**.002**
Linear-by-Linear Association	9.653	1	.002		
N of Valid Cases	100				

a. 0 cells (.0%) have expected count less than 5. The minimum expected count is 8.80.
b. Computed only for a 2x2 table.

A second assumption is that there is at least one observation in each cell of the table. If this is a problem then you may be able to solve it by collapsing categories, if the collapsed categories form meaningful categories themselves.

A third assumption is that the expected frequencies do not fall below five in more than 20% of the cells in the contingency table. Fortunately, there is an alternative test statistic that is not vulnerable to low expected frequencies; the Fisher's Exact test. SPSS calculates Fisher's Exact test as standard when calculating a χ^2 test of association. Using our original analysis from earlier in the chapter, we highlight the relevant output in Table 9.5.

One- and two- tailed significance testing is presented with the Fisher's Exact test results. The one-sided significance level would be the correct value to use if you had a one-tailed hypothesis (e.g. males will be more likely to have had a car crash than females). If your hypothesis was two-tailed (i.e. you had predicted gender and crash history were associated without specifying how) then you would use the two-sided probability. In this case the probability rounds to the same probability of .002 for both one- and two-sided calculations and also rounds to the same probability as shown on the top Pearson Chi-square line. There was no need to use Fisher's Exact test in this case because we had an expected frequency greater than 5 in all cells. SPSS has reported this for us in note *a* (in bold). This is where SPSS will warn you when you have too many cells with expected frequencies below 5. For example, if we had only been able to recruit 30 participants for our study of gender and crash history, we might have calculated the analysis in Screenshots 9.13 and 9.14.

The expected frequencies are low in the crash cells. SPSS warns us (in note *a*, Screenshot 9.14) that have 50% of cells with expected frequencies below five. Therefore, we should use Fisher's Exact test for this analysis.

Fisher's Exact test solves the problem of small expected frequencies when dealing with 2x2 tables, but it is not usually calculated for larger tables. When you have larger tables but small expected frequencies, you may be able to solve the problem by collapsing categories.

gender * crashhist Crosstabulation

| | | | crashhist | | Total |
			no crash	crash	
gender	women	Count	13	1	14
		Expected Count	10.3	3.7	14.0
		% within gender	92.9%	7.1%	100.0%
	men	Count	9	7	16
		Expected Count	11.7	4.3	16.0
		% within gender	56.3%	43.8%	100.0%
Total		Count	22	8	30
		Expected Count	22.0	8.0	30.0
		% within gender	73.3%	26.7%	100.0%

Screenshot 9.13

Chi-Square Tests

	Value	df	Asymp. Sig. (2-sided)	Exact Sig. (2-sided)	Exact Sig. (1-sided)
Pearson Chi-Square	5.117[a]	1	.024		
Continuity Correction[b]	3.416	1	.065		
Likelihood Ratio	5.660	1	.017		
Fisher's Exact Test				.039	.030
Linear-by-Linear Association	4.946	1	.026		
N of Valid Cases	30				

a. 2 cells (50.0%) have expected count less than 5. The minimum expected count is 3.73.

b. Computed only for a 2x2 table

Screenshot 9.14

THE χ^2 GOODNESS-OF-FIT TEST

The χ^2 statistic can also be useful if you only have one categorical variable and want to test whether the observed frequencies of each category are as expected. For example, you might be choosing which of four possible messages to discourage smoking (shown in Table 9.6) you will display in family doctor waiting rooms.

You ask a sample of 400 patients which they prefer (remember of course that the message people prefer has nothing to do with how effective the message will be in reducing smoking, but perhaps you want to balance providing an effective health message with providing a

Table 9.6

Smoking increases your chance of heart disease	Smoking increases your chance of cancer	Your family's health is at risk from breathing your smoke	Smoking makes your clothes smell
35	45	40	280

pleasant waiting room). If each message was preferred equally (the null hypothesis) then you would predict that an equal number of people would choose each one as their favourite: 400/4 = 100 each message. So 100 in each category are our *expected frequencies*. The observed frequencies are shown in Table 9.6. It looks like the smelly clothes message is more popular than the others; we have many more people choosing this message than expected by chance. Many fewer people choose the other messages than expected. However, you would not anticipate the observed frequencies to be exactly the same as the expected frequencies even if there was no difference between the messages. There would be some variation due to sampling error.

The one-variable χ^2 test helps us decide how likely the difference between observed and expected frequencies is to have arisen by chance. It is called a 'goodness-of-fit' test because it tests how well the observed frequencies fit to the expected values. The test statistic is calculated in a similar way to the χ^2 for association between two categorical variables, discussed above. For each category you identify the difference between the observed and expected frequencies, square this total and divide by the expected frequency. Then you add these figures up from each cell in the table to generate the χ^2 statistic. We will illustrate this calculation and running the analysis using SPSS below, with a slightly more complicated example.

The degrees of freedom for this test statistic are calculated as the number of categories minus 1 (3 in this case). For our example the χ^2 is 432.5 which is highly significant on three degrees of freedom. Therefore, we can reject the null hypothesis and conclude that there is a significant difference in preference for the messages. If we want to please the patients in the waiting room then we should display the smelly clothes smoking message.

The one-variable χ^2 test also allows you to define your own expected values for each category. For example, you might hypothesise that left handers are at greater risk of heart disease than right handers. To test this hypothesis you could take a random sample of people with heart disease and measure handedness. What would you expect to see if there was no association between handedness and heart disease? A 50:50 split between left and right handers? No, because left and right handers are not equally common in the general population. Let us assume 90% of the population are right handed. Therefore, if there was no association between handedness and heart disease you would expect 90% of heart disease patients to be right handed and 10% to be left handed. You might recruit a sample of 400 heart disease patients. You would therefore expect 90% (360) to be right handed and 10% (40) to be left handed. You might observe the data in Table 9.7.

Table 9.7

	Right handed	Left handed
Observed	305	95
Expected	360	40

Table 9.8

Men	Women
$(305-360)^2/360 = 8.40$	$(95-40)^2/40 = 75.63$

$\chi^2 = 8.40 + 75.63 = 84.03$

Again, the one-variable χ^2 statistic can be used to test whether these observed frequencies differ from the expected frequencies by more than chance would predict. The calculation is similar to the calculation you have just seen. For each cell the expected frequency is subtracted from the observed frequency and squared and then this is divided by the expected frequency. Then the values calculated for the two cells are added together to give the Pearson χ^2 statistic. The calculation is shown in Table 9.8.

The degrees of freedom are calculated as the number of categories minus 1 (which gives 1). A χ^2 of 84.03 on one degree of freedom is highly significant ($p < .001$). Therefore, this result shows that the frequency of left handers in heart disease patients is significantly greater than found in the general population.

RUNNING THE χ^2 GOODNESS-OF-FIT TEST USING SPSS

To run the analysis for the above example using SPSS the data sheet should look as shown in Screenshot 9.15.

The data need to be weighted to tell SPSS that frequency data has been entered. We covered this in the context of analysing 2×2 tables earlier in the chapter. Once the data are weighted, select *Analyze, Nonparametric Tests, Legacy Dialogs, Chi-square* (Screenshot 9.16).

In the dialogue box *gender* should be moved to the *Test Variable* list. Next look at the *Expected Values* box. You need to tell SPSS

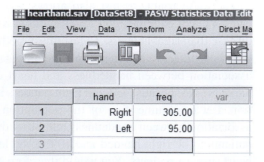

Screenshot 9.15

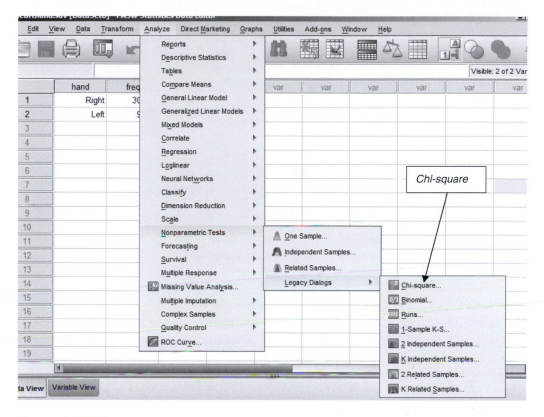

Screenshot 9.16

the values you expect for each category. If you expect the observations to be evenly spread across the categories by chance, as we did in the example about choosing the smoking message, then this can be left on the default setting of *All categories equal*. We cannot do this here though, as we do not expect equal proportions of left and right handers. First enter 360 – the expected frequency for right handers. This goes first as right handers are the lower coded of the handedness categories (right is coded 1, left is coded 2). Next press the *Add* button. Then enter 40 in the values box – the expected frequency of left handers and press *Add* again (Screenshot 9.17). Then press *OK*.

The results present two tables. The first (Screenshot 9.18) shows the observed and expected frequencies and also calculates the difference (the residual). We recommend checking that the expected frequencies have been allocated as you planned as the dialogue box above can be tricky to fill in.

The second table (Screenshot 9.19) shows the χ^2 statistic, the degrees of freedom and the probability. These are the same as the figures we found above. The χ^2 is 84.03 and this is highly significant on one degree of freedom. Note that the *p*-level should always be written as $p < .001$ when SPSS reports .000.

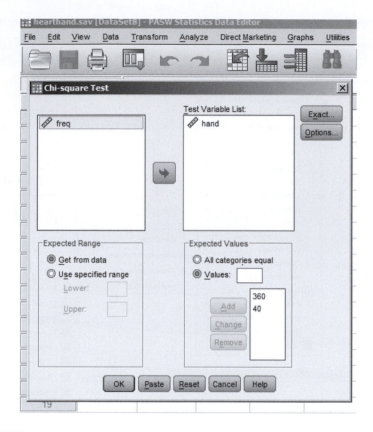

Screenshot 9.17

hand

	Observed N	Expected N	Residual
Right	305	360.0	-55.0
Left	95	40.0	55.0
Total	400		

Screenshot 9.18

Test Statistics

	hand
Chi-square	84.028[a]
df	1
Asymp. Sig.	.000

a. 0 cells (.0%) have expected frequencies less than 5. The minimum expected cell frequency is 40.0.

Screenshot 9.19

Summary

When testing the association between two categorical variables, a contingency table analysis with a χ^2 significance test is an appropriate choice. It is important that the categories are mutually exclusive so that each observation is only present in one cell of the table. The test also assumes less than 20% of cells have an expected count of five or less. If your data do not meet this assumption and you have a 2×2 table then you may use the Fisher's Exact test statistic instead. Where you are testing for associations between variables with three or more categories a contingency table analysis is appropriate if the above assumptions are met. Interpretation is usually more tricky in larger tables though, so you might want to collapse categories in variables with many categories to ease interpretation. This might also help if you are having problems with low expected frequencies.

A one-variable χ^2 goodness-of-fit test is very useful to test whether the distribution of participants across a single categorical variable is as expected. A significant χ^2 test indicates that the observed frequencies do not fit this expectation and the researcher will need to find a theoretical explanation for this.

MULTIPLE CHOICE QUESTIONS

1. A researcher wants to know whether equal numbers of undergraduates consume alcohol in three different categories. In which order should the categories be entered to ensure the χ^2 goodness-of-fit test can be correctly calculated?
   a) Teetotalers, healthy drinkers (less than 27 units per week), unhealthy drinkers (28 or more units per week)
   b) Unhealthy drinkers, healthy drinkers, teetotalers
   c) Healthy drinkers, teetotalers, unhealthy drinkers
   d) It does not matter

2. Fisher's Exact Test is used when:
   a) A relative of Ronald Fisher is looking over your shoulder
   b) You have a 2×2 table and all the cells have an expected frequency above 5
   c) You have a 2×2 table and one or more cells has an expected frequency below 5
   d) You have a larger contingency table (e.g. 4×3)

Questions 3 to 8 refer to the following output. This comes from a fictional study of gender and high blood pressure in middle-aged people.

		Female	Male	Total
Normal blood pressure	Observed	375	335	710
	Expected	355	?	
High blood pressure	Observed	125	165	290
	Expected	145	?	
Total	Observed	500	500	1000

Chi-Square Tests

	Value	df	Asymp. Sig. (2-sided)	Exact Sig. (2-sided)	Exact Sig. (1-sided)
Pearson Chi-Square	7.771[a]	1	.005		
Continuity Correction[b]	7.387	1	.007		
Likelihood Ratio	7.790	1	.005		
Fisher's Exact Test				.007	.003
Linear-by-Linear Association	7.763	1	.005		
N of Valid Cases	1000				

a. 0 cells (.0%) have expected count less than 5. The minimum expected count is 145.00.
b. Computed only for a 2x2 table

Symmetric Measures

		Value	Approx. Sig.
Nominal by Nominal	Phi	.088	.005
	Cramer's V	.088	.005
	N of Valid Cases	1000	

3. How should the contingency table be described?
   a) 1×1
   b) 1×2
   c) 3×2
   d) 2×2

4. How many females do not have high blood pressure?
   a) 375
   b) 335
   c) 355
   d) 125

5. What percentage of males have high blood pressure?
   a) $(165/1000)\times100 = 16.5\%$
   b) $(165/290)\times100 = 56.9\%$
   c) $(165/500)\times100 = 33.0\%$
   d) $(290/500)\times100 = 58\%$

6. Which pair of numbers should replace the question marks in the table (these are the expected frequencies for males in the each of the blood pressure categories)?
   a) 167.5 and 82.5
   b) 355 and 145
   c) 250 and 250
   d) None of the above

7. What should we interpret from this analysis?
   a) High blood pressure is significantly more common in males than females
   b) Males have lower rates of high blood pressure than females
   c) There is no association between gender and high blood pressure
   d) High blood pressure has different causes in males and females

8. How might the effect size of the relationship be measured?
   a) By how strongly the researcher feels about the project
   b) By the χ^2 of 7.77
   c) By the degrees of freedom (1)
   d) By the Cramer's V (.09)

9. What will the degrees of freedom be for a χ^2 test of a 3×4 contingency table?
   a) 12
   b) 4
   c) 6
   d) 11

10. What is meant by collapsing categories of a categorical variable?
    a) Combining two or more categories together
    b) The experimenter's theoretical model is unsound
    c) Hiding data that does not fit your hypothesis
    d) Removing observations that are outliers

11. In SPSS you calculate a χ^2 test for contingency tables via
    a) *Analyze, Descriptive Statistics, Crosstabs*
    b) *Analyze, Regression, Linear*
    c) *Analyze, Correlate, Bivariate*
    d) *Analyze, Compare Means*

12. A χ^2 goodness-of-fit test is so named because it
   a) Tests whether observed frequencies are a good fit to the experimenter's CV
   b) Tests whether the observed frequencies are a good fit to the specified expected frequencies
   c) Tests whether the experimenter's cardigan is the right size
   d) Tests whether the sample size is big enough to test the hypothesis

Questions 13–15 refer to the tables below. These results are from a fictional study examining whether Accident and Emergency doctors vary in their preference for which nights they want to work over the weekend. The following frequencies were observed:

Friday	Saturday	Sunday
140	70	10

Test Statistics

	Kotime
Chi-Square	1.155E2
df	2
Asymp. Sig.	.000

a. 0 cells (.0%) have expected frequencies less than 5. The minimum expected cell frequency is 73.3.

13. How many doctors participated in the study?
   a) 220
   b) 140
   c) 500
   d) 200

14. What are the expected frequencies for each day, under the null hypothesis that doctors do not have a preference?
   a) All 70.0
   b) All 33.3
   c) All 73.3
   d) 140, 70 and 10 respectively

15. How well do the observed frequencies fit the expected frequencies?
   a) Quite well, they don't look that different
   b) Not very well, they look a bit different
   c) They significantly differ, as shown by the residuals
   d) They significantly differ as shown by the χ^2

Measuring Agreement: Correlational Techniques

10

Overview

In this chapter you will learn about analysing the relations between variables. We start with the simplest of relationships – that of the relationship between two variables. This is called a bivariate relationship. Researchers hypothesise that there will be a significant relationship, or association, between two variables x and y. Mostly, the hypothesis will be directional, i.e. as x increases, y increases (a positive relationship), or as x increases, y decreases (a negative relationship). The null hypothesis is that any relationship between x and y is due to sampling error (chance). Correlational techniques are used to test the hypothesis that variables are related to each other. The conclusions drawn from a bivariate correlational analysis cannot be as strong as conclusions drawn from a study using an experimental design if the study involves questions of causality. Finding out that two variables are related is not the same as being able to state that x caused y.

It is also possible to find out the relationship between two variables, whilst controlling for the effect of a third. For instance, what is the relationship between *social*

(Continued)

(Continued)

support and *happiness* with *illness uncertainty* controlled for? This is explained on pages 309–311.

Correlational techniques are also used to measure agreement between ratings made by two different raters, and to test the reliability of questionnaires. These are advanced techniques and we briefly explain them, but do not cover them in detail.

From this chapter you will:

- Gain a conceptual understanding of correlational analysis
- Be able to decide when to use the parametric test, Pearson's *r*, and when to use the non-parametric equivalent, Spearman's rho
- Understand the situations under which you can suggest causality when using correlational analysis
- Learn how to carry out bivariate correlational analysis, and how to partial out covariates
- Learn the different ways correlational techniques can be applied
- Learn how to carry out correlational analysis in SPSS
- Learn how to interpret the findings of researchers who have used correlational analysis in their published articles

INTRODUCTION

Correlational analysis is used widely in the social and health sciences. Correlational techniques look at relationships, or associations, between variables. They do not look at differences between means. Correlational analysis is ideal when researchers are looking at naturally occurring behaviour. The researchers do not allocate people to groups, there are no 'independent' or 'dependent' variables, in the usual sense of the word (that is, we do not usually manipulate the variables). There are just variables, which traditionally we call *x* and *y*. If we took a sample of people and asked them to fill in questionnaires relating to a) stress and b) happiness, we could then enter the data into our statistical package and find out whether stress and happiness are related – or co-related (correlated), with each other. If we found that stress and happiness were highly associated, in that the tendency was for happier people to be less stressed and people who were not so happy were more stressed, we couldn't say whether low stress causes people to be happier, or whether being happier causes a person to be less stressed (in fact, a third variable, e.g. regularly eating chocolate, might cause people to both feel happy, and to feel less stressed, independently).[1] However, sometimes cause can be suggested. For instance if, in a clinical trial, a group of patients were given a dose-dependent drug on day 1, and severity of side-effects on day 3 was positively correlated with the dose of drug, it seems sensible to suggest that the dose of drug caused the side-effects, since causality doesn't go backwards (in the non-physics realm anyway).

BIVARIATE RELATIONSHIPS

A bivariate relationship is where one variable shows an association or correlation with a second variable. Bivariate correlational techniques assess the strength and magnitude of the association (relationship) between two variables, and the associated p-value shows us whether such a relationship is likely to be due to sampling error (or chance). Correlational techniques are not used to assess differences between variables.

When researchers have correlational hypotheses (i.e. they are looking for, or expecting there to be, a relationship between variables), then their study (or perhaps part of a study) is a correlational one. The hypotheses they have will be worded in such a way that it will be obvious that they are looking for an association between variables.

Here are some aims/hypotheses which show clearly the researchers are looking for associations between variables rather than differences.

- Bell and Belsky (2008) wanted to test the hypothesis that more supportive/less negative parenting is associated with lower resting blood pressure in children
- 'The aim of this study was to evaluate the correlation between the incidence of sporadic duodenal adenomas and colorectal neoplasias.' (Dariusz and Jochen 2009)
- A study by Mok and Lee (2008) examined the relationship between anxiety and pain intensity in patients with low back pain who were newly admitted to an acute care hospital setting

Hypotheses are often directional, i.e. 'we predict that high scores on the Medical Outcomes Scale Social Support will be associated with higher happiness scores'.

This means that the researchers have good reason to believe that people who score highly on *social support* will tend to score highly on *happiness* and that people who have lower scores on *social support* will tend to have lower scores on *happiness*.

Researchers test their hypotheses by carrying out an appropriate statistical test to determine whether any relationship between the variables is likely to be due to sampling error (or chance) (or whether it can be concluded that there is a meaningful relationship between the variables, see Chapter 4, pages 129–130). When researchers state a directional hypothesis, they are able to use a one-tailed level of significance when assessing results. If they simply predict a relationship, but haven't got any logical reason to predict the direction of the relationship, then they use a two-tailed level of significance (see Chapter 4, page 147).

Sometimes variables are related to each other (statistically) but the relationship doesn't mean much. For instance, the length of time the authors have been teaching shows a positive relationship with the number of students attending our three Universities. But the relationship between these two variables occurs just because of time – each year we have been at University the student numbers have increased, but the relationship doesn't have any importance! This is said to be a 'spurious' relationship.

Look at the Screenshot 10.1. For each participant, there is a score for the total of *social support* and a score for the total of *happiness*. What we want to know is: as scores in *social*

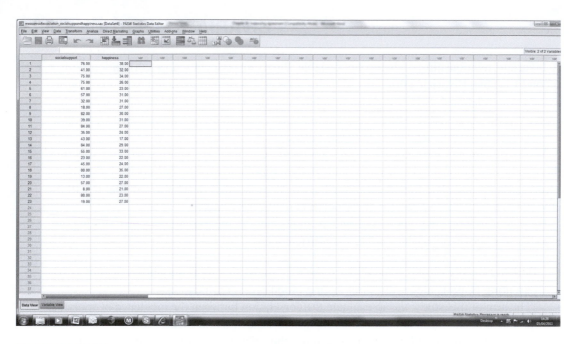

Screenshot 10.1

support increase, is there a tendency for scores in *happiness* to increase? Or, to put it the other way round, as scores in *social support* decrease, is there a tendency for *happiness* to decrease? You can't tell by simply looking at the data.

Looking at a scatterplot enables us to visualise the relationship between two variables. A scatterplot (sometimes called a scattergram) has a horizontal axis which we call *x* and a vertical axis which we call *y*. In Figure 10.1, the scores on the *x*-axis are *social support* (labelled 'Total of MOS social support') and the scores on the *y*-axis are *happiness* (labelled as 'Total of Oxford happiness').

Each datapoint represent *one* person's score. So Darren has scored 8 on *social support*, and 21 on *happiness*. Darren has low(ish) scores on these variables. We have shown these scores for Darren. To illustrate the point at which the datapoint is drawn, we have drawn a vertical line from 8 on MOS social support and a horizontal line from 21 on Oxford happiness. The datapoint is drawn at the place where the lines cross.

Husnara has high scores on both of these variables. The general pattern of the scores is from the left-hand bottom corner, to the right-hand top corner, which illustrates a positive relationship, i.e. here low scores on *social support* tend to be associated with low scores on *happiness*, and high scores on *social support* tend to be associated with high scores on *happiness*. There are always a few people who don't follow the general trend. What we are interested in, however, is the general pattern of results.

We could also predict a negative relationship:

We predict a negative relationship between social support and fatigue'.

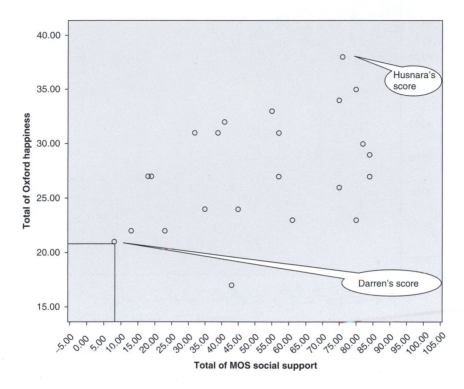

Figure 10.1   Scatterplot showing relationship between *social support* and *happiness*

This means we expect that people with low scores on *social support* would tend to score high scores on *fatigue*, and conversely, people who score highly on *social support* would tend to have low scores on *fatigue*.

As you can see (Figure 10.2) our prediction seems to be supported. Generally, low scores on *social support* are associated with high scores on the *fatigue* scale. Conversely, high scores on the *social support* scale are associated with low scores on the *fatigue* scale. The general pattern of scores goes from top left-hand corner to the bottom right-hand corner. Again, there may be some people who do not follow the general trend. But the negative relationship can be seen clearly: low scores on one variable are associated with high scores on the other. Here the pattern of datapoints is from the top left-hand corner to the bottom right corner.

Imagine a situation where there's no association whatsoever between variables. In this case, you would expect the scattergram to show no particular trend and the datapoints would be randomly distributed in the scattergram (Figure 10.3).

Here no trend is apparent.

When researchers carry out a correlational analysis, they usually look at the scatterplots to get a general idea of the relationships, although they often omit them in the articles which

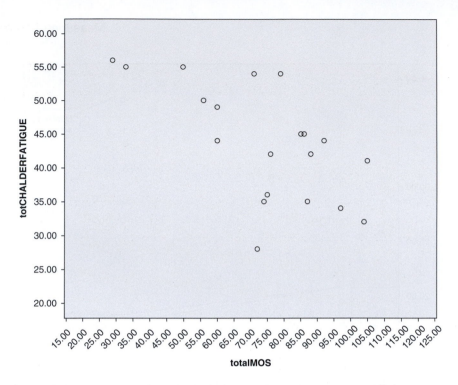

Figure 10.2 Scatterplot showing relationship between *social support* and *fatigue*

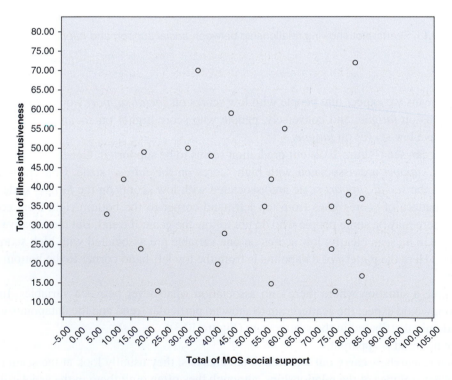

Figure 10.3 Scatterplot showing relationship between *social support* and *illness intrusiveness*

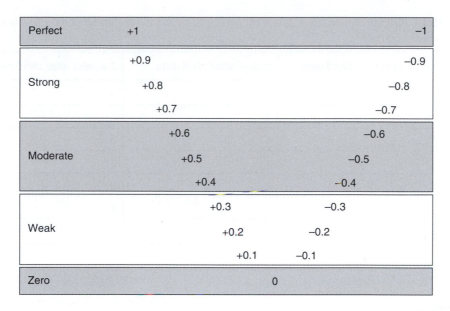

Figure 10.4   Strength of correlation coefficients

Source: Statistics without Maths for Psychology 5th Edition, Christine Dancey and John Reidy, © Pearson Education Limited 2007

they subsequently write. The strength of the relationship between the variables is assessed, not by the scatterplot, but by performing a statistical test. The parametric test which assesses correlational relationships is called 'Pearson's Product-Moment Correlation', which is called 'Pearson's r' for short. Parametric tests, as you know, are used when your data are normally distributed (see Chapter 4, page 140). If your data are skewed, we recommend that you use a non-parametric equivalent called Spearman's rho. We will be showing you how to obtain these statistics by using SPSS later in the chapter.

The strength of a correlational relationship is measured on a scale from 0 (no relationship) to +1 (perfect positive relationship) and from 0 (no relationship) to −1 (perfect negative relationship). The nearer to 1 (whether negative or positive), the stronger the relationship. The nearer to 0, the weaker the relationship (Figure 10.4).

If all the datapoints fall on a straight line then the relationship is said to be perfect. Pearson's r would then = 1.0.

It's almost impossible to find perfect relationships when carrying out real research (and when going on blind dates!). For instance, imagine that you gave your friends a simple

Table 10.1   Ratings of their blind date from participants, two days after blind date and two weeks after blind date[2]

Participant rating their blind date	2 days after blind date	2 weeks after blind date
Micky	3	3
Husnara	4	3
Sharon	4	5
Joy	1	1
Darren	2	3
Chung	3	2
Patricia	5	5

questionnaire about their blind date a couple of days after the date. You might just have a few simple questions (e.g. 'How much did you enjoy your blind date?') This could be rated on a five-point scale (e.g. 1 = 'I hated every second of it' to 5 = 'I loved every second of it'). Then you decide to ask them to rate their blind date again, two weeks later. Although in theory everyone *could* rate the blind date the same at both time points, it is highly unlikely. After two weeks had passed, some people might feel better (or worse) about their blind date (Table 10.1).

There is not a perfect correlation in this example. Figure 10.5 is the scatterplot relating to the blind date example.

There is a positive correlation between the two sets of scores, but it is not a perfect one.

PERFECT CORRELATIONS

A perfect correlation looks like Figure 10.6.

For every one-unit increase in x, y increases by a constant amount (by five in this case). This means all the dots fall on a straight line, and $r = +1$ (meaning this is a perfect positive correlation).

Figure 10.7 shows a perfect negative correlation.

We don't often find perfect negative relationships either. In this scatterplot, for every one-unit increase in the x scores, the y scores decrease by a constant figure (in this case five). You could draw a line through the datapoints, and every one of them would fall on the line. This shows that the relationship is perfect. A perfect negative relationship means $r = -1$.

The relationships we look at are usually imperfect relationships. Once we (or our statistical program) calculates r, then we tend to find values that are weak (.1 to .3); moderate (.4 to .6) or strong (.7 to .9) (see Cohen, 1988).

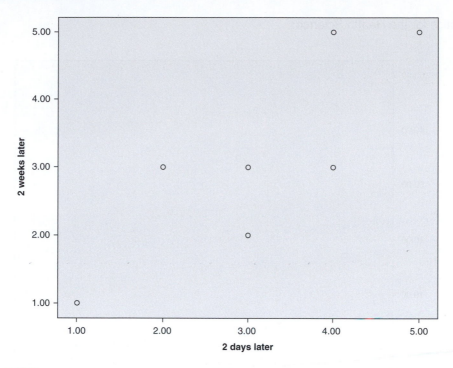

Figure 10.5 Scatterplot showing the relationship between two days after and two weeks after the blind date

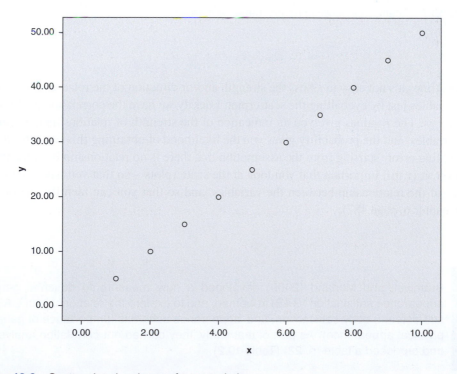

Figure 10.6 Scatterplot showing perfect correlation

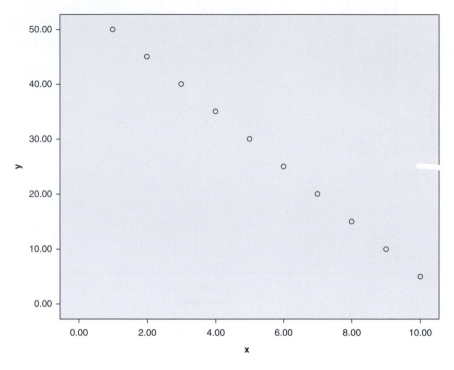

Figure 10.7 Scatterplot showing perfect negative correlation

Sometimes it's not easy to assess the strength and/or direction of the relationship between two variables just by eyeballing the scatterplot. Luckily we have the correlation coefficient r to assist us. The r-values give you an indication of the strength of relationship between the two variables, and the probability gives you the likelihood of obtaining this result by chance or sampling error (starting from the assumption that there is no relationship between them). However, it is still important that you look at the scatterplots – so that you have a complete picture of the relationship between the variables, and so that you can identify any outliers (see Chapter 6, page 187).

Activity 10.1

Bramwell and Morland (2009) developed a new measure to describe genital appearance satisfaction (GAS) in women, and to explore the relationship of GAS to self-esteem, body satisfaction, and 'appearance schemas' (importance of general physical appearance). As part of that study, they carried out correlation analyses, and produced a table (p. 22) (Table 10.2).

Table 10.2 Correlation coefficients for appearance schemas, body satisfaction, self esteem and genital appearance satisfaction

	Body satisfaction scale (BSS)	Self esteem scale (SES)	*Genital appearance satisfaction scale (GAS)*
Appearance schemas inventory	.46**	–.64**	*.28** *
Body satisfaction scale		–.55**	*.30** *
Self esteem scale			*–.41** *

**p < .01

It is important to realise that in this study the GAS was reverse scored, i.e. high scores on the GAS mean participants were *less* satisfied with their genital appearance.

a) Which relationship is the strongest? (Give name of both variables and the value of the correlation coefficient)

b) Which is the weakest correlation? (Give name of both variables and the value of the correlation coefficient)

c) Write a sentence explaining the relationship between self esteem and the GAS. Compare your results with ours at the end of the book

CALCULATING THE CORRELATION PEARSON'S *r* USING SPSS

We are going to use the data from *total of social support* and the *total of happiness*.

1) Click on *Analyze, Correlate, Bivariate* – the *Bivariate Correlations* dialogue box is obtained (Screenshot 10.2) .

2) Highlight the two variables that you wish to correlate (Screenshot 10.3).

3) Move the two variables over to the *Variables* box on the right-hand side.

   Notice that you can select different correlation coefficients, choose either a one-tailed or a two-tailed test, and choose to flag up statistically significant correlations. There is also an *Options* button on the right (Screenshot 10.4).

   You can allow SPSS to exclude cases pairwise, or listwise (see Chapter 6, page 191) and also obtain additional statistics.

4) Click on *Continue*.

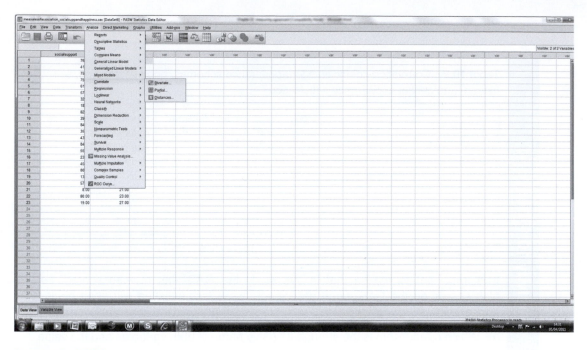

Screenshot 10.2

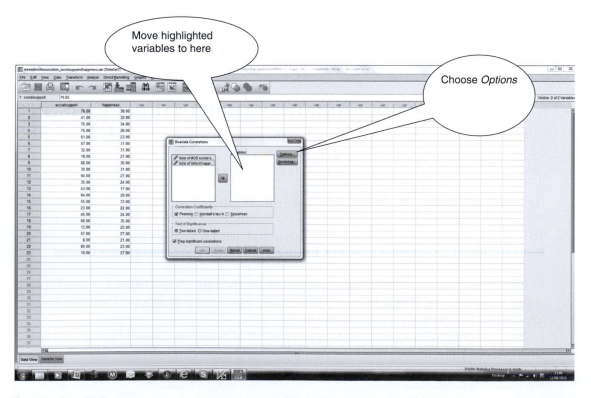

Move highlighted variables to here

Choose *Options*

Screenshot 10.3

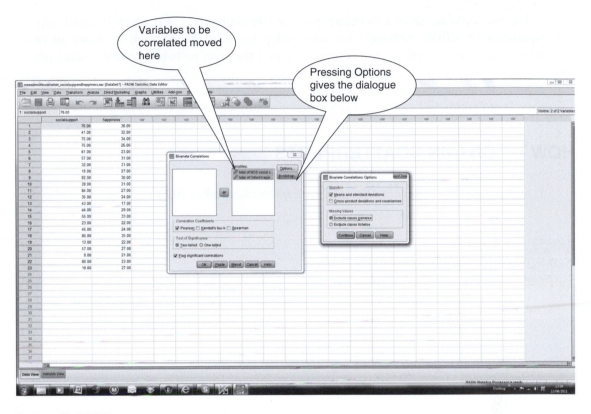

Screenshot 10.4

5)   Then click on *OK*.

Table 10.3 shows the output that will appear in the *Statistics Viewer*:

Table 10.3   Correlation coefficients between *social support* and *happiness*

Correlations			
		total of MOS social support	total of Oxford happiness
total of MOS social support	Pearson Correlation	1	.440*
	Sig. (1-tailed)		.018
	N	23	23
total of Oxford happiness	Pearson Correlation	.440*	1
	Sig. (1-tailed)	.018	
	N	23	23

*Correlation is significant at the 0.05 level (1-tailed).

The two variables show a moderate, positive relationship ($r = .44$) which is statistically significant ($p = .018$). Although this relationship has been flagged and is shown to be significant at the $p < .05$ level, it is better to report the exact probability value – since you have it – rather than reporting $p < .05$.

So from the above output, we could say: 'total social support and total happiness showed a moderate positive relationship which was statistically significant ($r = .440$, $p = .018$)'.

HOW TO OBTAIN SCATTERPLOTS

1) Click on *Graphs*, *Legacy Dialogs*, *Scatterplots* (Screenshot 10.5).

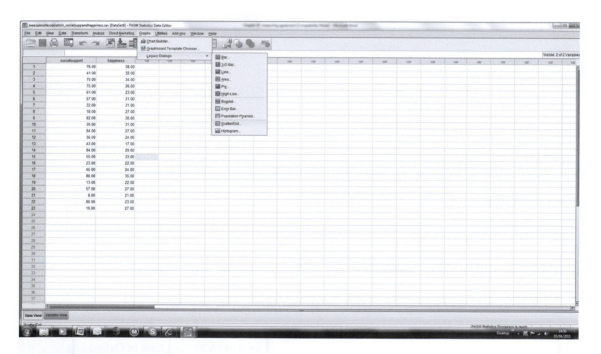

Screenshot 10.5

You will see Screenshot 10.6.
Click on *Simple Scatter* and then click on *Define*.

Move the two variables from the left-hand side to the right (Screenshot 10.7). Make sure the *x* variable (here *social support*) is moved to the *x* row, and the *y* variable (here *happiness*) is moved to the *y* row. You can also click on *Options* if you require these.

Then *Continue*, then *OK*. The output is as in Figure 10.8.

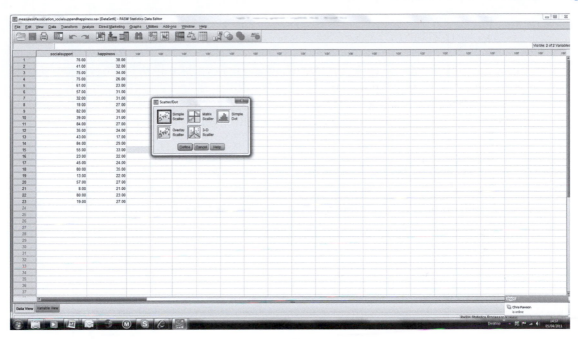

Screenshot 10.6

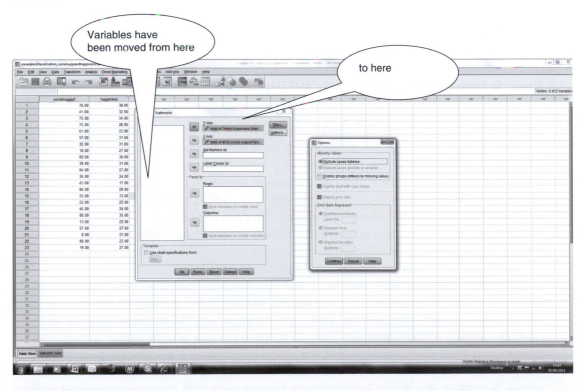

Screenshot 10.7

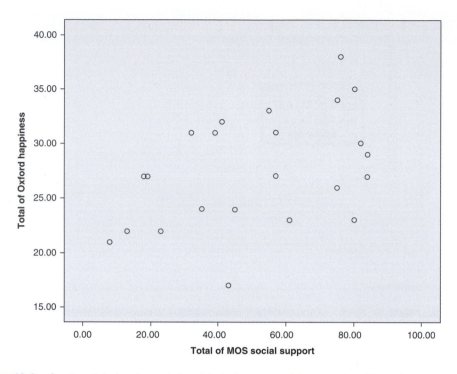

Figure 10.8 Scatterplot showing relationship between *social support* and *happiness*

Example from the Literature: Anxiety and Depression in Patients with Low Back Pain

Let's look at the study by Mok and Lee (2008), who we mentioned earlier in this chapter. They examined the relationship between anxiety, depression and pain intensity in patients with low back pain who were newly admitted to an acute care hospital setting. There were 102 participants in the study. They reported that anxiety was significantly positively related to pain ($r = .446$, $p < .005$) and also depression was significantly positively correlated with pain intensity ($r = .447$, $p < .0005$). Although they did not show scatterplots in their article, they kindly sent them to us. Figure 10.9 shows the one for anxiety with pain.

And Figure 10.10 shows the one for depression and pain.

We hope that you can see from the scatterplots that the relationships are positive – these are moderate correlations. Although the pattern of the results is from the bottom left-hand corner to the right-hand corner, the relationship is far from perfect – as would be expected. There are some people who have low depression scores and high pain intensity, but the trend is positive – in general people with lower scores on depression tend to have lower scores on pain intensity and vice versa. Normally you would expect some people with high depression scores and

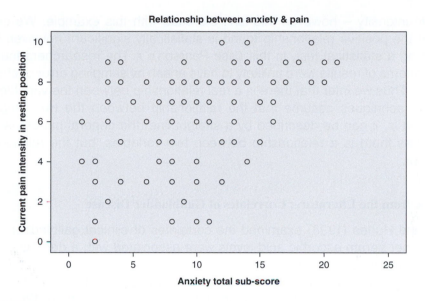

Figure 10.9   Scatterplot showing relationship between anxiety and pain

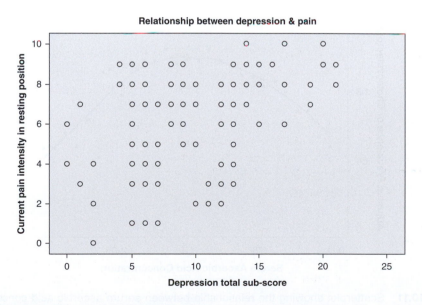

Figure 10.10   Scatterplot showing relationship between depression and pain

low pain intensity – however, this isn't the case with this example. We can't tell whether the positive relationship found is statistically significant however, without performing a statistical test, in this case Pearson's *r*. The researchers found that these patterns of results were unlikely to have arisen by sampling error or chance (*p* < .0005). Thus we infer that there is a real relationship between the variables.

These techniques assume that the relationship between the two variables is linear, that is, it can be described by a straight line (the general pattern is linear). Sometimes there is a relationship between two variables, but the relationship is non-linear.

Example from the Literature: Correlates of Gallbladder Disease

Simon and Hudes (1998) examined the correlates of clinical gallbladder disease and whether serum ascorbic acid levels were associated with a decreased prevalence of gallbladder disease.

They say 'an inverted U-shaped relation was found between serum ascorbic acid level and clinical gallbladder disease among women but not men' (p. 1208).

Figure 10.11 gives scattergram. You can see that the relationship is curvilinear, rather than linear.

This relationship is important, but Pearson's *r* or Spearman's rho would not be appropriate to test the relationship, since these tests assume linearity. If you did perform one of these tests, you would obtain a correlation coefficient, but it might not be statistically significant, or meaningful.

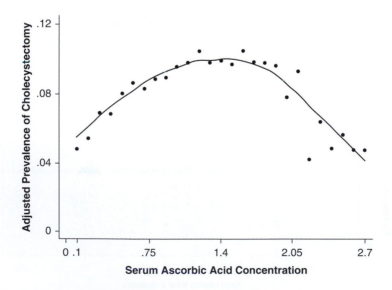

Figure 10.11   Scatterplot showing the relationship between serum ascorbic acid concentration (mg/dL) and prevalence of cholecystectomy among 4840 women

VARIANCE EXPLANATION OF *r*

Although *r* itself is a 'measure of effect', often researchers use r^2 ($r \times r$). r^2 is easy to hand-calculate. It tells us how much variance the variables share, in percentage terms.

So in this case, to find the amount of variance these two variables share we multiply .447 by .447 = .199. This means the two variables share 19.9% variance – in this case we would probably round this up and conclude that the variables share 20% of the variance.

This can be visualised by circles representing the variables. If depression and pain intensity were not related at all, the circles would be independent (Figure 10.12).

If they share variance, then there is some overlap between the circles (Figure 10.13).

Pearson's *r* is calculated by calculating a measure of the shared variance, and dividing this figure by a measure of the separate variances. This reflects the degree to which the two variables vary together.

In our example above *r* was calculated as .447. We then squared .447 ($.447^2 = .199$) We rounded this up, saying that 20% of the variation in scores in depression can be accounted for (or explained by) the variation in scores in pain intensity. Conversely, 20% of the variation in scores in pain intensity can be accounted for by depression. Having explained 20% of the variation in scores in this way, leaves 80% of the variation in scores to be explained by other factors. What other factors? Well, ones the researchers haven't measured – maybe current stress for instance, or lack of social support? There is no way of knowing without carrying out a study including these factors.

We can't say definitely whether depression and anxiety caused pain to become worse, or whether the pain caused the patients to be depressed. In fact, there could be a two-way relationship. Perhaps a third variable (personality factors, other pre-existing health conditions) could have caused both pain to increase, and depression and anxiety. In this study, the authors

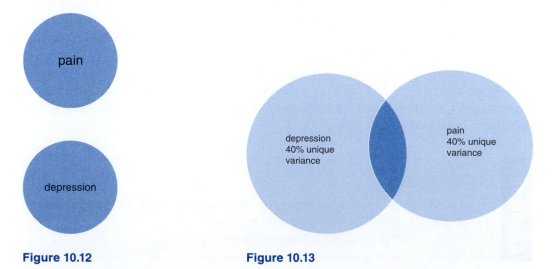

Figure 10.12   **Figure 10.13**

Table 10.4 Correlation coefficients between paternal parenting and cardiovascular activity for boys and girls

	Boys			Girls		
	Mean DBP	Mean SBP	Mean HR	Mean DBP	Mean SBP	Mean HR
Parenting early (54 months)						
Paternal sensitivity	−0.19**	−0.12*	−0.17**	−0.11	−0.06	0.04
Paternal closeness/conflict	0.01	−0.02	−0.01	−0.03*	−0.13*	0.01
Parenting intermediate (6 and 8 years)						
Paternal sensitivity	−0.13*	−0.08	−0.11*	−0.07	−0.02	−0.06
Paternal closeness/conflict	0.06	0.01	0.00	−0.07	−0.02	0.03
Parenting late (10 years)						
Paternal sensitivity	−0.06	0.04	−0.10	−0.13*	−0.06	−0.11
Paternal closeness/conflict	−0.02	−0.01	−0.04	−0.09	−0.01	0.02

*$P<0.05$; **$P<0.01$.
Blood pressure and heart rate data were averaged when the child was 9,10 and 11.
DBP, diastolic blood pressure; SBP, systolic blood pressure; HR, heart rate.

did not give a causal explanation, but they suggested that health professionals need to take depression and anxiety into consideration in any intervention for chronic back pain.

r and r^2 allow us to understand the strength of the relationship between the two variables. In Table 10.4 (Bell and Belsky 2008) we can see the r-values between two types of blood pressure (BP), heart rate and measures of parenting, for boys and girls separately. The probability values are given below the r-values, and the researchers have drawn our attention to the 'statistically significant' correlations using the asterisk. Some of these are quite weak. For instance the first row and column shows the boys mean diastolic BP correlates with paternal sensitivity – 0.19 (as you can see this is negative). The researchers hypothesised that more supportive parenting would be associated with lower heart rates – hence the negative correlation coefficient. Although this is statistically significant, it is a fairly weak relationship. As we said in Chapter 4, we can't just look at the p-value to make a judgement about whether results are important. Statistical significance does not necessarily equate to practical importance or clinical significance.

Activity 10.2

Look at Table 10.5.

a) What is the correlation coefficient for the mean diastolic BP with paternal sensitivity in girls? (parenting early 54 months)

b) Write a sentence interpreting this correlation coefficient

Example from the Literature

Meyer and Gast (2008) wished to investigate whether a relationship existed between peer influence and disordered eating behaviours in young people.

Pearson product-moment correlation coefficients were calculated. Weak–moderate positive correlations were found between the peer influence scores (IPIEC) and 'drive for thinness' subscale ($r = .598$, $p < .05$) and 'bulimia' subscale ($r = .284$, $p < .05$). Strong significant positive correlations were found between the IPIEC scores and the 'body dissatisfaction' subscale ($r = .658$, $p < .05$), p. 39.

OBTAINING CORRELATIONAL ANALYSIS IN SPSS: EXERCISE

Look at the following data (Screenshot 10.8), which is part of our dataset which was correlating fatigue with two measures of the SF-12 which gives two main measures of quality of life: the Physical Component Scale (PCS) and the Mental Component Scale (MCS).

Enter these data into SPSS, and check that you have obtained similar results to ours (Table 10.5).

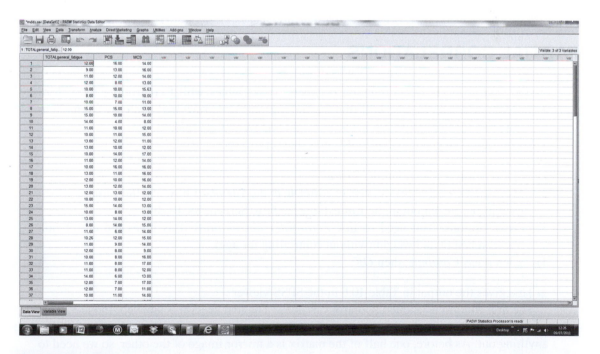

Screenshot 10.8

Table 10.5 Full correlations between fatigue, PCS and MCS

Correlations

		total of MFI general fatigue	total of physical component summary scales	total of mental component summary scales
total of MFI general fatigue	Pearson Correlation	1	−.069	−.196*
	Sig. (2-tailed)		.435	.025
	N	130	130	130
total of physical component summary scales	Pearson Correlation	−.069	1	.271**
	Sig. (2-tailed)	.435		.002
	N	130	130	130
total of mental component summary scales	Pearson Correlation	−.196*	.271**	1
	Sig. (2-tailed)	.025	.002	
	N	130	130	130

* Correlation is significant at the 0.05 level (2-tailed).
** Correlation is significant at the 0.01 level (2-tailed).

PARTIAL CORRELATIONS

Partial correlation is the correlation between two variables whilst controlling for a third (or more) variables. We also call this 'partialling out' or 'covarying'. An easy example to illustrate this is the relationship between height and weight in children.

Screenshot 10.9 gives a small illustrative dataset in SPSS.

1) Select *Analyze*, *Correlation*, *Partial*.
2) Move the two variables we wish to correlate to the *Variables* box, and the variable which we wish to partial out to the *Controlling for* box (Screenshot 10.10).
3) Press *Options*. You need to tick *Zero-order correlations* (this gives the correlation between height and weight (without controlling for age).
4) Then press *Continue*, then *OK*.

This gives the output in Table 10.6 in the SPSS viewer .

The first column is labelled 'Control variables'. The first section is labelled '-none-ª'. This means that the first section gives zero-order correlations, i.e. correlations without partialling anything out. As before, one half of the matrix is a mirror image of the other, so we need to read only one half. We have emboldened the relevant correlations.

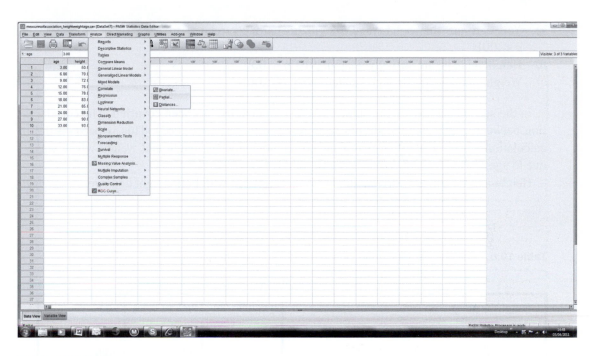

Screenshot 10.9

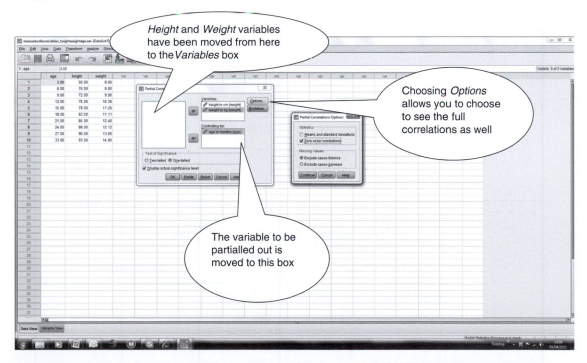

Height and *Weight* variables have been moved from here to the *Variables* box

Choosing *Options* allows you to choose to see the full correlations as well

The variable to be partialled out is moved to this box

Screenshot 10.10

a) You can see that height and weight are strongly related to each other: $r = .943$, $p < .001$
b) Height and age are strongly related: .919, $p < .001$
c) Weight and age are strongly related: .984, $p < .001$

In the second section we are shown that 'age in months' has been covaried. The correlation between height and weight has been reduced to .551 ($p = .062$). This is because the calculation has removed that part of the correlation between height and weight which was due to age.

Height and weight are correlated, but age is correlated with both height and age.

Table 10.6 Full and partial correlations for height and weight with age

Correlations

Control Variables			height in cm	weight in kg	age in months
-none-[a]	height in cm	Correlation	1.000	.943	.919
		Significance (1-tailed)	.	.000	.000
		df	0	8	8
	weight in kg	Correlation	.943	1.000	.984
		Significance (1-tailed)	.000	.	.000
		df	8	0	8
	age in months	Correlation	.919	.984	1.000
		Significance (1-tailed)	.000	.000	.
		df	8	8	0
age in months	height in cm	Correlation	1.000	.551	
		Significance (1-tailed)	.	.062	
		df	0	7	
	weight in kg	Correlation	.551	1.000	
		Significance (1-tailed)	.062	.	
		df	7	0	

a. Cells contain zero-order (Pearson) correlations

SHARED AND UNIQUE VARIANCE: CONCEPTUAL UNDERSTANDING RELATING TO PARTIAL CORRELATIONS

The diagram showing overlapping circles for each of our three variables is a simplified one, so that you can see clearly the relationships between them (Figure 10.14). It is not mathematically accurate, as in the interests of conceptual understanding, we lose mathematical accuracy.[3]

Weight is related to height (weight shares variance with height). This is represented by the overlapping circles. The shared variance between height and weight is represented by the areas a and b.

Age is related to (shares variance with) both height and weight. The relationship of age and height is represented by areas c and b. The relationship of age with weight is represented by areas b and d. Here we are talking of *shared* variance.

We also talk about *unique* variance. Area a shows the unique variance of weight on height (and vice versa). Area c illustrates the unique variance of age on height (and vice versa). Area d shows the unique variance of age and weight (and vice versa). Area b represents the part of the relationship between height and weight which is due to age. If the influence of age were removed (area b), the correlation between height and weight would go down, and it would then be represented by the area a only (Figure 10.15).

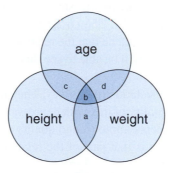

Figure 10.14   Diagram to illustrate shared and unique variance

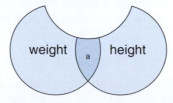

Figure 10.15   Relationship between weight and height with age partialled out

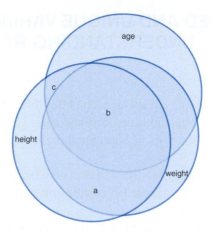

Figure 10.16

It is more difficult to illustrate our example because it is based on real data. Our circles don't neatly overlap each other in the way which our fictitious one on page 331 does.

In our real example, height and weight share variance ($.943 \times .943 = 89\%$); (age and height share variance ($.919 \times .919 = 84\%$) and age and weight share variance ($.984 \times .984 = 97\%$).

In the calculation, the shared variance of age with height and weight is removed (partialled out, held constant, covaried out).

Just as in the fictitious example, removing this shared variance will lead to a reduction in the shared variance of height and weight. The correlation between height and weight has reduced from .943 to .551. Thus we conclude that the relationship between height and weight is partially due to age. We doubt you will be able to see this so clearly in the depiction of our real data (Figure 10.16)!

Researchers often use partial correlation in this way. They might want to look at the relationship between symptoms and quality of life, with depression held constant (partialled out, covaried). If the correlation between symptoms and quality of life reduces after partialling out depression, then the conclusion is that part of the relationship between symptoms and quality of life is due to depression.

Activity 10.3

Gheissari et al. (2010) investigated the carotid intima-media thickness in children with end-stage renal disease on dialysis. As part of that study, they performed partial correlations.

Look at the following text:

After adjusting for age, partial correlation analysis showed significant correlation between carotid and bulb intima-media thickness (IMT-C) and n-PTH level (r = 0.85, p = 0.04) and serum alkaline phosphatase (r = 0.86, p = 0.02). p. 30

Which answer is *not* correct? (Answers are at the end of the book.)

a) The correlation between IMTC and serum alkaline phosphatase is significant, once age is partialled out
b) The correlation between n-PTH level and serum alkaline phosphatase is significant, once age is controlled for
c) The correlation between carotid and bulb intima-media thickness (IMT-C) and n-PTH level ($r = 0.85$, $p = 0.04$) and serum alkaline phosphatase ($r = 0.86$, $p = 0.02$) would not be statistically significant if age had not been partialled out

SPEARMAN'S rho

Quite often in the health sciences, researchers have small samples which are often skewed, hence the use of Spearman's rho is quite common. Non-parametric tests make no assumptions about normality, as you know. All things being equal, non-parametric tests are not as powerful as parametric ones. However, in circumstances where it is appropriate to use non-parametric tests, they can actually be more powerful.

A researcher has taken information about how many different medications 14 patients have taken in the past week, and correlated them with a measure of memory. From the literature he has read, he expects that the greater the number of medications, the worse the patients' memory will be, therefore he has used a one-tailed test. As there are only 14 patients in the study, he chooses Spearman's rho. The instructions for SPSS are exactly the same as for Pearson's *r*, until you obtain the *Bivariate Options* dialogue box (Screenshot 10.11).

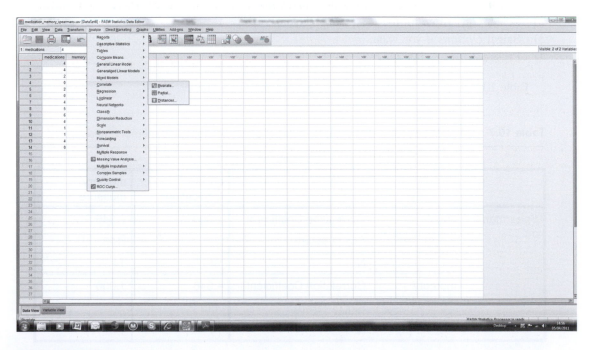

Screenshot 10.11

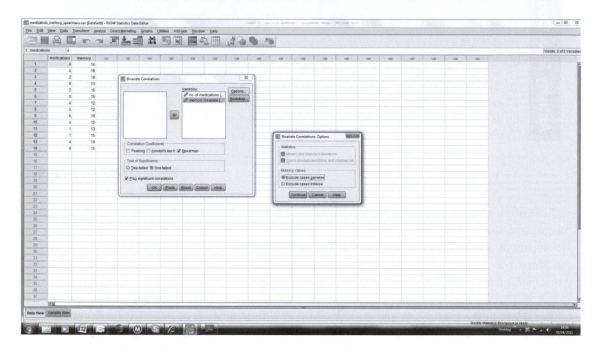

Screenshot 10.12

1) Select the *Spearman* option from the *Correlation Coefficients* choices (Screenshot 10.12).
2) Select *One-tailed* for the *Test of Significance*.
3) Select *Options* if you want.
4) Press *Continue*, then *OK*.

Table 10.7 gives the results that will appear in the SPSS viewer.

Table 10.7   Correlation coefficients (rho) for number of medications and memory measure

Correlations				
			no. of medications	memory measure
Spearman's rho	no. of medications	Correlation Coefficient	1.000	−.346
		Sig. (1-tailed)	.	.113
		N	14	14
	memory measure	Correlation Coefficient	−.346	1.000
		Sig. (1-tailed)	.113	.
		N	14	14

As you can see, this looks just like the table of correlations obtained for Pearson's r, and the figures are interpreted in exactly the same way.

The correlation coefficient is negative (as predicted) but it is weak and not statistically significant at any acceptable level of significance. Therefore the researcher concludes that the number of medications was not significantly related to poor memory

Example from the Literature: Arterial Blood Gas

Andrews and Waterman (2008) investigated whether patterns of arterial blood gas (ABG) sampling were influenced by values of fractional inspiratory oxygen (FiO$_2$), partial pressure of carbon dioxide (PCO$_2$) and oxygen saturation (%SaO$_2$). While it is common to give correlational results in a table, Andrews and Waterman have given this information in text form. A small part of this text from their results section is reproduced below:

> *Examining sampling patterns per day, the number of ABGs taken on day 1 correlated with high values of PCO$_2$ (p = 0.003; Sp (Spearman Rank Order Correlation Coefficient) = 0.3615) and low values of PO$_2$ (p = 0.002; Sp = −0.3758). p. 133*

Usually Spearman's correlation coefficient is written as 'rho'. In which case, you would write:

> *Examining sampling patterns per day, the number of ABGs taken on day 1 correlated with high values of PCO$_2$ (p = 0.003; rho = 0.3615) and low values of PO$_2$ (p = 0.002; rho = −0.3758).*

OTHER USES FOR CORRELATIONAL TECHNIQUES

Correlational techniques are used to assess the degree to which our measurements can be reproduced. These techniques are advanced techniques which, if you need to use them, we would refer you to Chapter 36 in Howitt and Cramer (2008) and to pages 368–378 of *SPSS for Psychologists* (Brace et al., 2009). As this is an introductory book, we do not seek to explain how you can use advanced correlational techniques for your own research. However, it is obviously important you have a basic awareness of such techniques, as you will want to understand them if you come across them in journal articles. So here we give a brief overview of the ways in which correlational techniques can be used. The statistics which are mentioned here – Cohen's kappa, Cronbach's alpha, etc., are all correlational coefficients and are interpreted in the same way as Pearson's *r*.

RELIABILITY OF MEASURES

In a healthy sample of individuals you would expect there to be a high association between body temperature today, and body temperature tomorrow. Or indeed, body temperature today, and body temperature in a week, or in a month. There will be variability of course, but you would expect this measure to have a high correlation. If the correlation coefficient were .90, this would indicate high reliability.

Questionnaires are more problematical – it could be that the relationship between stress and symptoms is strong – but if the questionnaires you use are not reliable, you could find that in your particular study, you don't find a strong association between these variables.

When designing questionnaires, researchers need to ensure their reliability. Part of the procedure is to give the questionnaires to people at time 1, and then to re-test them later. This kind of reliability is called test-retest reliability. The actual time difference varies, according to the study or experiment. The scores on the questionnaire(s) at time 1 and time 2 are correlated, and Pearson's r will show the degree of reliability. Often in journal articles you will see that the researchers give reliability measures. It is usual to accept .7 or above as being of good reliability.

Example from the Literature: Test-Retest Reliability of Scales of the Spiritual Well-Being Scale

In relation to this type of reliability, Arnold et al. (2007) wanted to find out the test-retest reliability of scales within the Spiritual Well-Being Scale (developed by Paloutzian and Ellison, 1982). Arnold et al. (2007) state:

> Test-retest reliability over 4 to 10 weeks ranges from 0.88 to 0.99 for Religious well-being, 0.73 to 0.98 for Existential well-being and 0.82 to 0.94 for Spiritual well-being. p. 4

This shows that the scales have reliability over the timescale specified.

INTERNAL CONSISTENCY

Sometimes, you might design a questionnaire with discrete scales incorporated into it. For instance, the Hospital Anxiety and Depression Scale (HADS) is composed of two scales – items relating to depression, and items relating to anxiety. In this case, the seven items relating to depression should show a high correlation between the depression items. The seven items relating to anxiety should also show a high correlation between the anxiety items.

This sort of reliability measures internal consistency. Cronbach's alpha is often reported when researchers want to give a measure of internal consistency. As with other correlation coefficients, a scale should have a value of >.7 in order to be considered reliable.

INTER-RATER RELIABILITY

This type of reliability measure is often used in observational studies, where two or more raters are observing behaviour of some sort. For instance, two or more different nurses may be observing patients and rating them on a particular questionnaire. If the questionnaire had 100% inter-rater reliability, anyone using the questionnaire and rating patients should give identical scores.

VALIDITY

Correlational analysis can also help with validity. One way to assess this is to correlate the questionnaire with other established questionnaires with known reliability. If you were to design a questionnaire measuring depression, for instance, you could give your questionnaire to participants, along with the HADS and/or the Center for Epidemiologic Studies Depression Scale (CES-D). If your questionnaire really measures depression, there should be a high degree of correlation between your newly designed questionnaire and these established questionnaires.

Example from the Literature: Nurses and Doctors using the Sedation-Agitation Scale

Ryder-Lewis and Nelson (2008) wished to discover whether nurses and doctors rated 69 patients (in intensive care units) similarly using the Sedation-Agitation Scale (SAS). The SAS assessed patients' behaviour from 1 (unrousable) to 7 (dangerous agitation). Nurse–doctor pairs – at the same time – rated each patient on this scale. They were not allowed to confer.

PERCENTAGE AGREEMENT

A simple percentage agreement is easily calculated. You simply count up the number of times the raters agreed and divide this by the total number of observations or codings, then multiply by 100. The authors in the above study state that the doctor and nurse raters selected the same scores on the SAS in 74% of the ratings. This indicates good agreement.

COHEN'S Kappa

A more reliable way to assess agreement than simple percentage agreement is Kappa. This uses a correlation coefficient as a measure for agreement. Kappa is more reliable because the formula corrects the percentage of agreement due to chance.

It does this by looking at the observed percentage of agreement and subtracting the percentage of agreements which would be expected by chance alone. The calculation involves dividing the resulting figure by 1 minus the percentage of agreements which would be expected by chance alone. Sometimes people say that Kappa is the 'chance-corrected percentage of agreement'.

In the example above, the researchers say 'The weighted kappa result of 0.82 indicated very good agreement (reliability)' (p. 215).

SPSS can calculate these statistics under the *Reliability Analysis* procedure. These are advanced techniques and we refer you to other books if you need to know about these.

Summary

Correlation analyses are useful for discovering the strength and magnitude of a relationship between two or more variables. Correlation coefficients, i.e. Pearson's *r* for data which meet the assumptions for parametric tests, or Spearman's rho for data which do not, range from 0 (no relationship) through to +1 (perfect positive relationship) or −1 (perfect negative relationship). A relationship between variables can be easily seen when a scatterplot has been drawn. Pearson's *r* and Spearman's rho assume there is a linear relationship between the variables; if a relationship is curvilinear, these tests are not appropriate. Partial correlations show the relationship between two variables when one (or more) variables are partialled out (held constant). There are other correlation coefficients (e.g. Cronbach's alpha, Cohen's kappa) which are used to measure reliability or agreement. Such measures are often used in questionnaire design. One cannot naturally assume causality when interpreting correlational analysis, although there are situations when causality can be suggested.

MULTIPLE CHOICE QUESTIONS

1. Look at the following scatterplot.

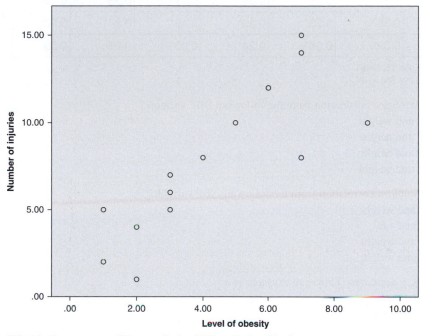

   What is the most sensible conclusion? The relationship is:
   a) Positive
   b) Negative
   c) Zero
   d) Non-linear

2. If you wish to test the relationship between *coping* and *quality of life*, with depression controlled for (co-varied out) you would use:
   a) Cronbach's alpha
   b) Cohen's kappa
   c) Partial correlation
   d) Bivariate correlation

3. Assume that general price rises and the consumption of bottled water is positively related. Which is the most sensible conclusion?
   a) Price rises lead to people drinking more bottled water
   b) Consuming a lot of bottled water leads prices to rise
   c) People drink more bottled water to help them cope with price rises
   d) There is a spurious relationship between consumption of bottled water and general price rises

Look at the following table, from a results section in an article by Patel (2009).

Explanatory variable	Systolic blood pressure (SBP)			Diastolic blood pressure (DBP)		
	Boys (n=250)	Girls (n=250)	Total (N=500)	Boys (n=250)	Girls (n=250)	Total (N=500)
Weight	0.32*	0.41*	0.34*	0.27*	0.33*	0.30*
Height	0.35*	0.33*	0.32*	0.19**	0.24*	0.22*
Age	0.32*	0.06*	0.24*	0.03	0.05	0.03

* Significant at the 1% level
**Significant at the 5% level

4. Which is the strongest correlation from the following DBP variable?
   a) Girls DBP and weight
   b) Boys DBP and height
   c) Girls DBP and height
   d) Boys DPB and weight

5. Which is the weakest correlation from the following SBP variable?
   a) Girls SBP and weight
   b) Girls SBP and age
   c) Boys SBP and weight
   d) Boys SBP and weight

6. As x increases, y decreases. This is an example of a:
   a) Positive relationship
   b) Negative relationship
   c) Zero relationship
   d) Non-linear relationship

7. Look at the following scatterplot. This is an example of a:
   a) Positive relationship
   b) Negative relationship
   c) Zero relationship
   d) Non-linear relationship

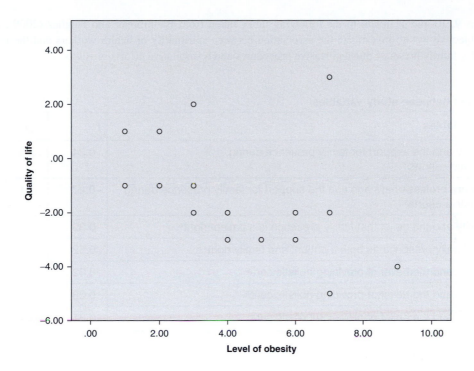

8. As *x* increases, *y* increases. This is an example of a:
   a) Positive relationship
   b) Negative relationship
   c) Zero relationship
   d) Non-linear relationship

Questions 9, 10 and 11 relate to the following table, taken from Baumhover and Hughes (2009), whose objective was to investigate the association between spirituality of health workers and their support for family presence during invasive procedures and resuscitative efforts in adults.

Correlation between study variables

Study variables	r	p
Spirituality and the support for family presence during resuscitative efforts[a]	0.24	.05
Health care professional's age and the support for family presence during resuscitative efforts[a]	−0.27	.01
Spirituality and the belief that family presence is a patient right[a]	0.33	.01
Viewing family presence as both a patient and family right[a]	0.52	.01
Spirituality and the belief of providing holistic care[a]	0.32	.01
Spirituality and the belief of providing holistic care[b]	0.28	>.05
Spirituality and the belief of providing holistic care[c]	0.31	.01

[a] All participants
[b] Physicians and physician assistants
[c] Nurses

9. Which group had the strongest correlation between spirituality and the belief of providing holistic care?
   a) All groups combined
   b) Physicians
   c) Physicians' assistants
   d) Nurses

10. Look at the relationship between the health care professional's age and support for family presence during resuscitative efforts. The association means that the higher the age of the health care professional, the:
   a) More support for family presence; this is statistically significant
   b) More support for family presence; this is not statistically significant
   c) Less support for family presence; this is statistically significant
   d) Less support for family presence; this is not statistically significant

11. Which of the following correlations is not statistically significant at any acceptable level of significance?
   a) Spirituality and the support for family presence during resuscitative efforts
   b) Viewing family presence as both a patient and family right
   c) Spirituality and the belief of providing holistic care (physicians and physician assistants)
   d) Spirituality and the belief of providing holistic care (nurses)

12. If, in a scatterplot, the datapoints are spread randomly, then the most likely correlation coefficient is:
    a) −.01
    b) −.35
    c) +.35
    d) −.46

13. Assume there is a significant correlation between coping strategies and quality of life (+ .76, $p < .001$). Assume self-efficacy is then partialled out, and the correlation reduces to .21 ($p = .70$). Which is the most sensible conclusion?
    a) The relationship between coping strategies and quality of life is spurious
    b) Self-efficacy shows no relationship between coping strategies and quality of life
    c) A small part of the relationship between coping strategies and quality of life can be explained by the relationship between self-efficacy and the other variables
    d) A large part of the relationship between coping strategies and quality of life can be explained by the relationship between self-efficacy and the other variables

Questions 14 and 15 refer to the following table.

Correlations

Control Variables			total of illness intrusiveness	total of illness uncertainty	total of self efficacy scale
-none-[a]	total of illness intrusiveness	Correlation	1.000	.283	-.582
		Significance (2-tailed)	.	.191	.004
		df	0	21	21
	total of illness uncertainty	Correlation	.283	1.000	-.251
		Significance (2-tailed)	.191	.	.249
		df	21	0	21
	total of self efficacy scale	Correlation	-.582	-.251	1.000
		Significance (2-tailed)	.004	.249	.
		df	21	21	0
total of self efficacy scale	total of illness intrusiveness	Correlation	1.000	.174	
		Significance (2-tailed)	.	.439	
		df	0	20	
	total of illness uncertainty	Correlation	.174	1.000	
		Significance (2-tailed)	.439	.	
		df	20	0	

a. Cells contain zero-order (Pearson) correlations.

14. What is the zero-order correlation between illness uncertainty and illness intrusiveness?
    a) +.283
    b) +.174
    c) + 1.00
    d) +.439

15. The relationship between illness intrusiveness and illness uncertainty, with self-efficacy partialled out, is:
    a) +.439
    b) +.174
    c) +.283
    d) −1.00

Notes

1   It works for us anyway.
2   This small dataset is for illustrative purposes only, normally we would have more participants in the study.
3   The actual formula for calculating partial correlations is given by $r^2 = a/(a + \text{height})$ or $a /(a + \text{weight})$.

Linear Regression

11

Overview

Linear regression is an extension of correlational analysis. In Chapter 10, you learned that when scores on *x* showed a linear relationship with *y*, Pearson's *r* or Spearman's rho produces a test statistic (*r* or rho respectively) which gave a measure of the strength of the relationship between them. What correlational analysis gives is a measure of how well the datapoints are clustered around an imaginary line. Linear regression analysis extends this by drawing a real line through the datapoints (this is called a line of best fit) and by giving a measure which shows how much the variable *y* changes as a result of a one-unit change in the variable *x*. We will give you a conceptual understanding of bivariate linear regression, and show you how to obtain the test statistics in SPSS, and how to interpret the output. We will also cover confidence intervals and effect sizes, in relation to linear regression. Linear regression answers the following questions: – How strong is the relationship between *x* and *y*? Is there a good fit between *x* and *y*? Or: from a knowledge of the *x* scores, can we predict what the *y* scores are likely to be?

(Continued)

(Continued)

From this chapter you will:

- Learn how to assess the relationship between two variables by using the line of best fit and associated statistics
- Understand the need to meet the assumptions of linear regression
- Learn how to predict an individual's score on *y* by a knowledge of his/her score on *x*
- Be able to construct a scatterplot with a line of best fit
- Understand how to interpret the test statistics: r, r^2 and b
- Have a knowledge of the ways in which linear regression can be used in research

INTRODUCTION

Linear regression is an extension of correlational analysis. Correlational analysis allows us to understand the relationship between one variable (traditionally called *x*) and another variable (traditionally called *y*). In order to carry out a correlational analysis (and, by extension, a bivariate linear regression analysis) we make the assumption that there is a linear relationship between them, i.e. that a straight line best describes the relationship between these variables. Just as in correlational analysis, where we look at a scatterplot to help us visualise the relationship between two variables, we can look at a scatterplot with a straight line drawn through the datapoints. Then we can see how closely the datapoints fit the straight line. The line is called a 'line of best fit' because it is drawn in the best place possible; a straight line drawn in any other place wouldn't describe the relationship so well. Linear regression leads to a mathematical equation (the regression equation) which allows researchers to predict *y* scores from the *x* scores. It is from the regression line (or more properly, from the equation which is used to draw this line) that we can predict a person's *y* score (called the dependent variable/criterion variable) from their *x* score (called the independent variable/predictor variable/explanatory variable). Note that in this chapter there are different names for some of the concepts. For instance, whilst researchers have moved on and now call what used to be 'research subjects', 'participants', SPSS still calls participants 'subjects'. Whilst researchers now use names like 'predictor variables and 'explanatory variables' for the *x* variables, SPSS still calls them 'independent variables'. Likewise, researchers now use the words 'criterion variable' to refer to the *y* variable. However, SPSS still calls this the 'dependent variable'. So it can get a bit confusing. However, the predictor variable is *x* and the criterion variable is *y*!

Most researchers use *multiple regression* (which uses two or more predictors, see Chapter 12) rather than linear regression, and so it is hard to find journal articles which we can use to illustrate bivariate linear regression. However, it is essential to understand bivariate linear regression before multiple regression, so we have taken a few liberties with the following hypotheses (i.e. we have mentioned just one predictor variable rather than the several used in the research reported below).

- Bruscia et al. (2008) computed a linear regression analysis to determine the extent to which length of illness in hospitalised cardiac and cancer patients could predict a sense of coherence
- Hanna et al. (2009) studied nurses. Their aim was to look to see whether the worry about the transmission of infection predicted the perceived importance of hand-washing

Example

Here is a simple example which illustrates linear regression. Figure 11.1 is a scatterplot showing the relationship between children's age (in months) and their height (in kilograms). As children get older, we obviously expect them in increase in weight, and this is what the scatterplot shows. This is an almost perfect positive correlation ($r = .969$).

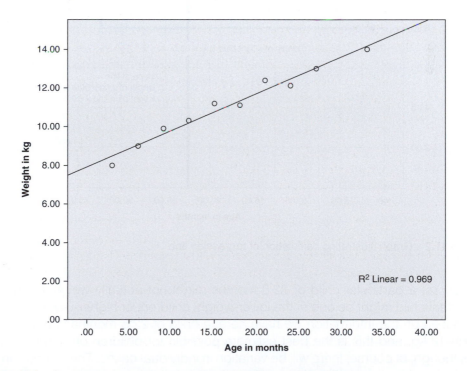

Figure 11.1   Scatterplot between age and weight with regression line

A correlational analysis shows us how closely the datapoints cluster around an imaginary straight line. But linear regression goes further – we draw a line of best fit, as shown. In this case, our statistical software does it for us.

We can use the regression line to predict what a child for whom we have only his or her age would weigh. For instance, imagine that we want to know how much a child is likely to weigh if s/he is 22.5 months old. We could then draw a vertical line upwards from 22.5 until we meet the regression line. Drawing a horizontal line from this point till it reaches the y-axis will show us what a child of 22.5 months is likely to weigh, which is just slightly over 12 kg (the bold line in Figure 11.2).

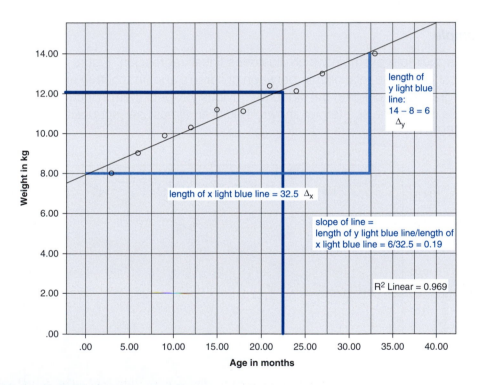

Figure 11.2 Graph illustrating calculation of regression line

Of course, a particular child of 22.5 months might not actually weigh 12 kg. That individual child might be one of the lower-weight children, or higher-weight children. But based on the information we have here, a child of 22.5 months is predicted to weigh 12 kg, and this is the best estimate possible for children of 22.5 months of age, though, of course, there will be variation in individual cases. The regression line is calculated by the statistical program, based on all the age and weight of all the children in our dataset, and is the line of best fit, that is, it is drawn in the best place possible, for this particular dataset. This line minimises the vertical distances between the datapoints and the line. The line is drawn according to a formula calculated by the statistical software. Instead of using the line of best fit to predict children with intermediate ages, we could use the formula instead.

The general formula for linear regression is:

$$\acute{y} = bx + a$$

or

$$\acute{y} = a + bx$$

$\acute{y}$ = the variable to be predicted (in this case weight, the one on the y-axis!).
b = a value representing the slope of the line – given by the statistical software.
x = the value of scores on the x-axis (in this case age).
a = the constant – the point at which the regression line crosses the y = axis.[1] This can be seen on the scatterplot, and the value is also given as part of the output.

How to Calculate the Regression Line

You simply take the distance between any two points on the x-axis (see lines in Figure 11.2) and calculate the length of this line. Draw a vertical line up until it meets the regression line, and calculate the length of this line in terms of the units being measured. Then simply divide the length of y line (labelled Δy) by the length of the x line (labelled Δ) in terms of the units being measured (x). The result is b, the slope of the line. The result by this method is .1846 (we have rounded this up in the scatterplot).

You can see from the scatterplot that a intercepts the y-axis at almost 8. The actual value, given by SPSS output, = 7.918. b is given as .190.

When a linear regression is carried out by statistical software, these values are given as part of the output.
So

$$\acute{y} = .190 \times age + 7.918$$

Let's use this formula to predict a particular child's score on y. Let's call her Jules. Jules' score on x (which is age, in this case) is 22.5. So the prediction for Jules is:

$$\hat{y} = bx + a \; (a = 7.918; \; b = .190; \; x = 22.5)$$
$$\hat{y} = .190 \times 22.5 + a = 4.275 + a$$
$$\hat{y} = 4.275 + 7.918$$
$$\hat{y} = 12.193$$

Thus the answer is 12.193.

This agrees with the prediction we obtained by using rulers and our regression line. Sometimes researchers use the equation from a linear regression line to predict new cases for which they have information on x, but not on y.

Mostly, however, researchers in the health sciences use the statistics obtained by linear regression to show how strongly the two variables (those on the x- and y-axes) are related. The slope of the line (the b-value) has a special meaning: for every one-unit increase in x, y changes by the value of b.

So in our case, for every one month of age, weight increases by .190 kg. This gives us a more concrete idea of how a change in one variable relates to a change in the other variable in terms of the respective units of measurement. The statistical software also gives us the usual information relating to statistical significance.

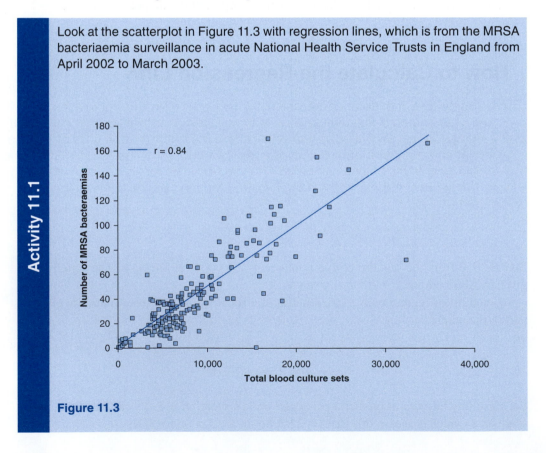

Activity 11.1

Look at the scatterplot in Figure 11.3 with regression lines, which is from the MRSA bacteriaemia surveillance in acute National Health Service Trusts in England from April 2002 to March 2003.

Figure 11.3

Activity 11.1

Give the following information:
a) The value of a
b) The value of r^2
c) For every increase in 10,000 of total blood culture sets, the number of MRSA bacteriaemias increases by approximately _____

LINEAR REGRESSION IN SPSS

We are now going to use two variables, age and weight, to illustrate a simple bivariate linear regression. In this case, we want to assess the relationship between age and weight. We hypothesise that age (of children) will predict their weight. Thus 'age' is the x variable, and 'weight' is the y variable.

1) Choose *Analyze*, *Regression*, *Linear* (Screenshot 11.1).

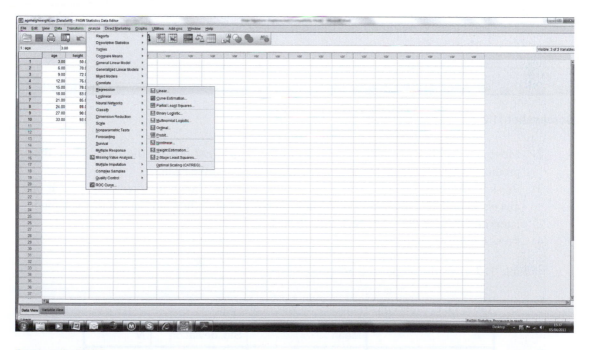

Screenshot 11.1

This gives a dialogue box (Screenshot 11.2).

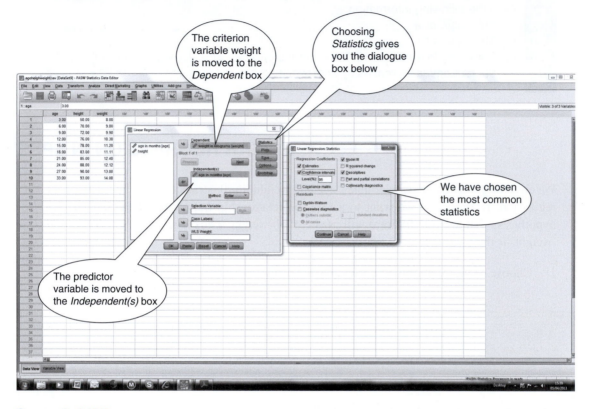

Screenshot 11.2

2) Move the criterion variable (*y*, weight) to the *Dependent* box on the right. Move the predictor variable (*x*, age) to the *Independent(s)* box on the right.
3) Press the *Statistics* button. This gives the dialogue box shown in Screenshot 11.2. It is always a good idea to obtain *Confidence intervals* around the regression line (explained later) and *Descriptives*, so check these boxes.
4) Press *Continue*, then *OK*.

Table 11.1 gives the output.

Table 11.1 Descriptive statistics for weight and age

	Mean	Std. deviation	*N*
Weight in kilograms	11.1030	1.85174	10
Age in months	16.8000	9.61249	10

This shows the means and standard deviations of both variables.

Table 11.2   Model summary for prediction of weight by age

Model Summary

Model	R	R square	Adjusted R square	Std. error of the estimate
1	.984[a]	.969	.965	.34852

a. Predictors: (Constant), age in months

The model summary (Table 11.2) shows you that *age in months* is the predictor variable. The *R*-value is simply Pearson's *r* for the two variables, *age in months* (*x*) and *weight in kilograms* (*y*). The *R*-value, as we already know, is very high (.984). R^2, as you know from Chapter 10, page 325, shows how much of the variation in scores on *y* can be accounted for by *x*. However, the results from a linear regression analysis fit the sample better than they would the population, so to reflect this rather optimistic result, SPSS adjusts R^2 downwards as a precautionary measure. Instead of reporting the R^2 result, it is usual to report the adjusted R^2 result. So in this case, rather than report the R^2 result, we would report that 96.5% (adj R^2) of the variation in *weight* can be explained by *age*.

Table 11.3   ANOVA for prediction of weight by age

ANOVA[b]

Model		Sum of squares	df	Mean square	F	Sig.
1	Regression	29.889	1	29.889	246.062	.000[a]
	Residual	.972	8	.121		
	Total	30.860	9			

a. Predictors: (Constant), age in months
b. Dependent Variable: weight in kilograms

Table 11.4 Coefficients for prediction of weight by age

Coefficients[a]

Model	B	Std. Error	Beta	t	Sig.	Lower Bound	Upper Bound
	Unstandardized coefficients		Standardized coefficients			95.0% confidence interval for B	
1 (Constant)	7.918	.231		34.274	.000	7.385	8.451
age in months	.190	.012	.984	15.686	.000	.162	.217

a. Dependent Variable: weight in kilograms

The ANOVA table (Table 11.3) tells us whether the regression analysis is statistically significant, or whether our results are due to chance, or sampling error. In this case the regression analysis is statistically significant ($F_{1,8} = 246.06$, $p < .001$).[2]

The coefficients table (Table 11.4) gives us the values of a (called the constant) and the values of b. These values are (perhaps confusingly) given under the column labelled *Unstandardized Coefficients, B*. The constant = 7.918 and b = .190. The b-value is unstandardised, that is, in the original units of measurement, in this case, *age in months*.

The output from SPSS also converts the original b-value (.190) into a standardized, z-score. The converted b value is called beta (β) and is interpreted in the same way as standard deviations (see Chapter 3, page 143). In this case, for every one standard deviation increase in age, weight increases by almost one standard deviation (.984). You will have probably noticed that .984 is identical to the R-value in this example – which means this information is somewhat redundant. That is always the case for a bivariate linear regression. However, in multiple regression (Chapter 12), where there are several x variables, the beta values will not be the same as R.

This table gives a t-value (15.686) and the associated significance level ($p < .001$) although as we have already reported an F-value and associated probability level, we do not need to report these results (again, this information is somewhat redundant in a bivariate linear regression, but it will be important in multiple regression).

The 95% confidence intervals allow us to state that although the slope of the regression line in the sample is .190, we can generalise to the population by saying that we are 95% confident that in the population the slope of the regression line is somewhere between .162 and .217.

We will talk more about the confidence intervals around b, and the output given by SPSS, later.

OBTAINING THE SCATTERPLOT WITH REGRESSION LINE AND CONFIDENCE INTERVALS IN SPSS

1) Click on *Graphs*, *Legacy Dialogs*, *Scatter/dot* (Screenshot 11.3).

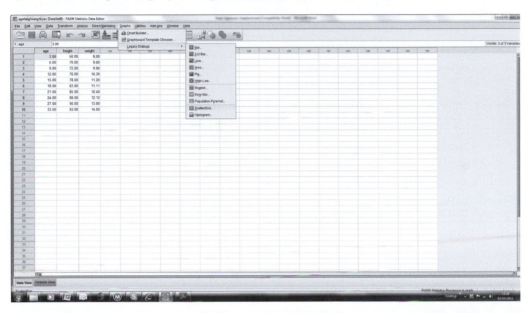

Screenshot 11.3

2) Select *Simple Scatterplot* and *Define* (Screenshot 11.4).

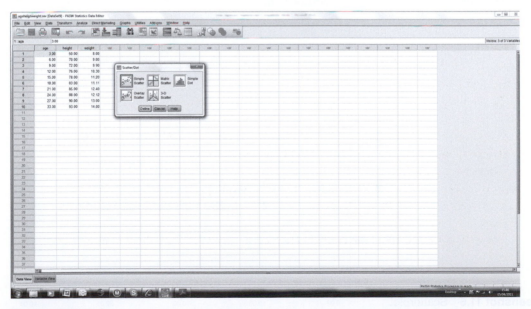

Screenshot 11.4

3)   Move the predictor variable *age* to the *x* row, and the criterion variable *weight* to the *y* row (Screenshot 11.5).

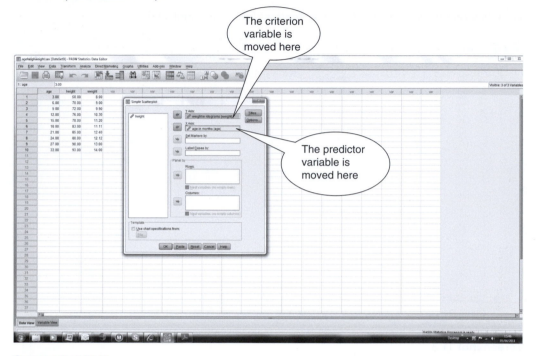

Screenshot 11.5

Then Press *OK*. This gives Screenshot 11.6.

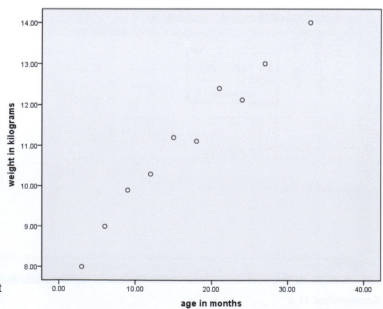

Screenshot 11.6   Scatterplot for age and weight

However, the *y*-axis starts at 8.00, which could be confusing. So we want to change this. Double click on the scatterplot, which will bring up the *Chart Editor* (Screenshot 11.7).

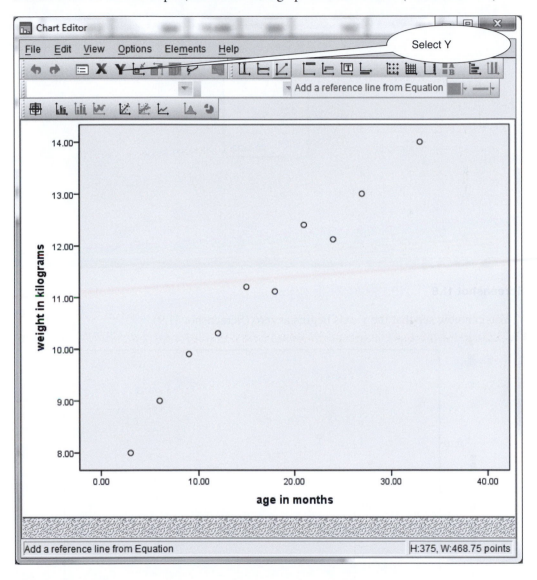

Screenshot 11.7

4) Select *Y*. This brings up the *Properties* box (Screenshot 11.8). You can then change the minimum value from 8.00 to 0. Press *Apply*.

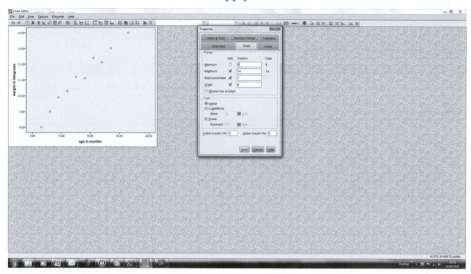

Screenshot 11.8

You can now see that the *y*-axis begins at zero (Screenshot 11.9).

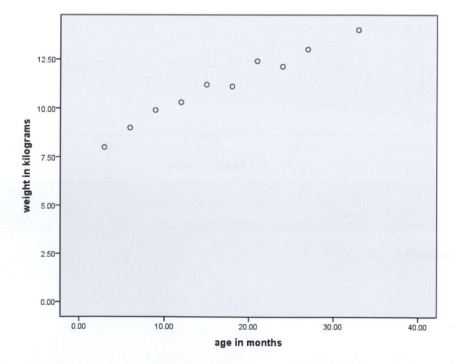

Screenshot 11.9

5) Then choose *Elements*, and *Fit Line at Total* (Screenshot 11.10).

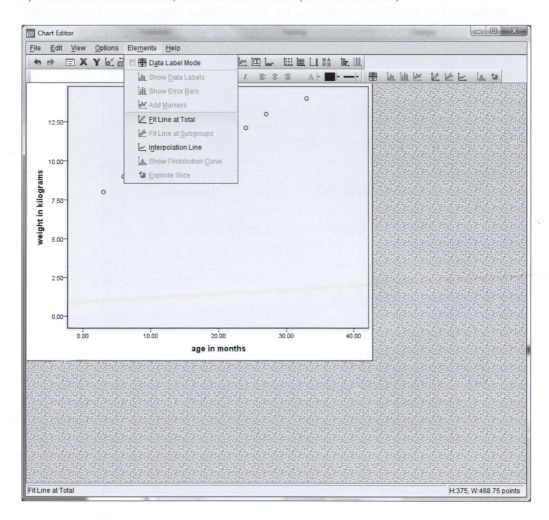

Screenshot 11.10

6) A dialogue box (Screenshot 11.11) also allows you to choose confidence intervals around the line of best fit. Choose *Individual* for the confidence intervals, and *Linear* for the properties.

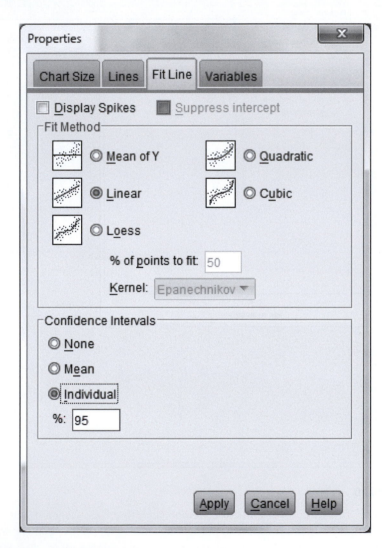

Screenshot 11.11

7) Press *Apply*.

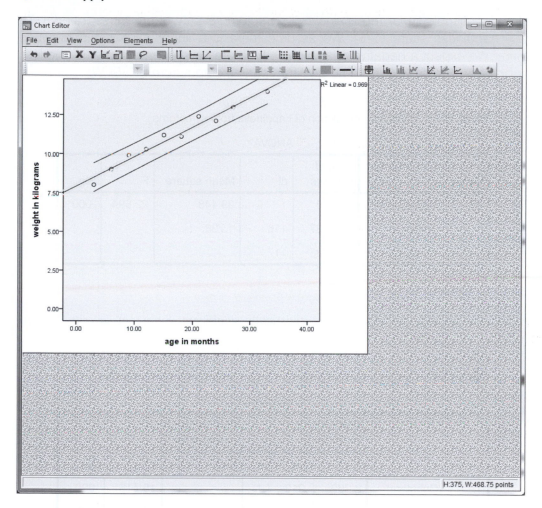

Screenshot 11.12

You can see (Screenshot 11.12) that the confidence intervals are shown around *b*, the slope of the line. So although our sample line is the best fit for our sample, we can generalise to the population and say that we are 95% certain that the true population regression line would be somewhere between the upper line and the lower line.

The examples above relate to positive relationships. When the relationship is negative, then as *x* increases by one unit, *y* will decrease by a certain amount. In this case, the value of *b* will be negative. Although the general formula is:

$$\acute{y} = bx + a$$

the value of *a*, or *b*, or both, can be negative.

Example

Here is a simple linear regression: x = symptom severity of an illness (rated 1–7), y = happiness score (1–5). We assume there is a linear relationship between them. We expect a negative relationship, the more severe the symptoms, the less happiness. Tables 11.5 and 11.6 give the (partial) output from SPSSFW.

Table 11.5   ANOVA for prediction of happiness from symptoms

ANOVA[b]

Model		Sum of squares	df	Mean square	F	Sig.
1	Regression	39.448	1	39.448	22.694	.000[a]
	Residual	201.637	116	1.738		
	Total	241.085	117			

a. Predictors: (Constant), symptoms
b. Dependent Variable: happiness

You can see that the regression is statistically significant. Symptom severity predicts happiness ($F_{1,116}$ = 22.69, p < .001).

Table 11.6   Coefficients for prediction of happiness by symptom severity

Coefficients[a]

Model		Unstandardized coefficients		Standardized coefficients	t	Sig.
		B	Std. error	Beta		
1	(Constant)	3.269	.212		15.415	.000
	symptoms	–.404	.085	–.405	–4.764	.000

a. Dependent Variable: happiness

The slope of the line is –.404. So for every one-unit increase in symptom severity, happiness goes down by .404 (almost half a happiness point!).
To predict an individual score for this study, the formula will be:

$$\acute{y} = 3.269 - .404$$

You might report the results in this way:

A linear regression analysis was performed in order to determine whether symptom severity was (negatively) related to happiness. The analysis showed that symptom severity predicted *happiness; this was statistically significant ($F_{1,116}$ = 22.69, p < .001). The slope of the regression line was −.404, showing that for every one unit increase in symptom severity, happiness decreased by almost half a happiness score.*

Or:

For every two-unit increases in symptom severity, happiness decreased by one point.

ASSUMPTIONS UNDERLYING LINEAR REGRESSION

In order to perform a bivariate linear regression, researchers must meet certain basic assumptions. This include the following:

* The relationship between *x* and *y* is linear (see Chapter 10, page 338)
* The criterion variable (DV) should be drawn from a normally distributed population of scores
* Outliers (extreme scores) may need to be considered for deletion

DEALING WITH OUTLIERS

When carrying out linear regression, it is sometimes the case that one or two datapoints are very different from the rest of the group. Researchers have debated whether or not someone who is very different from the general dataset should be allowed to have a disproportionate effect on the study. After all, what researchers are trying to do is to understand the general patterns of results. An outlier (someone who is very different from the rest of the group in terms of his/her *x* and *y* scores) can have a big influence on the regression line.

For instance, in a group of 15 scores where *b* = 2.179, the presence of a single outlier can 'move' the line towards the outlier, such that *b* = 3.965.

Researchers shouldn't, however, just remove an outlier without due consideration. If the outlier really is different from the rest of the group, especially if s/he is different from the rest on other variables as well, then perhaps it is sensible to remove the outlier. Although it is not usual for undergraduates to have to deal with these sorts of problems, we bring them to your attention because you will see that this is fairly common practice in studies using regression. Researchers should always state that they have done this, just as the following researchers have done.

Example from the Literature: Nurses Handwashing Behaviour

Hanna et al. (2009) carried out a study looking at the psychological processes underlying nurses' behaviour. They carried out linear regression analysis. First, they checked the assumptions of linear regression were met. They say:

The data were checked to ensure that the assumptions of linear regression were met. One of the assumptions underlying regression analysis is that no single data point has an undue influence on the outcome of the analysis. These are known as leverage points. In our analysis we found a single leverage point, i.e. one case that behaves differently from the remainder of the sample. As the purpose of the analysis is to summarise the relationships between variables within a group, then any case that does not conform to the remainder of the group is best removed, in order for the analysis to represent the sample ... one case was removed for being an extreme outlier. p. 92

Their aim was to look to see whether self-efficacy, perceived risk, perceived susceptibility and psychological distress (specifically occupational stress) predicted the 'perceived importance of handwashing'. Although Hanna et al. used multiple regression for their analyses, we asked them for their dataset so that we could illustrate bivariate linear regression for us. They kindly sent us their data. The following output was obtained using a variable 'worry about the transmission of infection (x)' to predict perceived importance of handwashing (y). The hypothesis was that worry about transmission of infection would be positively related to the perceived importance of handwashing.

The output (from SPSS, Table 11.7) shows that (worry about) 'transmission of infection' was entered into the equation, i.e. *transmission of infection* is the predictor/explanatory variable in a standard linear regression. It confirms that the dependent variable (i.e. the criterion variable) is *perceived importance of handwashing*.

Table 11.7 Variables in the equation

Variables Entered/Removed[b]

Model	Variables entered	Variables removed	Method
1	transmission of infection[a]	.	Enter

a. All requested variables entered.
b. Dependent Variable: Perceived importance of hand-washing

The model summary (Table 11.8) shows that the R-value between the predictor variable (worry about transmission of infection) and the criterion variable (perceived importance of handwashing) is .437. This is Pearson's r. This is therefore a moderate correlation. R^2 (.437 × .437) is .191. Thus 19% of the variation in the scores of perceived importance of handwashing can be explained by the variation in scores in the fear of transmission of infection. This figure is, however, specific to the sample of 76 people that Hanna et al. had in their study. In generalising to the population, the .191 has been adjusted downwards (the figure of .191 is too optimistic). Thus we would report the adjusted R^2 value (18%) rather than the 19%. The last column includes information on the standard error (a measure of variability applied to sample means).

Table 11.8 Model summary for prediction of handwashing by worry about transmission of infection

Model Summary

Model	R	R Square	Adjusted R square	Std. error of the estimate
1	.437[a]	.191	.180	1.13846

a. Predictors: (Constant), transmission of infection

The ANOVA output (Table 11.9) shows us how likely it is that our results were obtained by sampling error (chance). $F_{1,75} = 17.49$, $p < .001$. Thus, these results are highly unlikely to have arisen by chance, if there were really no relationship between them. This means that the explanatory variable, the worry about transmission of infection, significantly predicted the perceived importance of handwashing. The hypothesis is therefore confirmed.

Table 11.9 ANOVA for the prediction of perceived importance of handwashing by fear of the transmission of infection

ANOVA[b]

Model		Sum of squares	df	Mean square	F	Sig.
1	Regression	22.665	1	22.665	17.488	.000[a]
	Residual	95.910	74	1.296		
	Total	118.576	75			

a. Predictors: (Constant), transmission of infection
b. Dependent Variable: perceived importance of hand-washing

Table 11.10 shows the important regression statistics as well as *t*-values and the associated statistical significance. This shows that for every one-point increase in the score of (fear of) *transmission of infection*, the perceived importance of hand-washing increases by .735 (this is *b*, the slope of the line). We know it increases (rather than decreases) because .735 is positive. The unstandardised slope of the line (.735) has been converted to a standardised score called beta. These can be interpreted exactly as you have learned for *z*-scores (see Chapter 4, page 143).

In this case, for every one standard deviation increase in x (worry about transmission of infection), y (perceived importance of handwashing) increases by .437 of a standard deviation. The t-value is 4.182, and the associated p value < .001. The 95% confidence intervals are given around the *unstandardized* slope. So b, the slope of the line, for this sample, is .735. However, generalising to the population, we would expect that b would fall somewhere between .385 and 1.086.

Table 11.10   Coefficients for the prediction of perceived importance of handwashing by fear of the transmission of infection

Coefficients[a]

Model		Unstandardized coefficients		Standardized coefficients	t	Sig.	95.0% confidence interval for B	
		B	Std. Error	Beta			Lower Bound	Upper Bound
1	(Constant)	2.330	1.725		1.351	.181	−1.107	5.767
	transmission of infection	.735	.176	.437	4.182	.000	.385	1.086

a. Dependent Variable: perceived importance of hand-washing

In case you have forgotten what the constant is, this is the value of a, the intercept. The only reason you might want to know the value of a (2.330) is to be clear about the regression equation, which could be used to predict the score of someone for whom you had information on x, but not on y.

Here the formula is:

Perception of the importance of handwashing =
(.735 × scores on worry about transmission of infection) + 2.330

Activity 11.2

If someone scored 8 on 'worry about transmission of infection', what would be his/her predicted score for the 'perception of the importance of handwashing?'

Example

We carried out a study investigating variables contributing to happiness in people with Irritable Bowel Syndrome. As part of this study, we looked at whether self-efficacy could predict happiness. The hypothesis was that self-efficacy would be positively related to happiness.

Figure 11.4 gives the scatterplot with regression line and 95% confidence limits around the line.

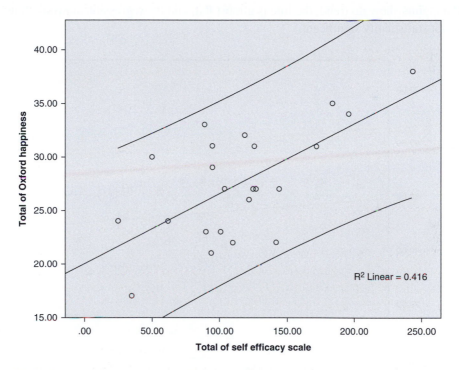

Figure 11.4 Scatterplot between self-efficacy and happiness with 95% confidence limits

We found that self-efficacy significantly predicted happiness ($F_{1,21}=14.97$, $p < .001$), explaining 42% of the variance. The *b*-value was .07, showing that for every one-unit increase in self-efficacy, happiness increased by .07. Generalising to the population, confidence intervals show that we are 95% confident that the true population regression line falls between .03 and 1.00. The hypothesis was therefore confirmed.

WHAT HAPPENS IF THE CORRELATION BETWEEN *X* AND *Y* IS NEAR ZERO?

As you know from correlational analysis, if the correlation is zero or near zero, the data-points will show no discernible trend – they will be scattered about randomly. In this case, $b = 0$ (or near it) because the regression line will be flat, or almost flat. Look at the scatterplot in Figure 11.5 with regression line.

The statistics for the dataset – shown in the form of a scattergram, show that $b = -.034$. The datapoints show no trend, the line is almost flat, and the regression analysis shows that this is not statistically significant.

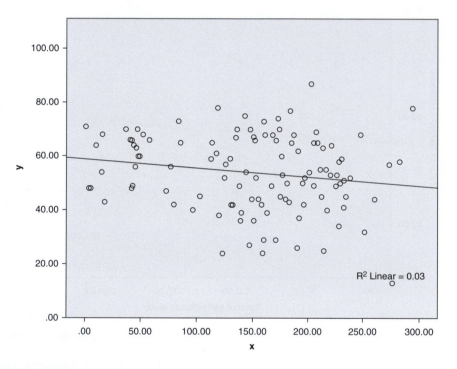

Figure 11.5   Scatterplot showing no relationship between *x* and *y*

Example from the Literature

Bize and Plotnikoff (2009) looked at the relationship between a short measure of health status and physical activity in a workplace population. As part of that study, they looked at the way in which health status related to physical activity. Physical activity (energy expenditure) was calculated by a formula which resulted in an average score called MET minutes. The researchers used simple linear regression to determine whether health status predicted MET. They produced a table (Table 11.11).

Table 11.11   Coefficients from Bize and Plotnikoff data

	Unstandardised coefficients		Standardised coefficients	t	Sig.
	b	SE	β		
Constant	−95.073	259.540		−0.366	0.714
Health status	374.822	68.338	0.224	5.485	<0.001

Adjusted R^2 = 0.048

The authors say:

> *Health status predicted energy expenditure (p < 0.001) ... each unit increase in health status level translated in a mean increase of 375 MET minutes in energy expenditure. Health status level explained five percent of the variance (adj R^2 = 0.05) for energy expenditure.*

Note that in the interpretation of the results, Bize and Plotnikoff have rounded up the health status score from 374.822 to 375, and the variance explained from 0.048 to 0.05. The scores for health status and MET minutes are positive, so that for every one-unit increase in health status, MET minutes increase by 375. This was statistically significant at $p < .001$. Although health status explains 5% of the variation in MET minutes, and is statistically significant, it's hard to know whether this is practically/clinically important. With large participant numbers, small effects may lead to results like this being declared statistically significant. In this study, there were 573 people.

USING REGRESSION TO PREDICT MISSING DATA IN SPSS

In Chapter 6 on data screening and cleaning, we said that regression analysis could be used to predict the value of missing scores. We will illustrate how this is done by using part of a dataset which we are working on at the moment. We have many variables in this dataset, but the two we are focusing on now is *cognitive failures* (measured by the Cognitive Failures Questionnaire CFQ) and the Prospective Memory Questionnaire (PMQ).

There are 44 participants, and three of them have missing scores on the CFQ, whereas all have scores on the PMQ.

These are the steps in order to use regression analysis to predict scores which might be missing.

1) Carry out a regression analysis using PMQ as the predictor variable and CFQ as the criterion variable
2) Use the output to obtain the regression equation
3) Use the regression equation to predict the missing values. Here we show you how to do this:

Choose *Analyze*, *Regression*, *Linear* (Screenshot 11.13).

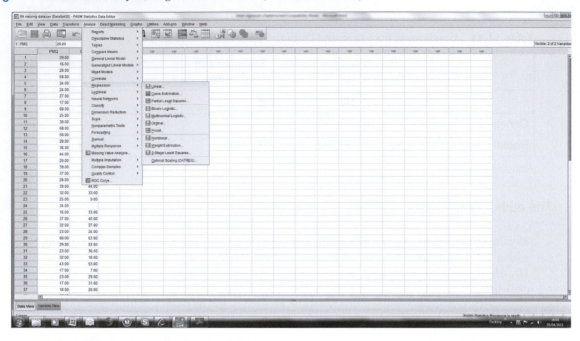

Screenshot 11.13

This gives Screenshot 11.14.

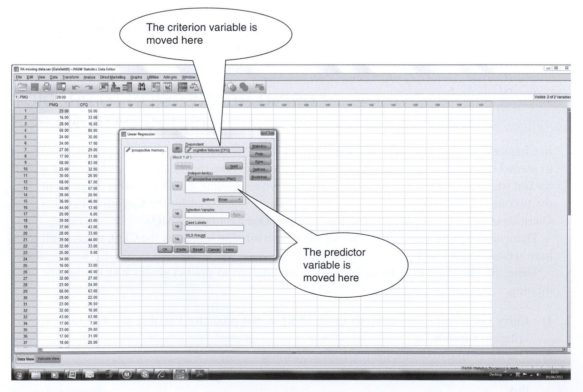

The criterion variable is moved here

The predictor variable is moved here

Screenshot 11.14

Move the predictor variable to the *Independent(s)* box on the right, and the criterion variable to the *Dependent* box on the right. Click *OK*.

Tables 11.12–11.14 give the output.

Table 11.12 Model summary for prediction of cognitive failures by prospective memory scores

Model Summary

Model	R	R square	Adjusted R square	Std error of the estimate
1	.771[a]	.594	.584	12.34697

a Predictors: (Constant), prospective memory

This shows that the correlation between the two variables is strong ($r = .771$).

Table 11.13 ANOVA for prediction of cognitive failures by prospective memory scores

ANOVA[b]

Model		Sum of squares	df	Mean square	F	Sig.
1	Regression	8696.915	1	8696.915	57.048	.000[a]
	Residual	5945.463	39	152.448		
	Total	14642.378	40			

a Predictors: (Constant), prospective memory
b Dependent Variable: cognitive failures

The analysis is statistically significant: $F_{1,39} = 57.05$, $p < .001$. This means that as we are certain that prospective memory is a good predictor of cognitive failures, we can use the regression equation to predict new cases, or cases with missing values on cognitive failures.

Table 11.14 Coefficients for the prediction of cognitive failures by prospective memory scores

Coefficients[a]

Model		Unstandardized coefficients		Standardized coefficients		
		B	Std. error	Beta	t	Sig.
1	(Constant)	−1.655	5.138		−.322	.749
	prospective memory	1.116	.148	.771	7.553	.000

a. Dependent Variable: cognitive failures

The formula is:

$$\text{Cognitive failures} = (b_1 x_1) - a$$

The figures, taken from Table 11.14, is:

$$\text{cognitive failures} = (1.116 \times \text{score on prospective memory}) - 1.655$$

Now we know the formula, we can use this to predict the missing scores on cognitive failures (Table 11.15).

Table 11.15   Regression means for scores on cognitive failures and prospective memory

Regression Means[a]

CFQ	PMQ
34.1732	32.1591

a. Residual of a randomly chosen case is added to each estimate.

PREDICTION OF MISSING SCORES ON COGNITIVE FAILURES IN SPSS

Choose *Transform*, *Compute Variable* (Screenshot 11.15).

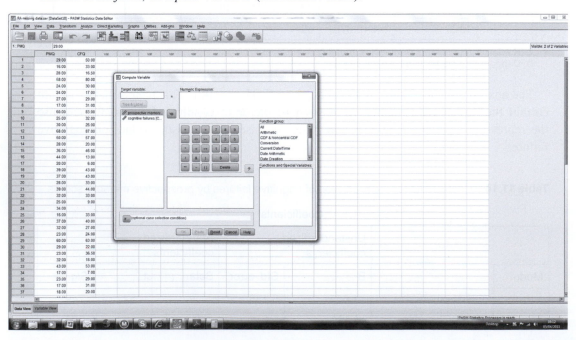

Screenshot 11.15

You then choose the name for the predicted variable. We have chosen *predictedCFQ* – this is typed into the *Target Variable* box on the left (Screenshot 11.16).

You then put the regression equation into the *Numeric Expression* box on the right. You choose the '( )' from the numerical keypad, and type in 1.116*, then you move the predictor variable from the left to the *Numeric Expression* box. Then move '-' to the *Numeric Expression* box and finally, 1.655.

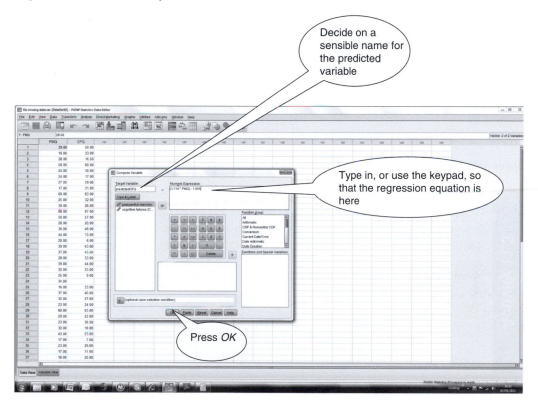

Screenshot 11.16

Press *OK*.

If you look at your dataset, you will see a new variable added – the *predictedCFQ* (Screenshot 11.17).

The first missing score is for case 24, which has a missing score on CFQ. The predicted CFQ score is 36.29. We could therefore use this score to replace the missing score. However, as the scores on CFQ are whole numbers, we may want to correct to the nearest number. In this case, we would replace the missing values with 36.

RA missing data.sav [DataSet1] - PASW Statistics Data Editor

File Edit View Data Transform Analyze Graphs Utilities Add-ons Window Help

1 : PMQ   29.00   Visible: 2 of 2 Variables

	PMQ	CFQ	var	var	var	var	var	var	var	var	var	var	var	var	var	var	var	var	var	var
8	17.00	31.00																		
9	60.00	83.00																		
10	25.00	32.00																		
11	30.00	26.00																		
12	68.00	87.00																		
13	50.00	57.00																		
14	28.00	20.00																		
15	36.00	46.00																		
16	44.00	13.00																		
17	20.00	6.00																		
18	39.00	43.00																		
19	37.00	43.00																		
20	28.00	33.00																		
21	39.00	44.00																		
22	32.00	33.00																		
23	25.00	9.00																		
24	34.00																			
25	16.00	33.00																		
26	37.00	40.00																		
27	32.00	27.00																		
28	23.00	24.00																		
29	60.00	63.00																		
30	29.00	22.00																		
31	23.00	36.50																		
32	32.00	18.00																		
33	43.00	53.00																		
34	17.00	7.00																		
35	23.00	29.00																		
36	17.00	31.00																		
37	18.00	20.00																		
38	25.00																			
39	33.00	22.00																		
40	49.00	26.00																		
41	40.00	43.00																		
42	35.00																			
43	28.00	35.00																		
44	17.00	16.00																		

Data View Variable View

PASW Statistics Processor is ready

Screenshot 11.17

Activity 11.3

Fill in the Case Numbers, Predicted CFQ and the score you would enter instead of the missing score for the two other missing scores (this information is extracted from Screenshot 11.17. Answers are at the end of the book.

Case	Predicted CFQ	Score you would enter instead of missing score
24	36.29	36

Summary

Linear regression is an extension of correlational analysis. It allows us to determine the strength of an association between the independent variable, called the explanatory or predictor variable and the dependent variable, called the criterion variable. The slope of the line of best fit (b) shows how much y changes as a result of an increase in x. This allows us to predict scores from x, on a sample where y is unknown. A scatterplot with the line of best fit, and confidence intervals around the line, gives us a way of generalising to the population. Inferential statistics show whether the line of best fit is likely to have arisen by sampling error or not. Linear regression, or more usually multiple regression, is a correlational technique very much suited to the investigation of naturally occurring phenomena.

MULTIPLE CHOICE QUESTIONS

Questions 1–3 relate to the following scatterplot with regression line:

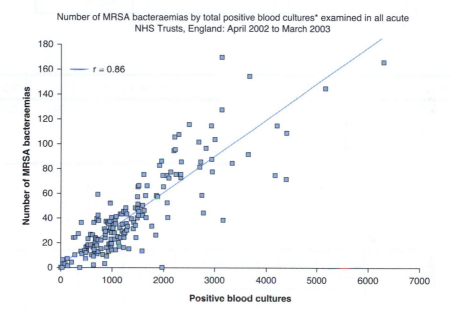

Number of MRSA bacteraemias by total positive blood cultures* examined in all acute NHS Trusts, England: April 2002 to March 2003

1. The value of *a* is:
   a) 0
   b) 1000
   c) 7000
   d) Cannot tell

2. Calculate the slope of the line using the regression line in the scattergram above. The slope of the line, *b*, is approximately:
   a) 0.33
   b) 0.55
   c) 0.66
   d) 0.77

3. For a value of 5500 blood cultures, what is the (approximate) number of predicted MRSA bacteraemias?
   a) 100
   b) 120
   c) 140
   d) 160

Questions 4–8 relate to the output below, relating to a linear regression between social support (x) and happiness (y).

Model Summary

Model	R	R square	Adjusted R square	Std. error of the estimate
1	.440[a]	.194	.155	4.74225

a. Predictors: (Constant), total of MOS social support

ANOVA[b]

Model		Sum of squares	df	Mean square	F	Sig.
1	Regression	113.384	1	113.384	5.042	.036[a]
	Residual	472.268	21	22.489		
	Total	585.652	22			

a. Predictors: (Constant), total of MOS social support
b. Dependent Variable: total of Oxford happiness

Coefficients[a]

Model		Unstandardized coefficients		Standardized coefficients			95.0% Confidence Interval for B	
		B	Std. Error	Beta	t	Sig.	Lower Bound	Upper Bound
1	(Constant)	22.929	2.289		10.016	.000	18.169	27.690
	total of MOS social support	.090	.040	.440	2.245	.036	.007	.174

a. Dependent Variable: total of Oxford happiness

4. We are 95% confident that the true population regression line will fall between:
   a) 18.169 and 27.690
   b) .007 and .174
   c) 2.245 and 27.690
   d) None of the above

5. What is the correlation coefficient for the two variables?
   a) .440
   b) .194
   c) .155
   d) 4.74

6. Which statement is correct?
   a) The regression analysis is statistically significant ($F_{1,22} = 5.042$, $p = .036$)
   b) The regression analysis is statistically significant ($F_{1,21} = 5.042$, $p = .036$)
   c) The regression analysis is not statistically significant ($F_{1,22} = 5.042$, $p = .036$)
   d) The regression analysis is not statistically significant ($F_{1,21} = 5.042$, $p = .036$)

7. The regression equation is $\hat{y} =$
   a) $2.289x + .040$
   b) $22.929x + .09$
   c) $.09x + 22.929$
   d) None of the above

8. The standardised b weight is:
   a) .090
   b) .040
   c) .440
   d) 2.245

9. Which of the following is *not* true?
   a) The regression line is known as the line of best fit
   b) b is the slope of the regression line
   c) a is the constant
   d) b is a standardised score

10. A predictor variable is also known as
    a) The explanatory variable
    b) The criterion variable
    c) a) and b) above
    d) Neither a) nor b)

11. Which of the following is *not* true in respect of a bivariate linear regression?
    a) The relationship between x and y should be linear
    b) The criterion variable should be drawn from a normally distributed population of scores
    c) The predictor variable should be drawn from a normally distributed population of scores
    d) Outliers may need to be considered for deletion

12. The general equation for a bivariate linear regression is: $\hat{y} =$
    a) $bx + a$
    b) $ax + b$
    c) $a \div bx$
    d) None of the above

13. The slope of the regression line can be calculated by:
    a) $\Delta x \div \Delta y$
    b) $\Delta y \div \Delta x$
    c) $\Delta y + \Delta x$
    d) $\Delta x - \Delta y$

14. The constant is:
    a) The point at which the regression line crosses the x-axis
    b) The point at which the regression line crosses the y-axis
    c) The slope of the regression line
    d) None of the above

15. b means that: for every one-unit increase in
    a) y, x changes by one standard deviation
    b) x, y changes by one standard deviation
    c) x, y changes by a certain constant amount
    d) y, x changes by a certain constant amount

Notes

1   Note that SPSS scatterplots often don't have the edge of the graph positioned on the y-axis (as we have done).
2   As shown in Chapter 8, page 255, the df are reported for F-values. The df are obtained from the ANOVA table. Report df for the regression, and df for the residual, i.e. in this case 1,8.

Standard Multiple Regression

12

Overview

Multiple regression is an extension of correlational analysis and bivariate linear regression. In multiple regression, researchers use several predictor variables in order to see how they relate to, or predict, a criterion variable. Multiple regression allows us to determine how much variance is accounted for by the predictor variables, together and separately. Once you have understood bivariate linear regression, then multiple regression is not so difficult. The experimental hypothesis is formulated to answer one or more of these questions – how strong is the relationship between all the explanatory/predictor variables x's and the criterion variable, y? Is there a good fit between the combined x variables, and y? Or: From a knowledge of the x scores together, can we predict what the y scores will be? Multiple regression is a common technique in the social sciences – often researchers want to understand the way in which several variables influence a criterion variable, rather than looking at just one variable (bivariate linear regression).

(Continued)

(Continued)

From this chapter you will be able to:

- Learn how to assess the relationship between a set of *x* variables and *y*
- Understand the need to meet the assumptions of multiple regression
- Learn how to predict an individual's score on *y* by a knowledge of his/her scores on the predictor variables
- Understand how to interpret the test statistics: multiple R, r^2, adjusted r^2, the *b* weights (unstandardised) and the beta weights (standardised)
- Have a knowledge of the ways in which multiple regression can be used in research

INTRODUCTION

Multiple regression, being an extension of correlational analysis and bivariate linear regression, allows researchers to assess the relationships between a set of predictor variables $(x_1, x_2, x_3 \ldots)$ and a criterion variable (y).

So now we can use the examples from the last chapter, showing how the researchers used multiple regression to answer their research questions.

- Bruscia et al. (2008) computed a multiple regression analysis to determine the extent to which six variables (age, gender, diagnosis, race, length of illness and education) could predict a sense of coherence in hospitalised cardiac and cancer patients
- Hanna et al. (2009) wanted to determine whether four variables (perceived importance of handwashing, perceived risk to self, perceived risk to others and workplace assististance for handwashing) predicts handwashing behaviour in nurses
- Unwin et al. (2009) wanted to examine the influence of demographic, amputation and psychosocial variables on positive psychological adjustment outcomes for lower limb amputees

In order to perform a multiple regression, researchers must meet certain basic assumptions:

- The relationship between the predictor/explanatory variables (the *x*'s) and *y* is linear (see Chapter 10, page 324 and Chapter 11, page 346)
- Multivariate outliers (extreme scores on several variables) may need to be considered for deletion
- You need to have far more participants than variables. A good formula is given by Tabachnick and Fidell (2007) ($N > 104 + 8m$, where m = number of explanatory variables)

The general formula for multiple regression is:

$$\acute{y} = (b_1x_1) + (b_2x_2) + (b_3x_3) \cdots + a$$

The formula can also be written like this:

$$\acute{y} = a + (b_1x_1) + (b_2x_2) + (b_3x_3) \cdots$$

($\acute{y}$ is called 'y hat', and the hat above the y means 'predicted y' – as opposed to y, which means the 'actual value of y'.

y = the variable to be predicted (in this case weight, the one on the y-axis!)

b = a value representing the slope of the line for each predictor variable – given by the statistical software.

a = the constant – the point at which the regression line crosses the y-axis.[1]

This builds on what you have learned in the last chapter.

Example from the Literature

To illustrate multiple regression, we are going to use the example from the last chapter, which is Hanna et al.'s (2009) data on handwashing in nurses. For one of their analyses, they used four variables as predictor variables (the perceived importance of handwashing to the nurses, the perceived risk to themselves in relation to infection, the perceived risk to others in relation to infection, and the degree to which the nurses thought their workplace assisted them in handwashing.

These are the predictor variables (x_1, x_2, x_3 and x_4). The criterion variable (y) is how often the nurses washed their hands (frequency of handwashing).

MULTIPLE REGRESSION IN SPSS

As Hanna et al. kindly sent us their dataset (only part of which we reproduce below), we are going to illustrate multiple regression by using their data. Our results differ slightly from theirs, as we haven't removed the influence of outliers.

1) Click on: *Analyze Regression, Linear* (Screenshot 12.1).
2) This gives Screenshot 12.2.
3) Move the predictor variables from the left into the *Independent(s)* box, using the button. Move the criterion variable (frequency of handwashing) from the left to the *Dependent* box, using the button. Then click on *Statistics*. This gives Screenshot 12.3.

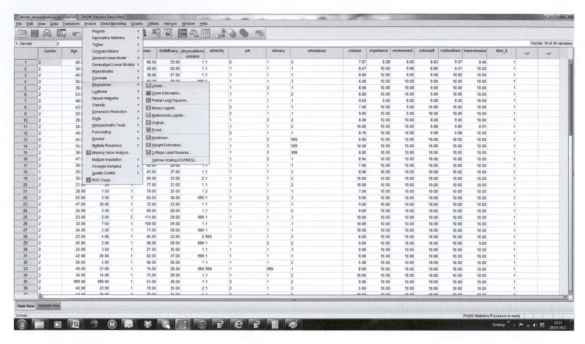

Screenshot 12.1

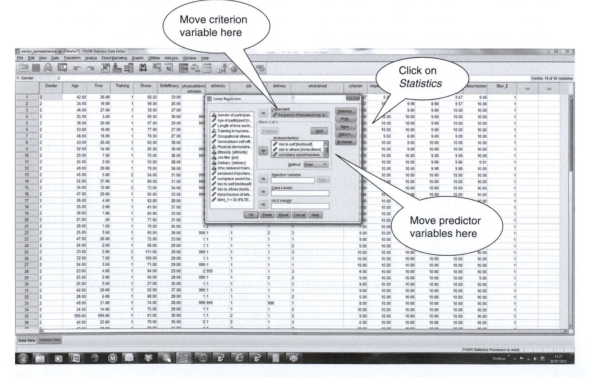

Screenshot 12.2

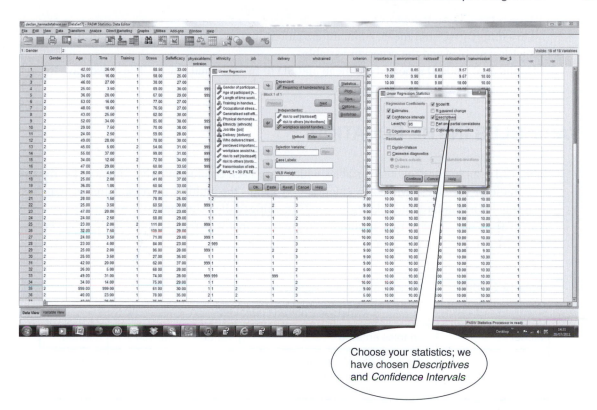

Choose your statistics; we
have chosen *Descriptives*
and *Confidence Intervals*

Screenshot 12.3

We have selected *Descriptives* and *Confidence Intervals*. Click on *Continue*, then *OK*.
SPSS can give you a variety of outputs. Table 12.1 gives the most important. Most research-ers include in their write up simple descriptive statistics. However, they wouldn't simply copy the output from SPSS. It is not usual, for instance, to give a table of descriptive statistics using so many decimal places. Most researchers would round to two decimal places. It also wouldn't be necessary to have a column labelled *N*, as each of the *N*s are the same.

Table 12.1 Descriptive statistics for handwashing and risk

Descriptive Statistics

	Mean	Std. Deviation	N
frequency of handwashing	7.6935	2.04361	76
perceived importance of handwashing	9.5222	1.25738	76
risk to self	8.7373	1.62950	76
risk to others	9.4674	1.06901	76
workplace assist handwashing	8.9633	2.03099	76

This simply gives the mean, standard deviations and number of participants for the four predictor variables and the criterion variable.

Hanna et al. (2009) reported the mean and SD to two decimal places. They also gave the median, the range and the potential range.

VARIABLES IN THE EQUATION

Table 12.1 simply confirms the variables which have been entered into the equation, i.e. the four predictor variables. 'Method = enter' simply means the multiple regression that is being performed is a standard multiple regression (sometimes called simultaneous multiple regression). This is the simplest type of multiple regression, that we are describing in this chapter, and is the default in SPSS. Hanna et al. (2009) used this.

Table 12.2   SPSS output: variables in the regression equation

Variables Entered/Removed[b]

Model	Variables entered	Variables removed	Method
1	workplace assist handwashing, risk to self, perceived importance of handwashing, risk to others[a]		Enter

a. All requested variables entered.
b. Dependent Variable: frequency of handwashing

Table 12.2 confirms a) the 'variables entered' (i.e. the predictor variables) and b) the dependent variable (which we call the criterion variable). Researchers would not use this table when reporting their results.

Multiple *R*

This table (Table 12.3) is important, as it shows us the correlation between the predicted scores and the actual scores. *R* can be seen to be .638, which is a strong correlation.

Table 12.3   SPSS output: model summary

Model Summary

Model	R	R square	Adjusted R square	Std. error of the estimate
1	.638[a]	.407	.373	1.61770

a. Predictors: (Constant), workplace assist handwashing, risk to self, perceived importance of handwashing , risk to others

R^2

R^2 (.638 × .638) is given as .407. This shows that nearly 41% of the variance in scores on 'frequency of handwashing' can be explained by the variation in scores on the four predictor variables.

Adjusted R^2

However, as we have seen in the previous chapter, R^2 refers to the sample ($N = 76$) which Hanna et al. had, and in order to generalise to the population, we need to adjust R^2. The formula for adjusted R^2 takes into account the number of variables and sample size, and adjusts R^2 downwards. So now we can say that we expect approximately 37% of the variance in frequency of handwashing to be explained by the four predictor variables.

Output Tables

Researchers would not reproduce Table 12.3 in their results – they normally report the test statistics as text.

The ANOVA Table

Table 12.4 ANOVA Table

ANOVA[b]

Model		Sum of squares	df	Mean Square	F	Sig.
1	Regression	127.421	4	31.855	12.173	.000[a]
	Residual	185.803	71	2.617		
	Total	313.224	75			

a. Predictors: (Constant), workplace assist handwashing, risk to self, perceived importance of handwashing, risk to others
b. Dependent Variable: frequency of handwashing

Researchers generally report the F-value, the degrees of freedom, and the probability value – as text, rather than in a table.

The ANOVA (Table 12.4) shows us that the prediction is significantly greater than would be expected by chance, i.e. the four predictor variables together significantly predict frequency of handwashing behaviour in nurses ($F_{4,71} = 12.173$, $p < .001$).

So we know the combined effect of the predictor variables on the criterion variable. Now we might want to see the separate effects of the predictor variables on the criterion variable.

Individual Coefficients

Table 12.5   Coefficients[a]

Model		Unstandardized coefficients		Standardized coefficients			95.0% confidence interval for B	
		B	Std. error	Beta	t	Sig.	Lower bound	Upper bound
1	(Constant)	−5.397	2.009		−2.686	.009	−9.403	−1.391
	perceived importance of handwashing	.403	.160	.248	2.523	.014	.084	.721
	risk to self	.215	.134	.171	1.602	.114	−.052	.482
	risk to others	.453	.211	.237	2.147	.035	.032	.874
	workplace assist handwashing	.345	.095	.343	3.630	.001	.156	.535

a. Dependent Variable: frequency of handwashing

Sometimes researchers report the coefficients and associated statistics in a table – although generally not all the information is reported. It is useful when the researchers report the confidence intervals around the slope of the line, as this gives us an idea of how well the regression results are likely to generalise to the population.

For instance, in Hanna et al.'s journal article, they report both the unstandardised and standardised coefficients, with the standard error, the *t*-values, and the exact probability levels.

The Constant, *a*

Table 12.5 shows us the value of the constant, *a* (confusingly under the *b* column). This is −5.397. This is not of great interest to us, unless we want to use the regression formula to predict scores in a new sample of people.

Unstandardised *b* weights

Let's look at the 'perceived importance of handwashing'. The unstandardised coefficient, *b*, is .403. This means that for every one unit increase in perceived importance of handwashing (x_1), the predicted frequency of handwashing rises by .403 (*y*). Thus, for every one point increase on 'perceived importance of handwashing' the frequency of handwashing rises by almost a half a point.

Beta, the Standardised Weights

Beta is the standardised *b* weight, i.e. the original unstandardised *b* weight (in this case .403) is converted to a standardised score (a *z*-score, see Chapter 4, page 143). The standardised score is .248. Thus for every one standard deviation increase in perceived importance of handwashing, the frequency of handwashing increases by .248 of a standard deviation (approximately a quarter of a standard deviation. The t-value = 2.523, and this is statistically significant (p = .014). The confidence intervals relate to the unstandardised b weights. So although, in Hanna et al.'s sample, b = .248, in the general population we would expect, with a 95% likelihood, that the true value of b would fall somewhere between .084 and .721.

The perceived importance of handwashing isn't the strongest predictor though. The strongest predictor is found by looking at the standardised beta weights. If you look at the table, you will see that the strongest predictor is the perception of the degree to which the nurses thought their workplace assists handwashing (workplace assists handwashing), as this has a beta weight of .343. The 'perceived risk to self', on its own, is not significantly significant, i.e. it does not predict the frequency of handwashing.

Activity 12.1

How would you explain the relationship of the perceived 'risk to others' and 'frequency of handwashing'? In your explanation, make sure you talk about the unstandardised b weights, the standardised b weights, and the associated statistics. Compare your explanation to ours at the end of the book.

THE REGRESSION EQUATION

The regression equation is not usually reported in the results sections of journal articles, as it is not usually relevant.

The generic multiple regression equation, as we have seen is

$$Y = (b_1 \times x_1) + (b_2 \times x_2) + (b_3 \times x_3) + (b_4 \times x_4) \cdots + a$$

So in this case it is:

Predicted frequency of handwashing =
(x_1 × perceived importance of handwashing) + (x_2 × risk to self)
+ (x_3 × risk to others) + (x_4 × workplace assists handwashing) + a

This means we simply find the appropriate unstandardised b weights and put them into the equation, along with a, which in this case is negative:

Predicted frequency of handwashing =
(.403 × perceived importance of handwashing) + .215 × risk to self)
+ (.453 × risk to others) + (.345 × workplace assists handwashing) − 5.397

PREDICTING AN INDIVIDUAL'S SCORE

Assume that a new participant, Imogen, has scores on the predictor variables, but that we have no information on the frequency of her handwashing. We can predict (estimate her likely) score on the frequency of her handwashing, by using her x scores:

Perceived importance of handwashing = 9

Risk to self = 8

Risk to others = 8

Perception of the degree to which the nurses thought their workplace assists handwashing (workplace assists handwashing) = 10

$$\text{Predicted frequency of handwashing} = (.403 \times 9) + (.215 \times 8) =$$
$$(.453 \times 8) + (.345 \times 10) - 5.397$$
$$= \text{Predicted frequency of handwashing} = (3.627 + 1.72 + 3.624 + 3.45) - 5.397$$
$$= \text{Predicted frequency of handwashing} = 12.421 - 5.397$$
$$= \text{Predicted frequency of handwashing} = 7.024$$

Participant 50 in Hanna et al.'s dataset actually had these set of scores, and s/he scored 7 on the frequency of handwashing. So the prediction was really good.

HYPOTHESIS TESTING

In relation to hypothesis-testing, multiple regression is often used in an exploratory-type way, so that researchers do not formulate a formal hypothesis. For instance, in the above study the researchers say 'This study explored the association between a range of psychological variables and self-reported handwashing in a sample of nurses who work in a large general hospital' (p. 1). Whilst they obviously expected their explanatory variables to relate to handwashing, they did not specify which of their variables would be more important. As they did not state a formal hypothesis, the researchers cannot confirm or reject any hypotheses. The results, however, are important as they tell us that certain variables are able to predict nurses' handwashing behaviour quite well, and thus hospitals can change procedures so that nurses are more likely to wash their hands, thus reducing the potential for transmission of infections.

Example from the Literature

Bruscia et al. (2008) studied a Sense of Coherence (SOC) in patients who were in hospital for cancer or cardiac problems. They wanted to find out whether age, gender, diagnosis, race, education and length of illness predicted SOC. Note here too, that the researchers have not given a formal hypothesis which they can confirm or reject. The study was an exploratory one, as they wanted to 'assess and compare the SOC scores' and to determine whether the variables they chose are significant predictors of the SOC in their patient group (p. 3) The authors reduced the probability of a Type I error by using an alpha level of .01. This is referred to as a Bonferroni correction. There were 172 patients. Quite often researchers report results of a multiple regression in a table, but Bruscia et al. reported them as text.

> *The analysis revealed the multiple* R *to be .27; the six variables accounted for .07* (R²) *of the variance in the SOC. An ANOVA showed that, when the Bonferroni correction* (p < .01) *was applied, these six variables, taken together, were not significant predictors of the SOC* (F = 2.2, df = 6, p = .04).
>
> *Standardized beta coefficients showed that two variables contributed most to the prediction of the SOC, length of illness* (β = .20, p < .01) *and age* (β = .16, p < .05). p. 289

The authors therefore show us that the six variables they used as predictors were poor predictors of SOC, explaining only 7% of the variance in scores of SOC, and that length of illness and age contributed most to the prediction.

Example from the Literature

Unwin et al. (2009) looked at factors which they believed might predict adjustment outcome for lower limb amputees. Several measures were used – the Hope Scale, the Multidimensional Scale of Perceived Social Support (MSPSS), the Trinity Amputation and Prosthetic Experiences Scale (TAPES pain subscale and the Positive and Negative Affect Scale (PANAS). These measures were taken at referral and six months later. Two multiple regression analyses were carried out. The first used the PANAS as the criterion variable, and seven variables as the predictor (explanatory) variables. Table 12.6 is the table they produced (p. 1047).

Table 12.6 Multiple regression analysis for positive mood (PANAS subscale)

	b	SE B	*Beta*
(Constant)	1.945	9.589	
Phantom intensity (TAPES)	0.334	0.830	*0.04*
Age	–0.020	0.073	*–0.03*
Gender	1.705	2.457	*0.07*
Level of amputation	2.597	1.772	*0.16*
Cause	–0.427	2.085	*–0.02*
MSPSS	0.080	0.060	*0.15*
*Hope Scale***	0.761	0.227	*0.38*

R^2 = .22 for model, **p < .001

There are seven predictor variables, which means the number of participants, according to Tabachnick and Fidell (2007) should be $104 + 8m = 160$. This study had 99 participants who participated at both timepoints, but the number of participants fell short of the guidelines above. Why does it matter? Because if you have many variables and not enough participants, the statistics obtained will be 'optimistic'. Just as, in bivariate linear regression, the mathematical procedure gives the line of best fit, multiple regression is a mathematical procedure which gives the best 'plane of best fit' (because there are more than two variables) so the statistics fit the sample very well, but may not generalise to the population. Having too few participants for the number of variables leads to 'overfitting'. This means that the results fit the sample far better than they do the population.

Note some of the *b* and beta weights are negative. These are interpreted just like negative correlations. However, as neither of the negative *b* weights are strong it doesn't make sense to interpret them. Although the authors haven't given probability levels for the non-significant variables, we can see from the beta weights that the lines of best fit are near zero.

In Table 12.6, it can be seen that only 22% of the variation in scores on 'positive mood' can be explained by the seven predictors/exploratory variables in the model (notice the authors have not reported the adjusted R^2, which would be smaller than this). Only one individual explanatory variable (Hope) is able to significantly predict positive mood ($p < .001$). We can interpret this variable by looking at the *b* or beta coefficients. Choosing the standardised weight (beta), we can say that for every one standard deviation increase in Hope, positive mood increases by .38 of a standard deviation. Although this is a fairly weak effect, it is statistically significant.

Activity 12.2	The above researchers produced a similar table using General Adjustment (a subscale of TAPES) as the criterion variable and seven explanatory (predictor) variables. Look at Table 12.7, and write a brief paragraph explaining the results. If you have understood the above paragraph, you shouldn't have too much trouble interpreting this table (Unwin et al., 2009, p. 1048). You can check your results with ours at the end of the book.

Table 12.7 Multiple regression analysis for general adjustment (TAPES subscale)

	b	**SE B**	*Beta*
(Constant)	5.153	4.826	
Phantom Intensity	−0.006	0.512	−0.011
Age	−0.019	0.038	−0.058
Gender	1.027	1.232	0.087
Level of amputation	−0.805	0.897	−0.094
Cause	0.652	1.064	0.070
Social Support**	0.102	0.030	0.363
Hope Scale*	0.146	0.054	0.293

$R^2 = 0.29$ for model, *p < 0.01, **p < 0.001

Example from the Literature

Farren (2010) examined the contribution of power, uncertainty, and self-transcendence to the quality of life in breast cancer survivors. Farren reported the results of her analysis as text. Here is just one part of the results:

> *Simultaneous multiple regression analysis was conducted to determine the extent to which variance in quality of life could be explained by power, uncertainty, and self-transcendence when considered together. The model explained 39%, F = (3,100) 21.411, p = .000² (adj. R²= .373) of the variance in quality of life. However, standardized regression co-efficients show that while uncertainty (beta = −.174, t = −2.076, p = .040) and self-transcendence (beta = .551, t = 5.988, p = .000) made a statistically significant contribution to the explained variance, power did not (p = .898). p. 68*

This shows us that the variables together explain 37.3% of the variation in scores of quality of life (we have used the adjusted R^2). Farren has explained that uncertainty and self-transcendence made a statistically significant contribution to the prediction of quality of life, whereas power did not. However, you should be able to see that uncertainty was a weak predictor (as uncertainty rises by one standard deviation, quality of life reduces by .17 of a standard deviation), but that self-transcendence is a much stronger predictor. As self-transcendence rises by one standard deviation, quality of life rises by .55 of a standard deviation, significant at $p < .001$. .5 is considered a moderate effect (Cohen, 1988).

OTHER TYPES OF MULTIPLE REGRESSION

There are two other types (models) of multiple regression. They differ in the way that the variance is allotted. You have already come across using overlapping circles to represent shared and unique variance in Chapter 10 – but a bit of repetition is a good thing!

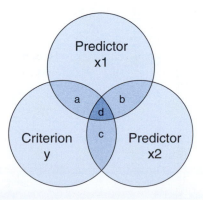

Figure 12.1 Overlapping areas of variance[3]

Researchers talk about variance in terms of percentages. As you will know from Chapters 10 and 11, in order to obtain a measure of effect, we square r (or in multiple regression, R) in order to give an easily understood measure of relationship between them. If $R = .50$, then $R^2 = .25$ ($.50 \times .50$). We can then say that 25% of the variation in scores on one variable is explained, or accounted for, by the variation in other scores. This is called the 'variance explained'. Figure 12.1 shows the overlapping areas of variance, and the areas a, b, c and d are all areas of shared variance[4]. What it shows is that predictor $x1$ shares unique variance with the criterion variable y (area a) and unique variance with predictor $x2$ (area b). In addition, predictor $x2$ shares variance with the criterion variable y (area c). The shared variance for $x1$ $x2$ and the criterion is illustrated by area d in the middle. Multiple R represents all the shared variance between the predictor variables and the criterion. So the variance represented in multiple R contains areas a, d and c.

When you look at the individual results for each variable, the results represent the unique variance only. So in the example above, the variance of $x1$ on y is represented by area a; the variance for predictor $x2$ on y by area c.

This means that if there are a lot of predictor variables, all highly correlated, Multiple R might be large and statistically significant, whereas the individual predictors may show up as being not very important at all, individually.

Example

Look Screenshot 12.4, which are for six symptoms of Irritable Bowel Syndrome (IBS). We want to see how much variance in 'depression' is accounted for (y, the criterion variable) by the IBS symptoms ($x1$ to $x6$). We therefore carry out a standard multiple regression analysis.

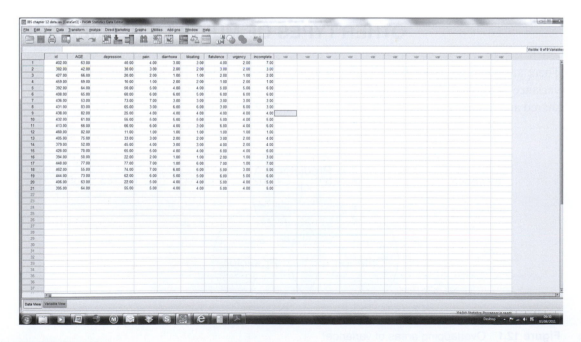

Screenshot 12.4

Table 12.8   Model summary

Model	R	R square	Adjusted R square	Std. error of the estimate
1	.881[a]	.776	.680	12.31674

a. Predictors: (Constant), incomplete, urgency bowel movement, bloating, abdominal pain, diarrhoea, flatulence

Wow! look at this! In the sample, this means we've explained 78% of the variance, i.e. 78% of the variation in depression scores is accounted for by the six symptoms of IBS. We can see that this is significant ($F_{6,14}$=8.08, p = .001) (Tables 12.8 and 12.9).

Table 12.9   ANOVA[b]

Model		Sum of squares	df	Mean square	F	Sig.
1	Regression	7352.457	6	1225.409	8.078	.001[a]
	Residual	2123.829	14	151.702		
	Total	9476.286	20			

a. Predictors: (Constant), incomplete, urgency bowel movement, bloating, abdominal pain, diarrhoea, flatulence
b. Dependent Variable: depression

Now we think, great, let's look at the individual predictors (Table 12.10).

Table 12.10   Coefficients[a]

Model		Unstandardized coefficients		Standardized coefficients		
		B	Std. error	Beta	t	Sig.
1	(Constant)	.203	7.973		.026	.980
	abdominal pain	8.589	3.016	.742	2.848	.013
	diarrhoea	−.831	4.502	−.064	−.185	.856
	bloating	4.603	3.423	.345	1.345	.200
	flatulence	−2.166	5.716	−.172	−.379	.710
	urgency bowel movement	.672	4.062	.050	.166	.871
	incomplete	.373	4.021	.031	.093	.927

a. Dependent Variable: depression

Hmm. Apart from abdominal pain, none of the explanatory variables seem to explain anything! Well, that's an important finding in itself, because it means that each symptom, on its own (apart from abdominal pain) isn't that important to depression – it's the *combined symptoms* that matter.

The reason why we have such a high R^2 is that R^2 includes all the variance – both unique and shared. However, the individual results include only the **unique** variance. Because the symptoms are highly correlated with each other, as you would expect, the unique variance is low.

The standard model of multiple regression is the one we recommend you use, as it is the 'safest', in terms of overfitting (see page 547), and it allows you to see the unique contribution made by the explanatory variables, to the criterion variable.

However, there are two other models known as *statistical or stepwise regression*, and *hierarchical regression*. Hierarchical regression tends to be used more often than statistical regression, and so what follows now is a very brief introduction to hierarchical regression, as you are likely to come across this type of regression in journal articles.

HIERARCHICAL MULTIPLE REGRESSION

Whereas in standard multiple regression, all the predictor variables are entered into the equation (statistical program) simultaneously, in hierarchical multiple regression, the researchers can control the order of entry. Researchers use this type of regression when they have good theoretical reasons for entering variables in a specified order. Often, researchers want to co-vary social, demographic or other variables. These are entered into the program first, to 'get them out of the way' and to see how much extra variance is accounted for by their variables of interest (Figure 12.2).[5]

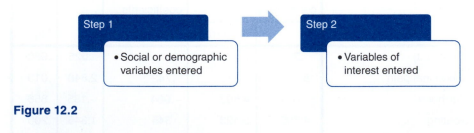

Figure 12.2

Example

Let us assume researchers are carrying out a study to determine whether physiological measures (such as blood pressure) predict cognitive decline. The researchers might already know, from the literature, that age or alcohol use is a good predictor of cognitive decline. In this case they might want to enter 'age' and a measure of alcohol use into the program first, at Step 1. At Step 2, they would enter their variables of interest, e.g. blood pressure measure. This would show them how much extra variance the blood pressure measure explains, once age and alcohol are taken into account (covaried, partialled out).

They might find, for instance, that age and alcohol use account for 10% of the variation in scores on the cognitive measure. At Step 2, they might find an extra 20% of the variance could be explained by the blood pressure measure (Figures 12.3 and 12.4).

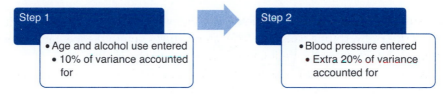

Figure 12.3

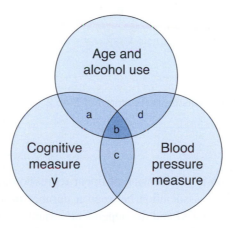

Figure 12.4   Diagram showing overlapping variance between $x1$, $x2$ and y

As age and alcohol use have been entered first, at Step 1, age and alcohol use are entered into the program (Figure 12.5).

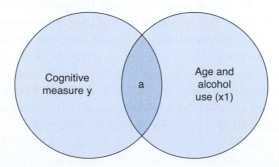

Figure 12.5   Age and alcohol entered at Step one: full correlation between $x1$ and y

So the contribution of age and alcohol use is represented by the area a, and has credit for this amount of variance.

Once the blood pressure measure is entered, it accounts for only the *extra* amount of variance, that is, only the unique variance of *x2* and *y* (the lower part of the area b, Figure 12.6).

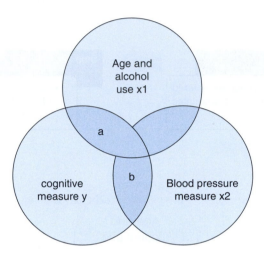

Figure 12.6   Blood pressure measure (*x2*) entered at Step 2

Summary

Standard multiple regression is an extension of linear regression analysis. It allows us to determine the strength of an association between a number of *x* variables (called the explanatory or predictor variables) and the dependent variable, called the criterion variable. The analysis can answer the question 'How much of the variation in scores on the criterion variable is accounted for by all the explanatory variables together?' (this is R^2). The ANOVA table shows us whether the prediction is statistically significant.

Standard multiple regression also allows us to look at the unique contribution of each separate explanatory variable on the criterion variable (the coefficients table). This shows us each individual slope of the line of best fit (*b*) and the *t*-value shows us the statistical significance of each one. Confidence intervals around the slope of the line can also be obtained. Each explanatory variable is assessed as if all the other variables had been entered first, i.e. it shows the unique variance accounted for by each individual explanatory variable. The standardised beta weights allow a like-for-like comparison of each of the individual explanatory variables. Multiple regression is a correlational technique very much suited to the investigation of naturally occurring phenomena.

MULTIPLE CHOICE QUESTIONS

1. $\acute{y}$ =value of:
   a) The criterion variable
   b) The predicted criterion variable
   c) The predictor variable
   d) Value of b

2. Which is not true? The predictor variables are also called the:
   a) Explanatory variables
   b) Criterion variables
   c) Independent variables
   d) x variables

3. Which of these is not true?

   Researchers use hierarchical multiple regression when they:
   a) Want to control the order of entry
   b) Want to enter covariates into the model
   c) Have theoretical reasons for entering variables into the programme in a specific order
   d) Want to enter all the variables into the equation simultaneously

   Questions 4–6 relate to a study of people with Menière's Disease. The criterion variable is *depression*, and the predictor variables are *general self-efficacy*, *Dizziness Handicap Scale* and *illness uncertainty*.

   Look at the following model summary.

Model Summary

Model	R	R square	Adjusted R square	Std. error of the estimate
1	.557ª	.310	.281	12.48793

a. Predictors: (Constant), total of general self-efficacy, total of the dizziness handicap scale, total of illness uncertainty

4. How much of the variation in depression scores can be accounted for by the predictor variables, in this particular sample?
   a) 56%
   b) 31%
   c) 28%
   d) 12%

Coefficients[a]

Model		Unstandardized coefficients		Standardized coefficients		
		B	Std. error	Beta	t	Sig.
1	(Constant)	70.267	12.577		5.587	.000
	total of the dizziness handicap scale	.540	.158	.350	3.429	.001
	total of illness uncertainty	.144	.089	.166	1.615	.111
	total of general self-efficacy	−.607	.223	−.282	−2.720	.008

a. Dependent Variable: total of CESD depression

5. Which is the strongest predictor of depression?
   a) Dizziness Handicap Scale
   b) Illness uncertainty
   c) General self-efficacy
   d) All are equal in strength

6. Which of the following is true?
   a) As general self-efficacy rises by one SD, depression decreases by .607
   b) As illness uncertainty rises by one unit, depression decreases by .144
   c) As scores on the Dizziness Handicap Scale increase by one unit, depression increases by .54 of a unit
   d) As scores on the Dizziness Handicap Scale increase by one SD, depression increases by .54 of a SD

Questions 7 and 8 relate to the following:

Look at the following text from Dingle and King (2009). They were looking at the impact of several variables on the outcome from a private hospital drug and alcohol treatment programme. As part of that study, they carried out a standard multiple regression to predict follow up % days abstinent (from substance use) from the following scores: depression, anxiety, stress, number of co-occurring mental disorders at admission (0 to 4).

They say 'The overall regression model was highly significant ($R^2 = .42$; $F = 12.1$, $p < .001$). However, the number of co-morbid diagnoses patients were given at admission was not related to follow-up abstinence. Again, only … depression symptoms were a significant univariate predictor in the model ($\beta = .713$, $t = 6.52$, $p < .001$).' (p. 19).

7. How much variation in the scores on % days abstinent is accounted for by the predictors in their analysis? (figures rounded to nearest whole number)
   a) 18%
   b) 12%
   c) 42%
   d) 72%

8. As scores on depression rises by one standard deviation, the % days abstinent:
   a) Increases by .71 of a standard deviation
   b) Decreases by 6.52 standard deviations
   c) Decreases by .71 of a standard deviation
   d) Decreases by 6.52 standard deviations

9. If a researcher has ten predictor variables, how many participants (approximately) should s/he have?
   a) 480
   b) 380
   c) 280
   d) 180

Questions 10–11 relate to a study by Bramwell and Morland (2009) who studied genital appearance and satisfaction in women. As part of that study, they used a multiple regression to determine the contribution of appearance schemas, (a self-report measure relating to the importance of physical appearance in general), body satisfaction and self-esteem to Genital Appearance Satisfaction (GAS – a new questionnaire developed by the authors). The following table is reproduced from the authors' article (p. 22). The higher the score on the GAS, the less satisfied the women were.

Regression of GAS onto the appearance schemas inventory, body satisfaction and self-esteem

Independent variables	Standardised coefficient	p
Appearance schemas	−0.02	.85
Body satisfaction	0.07	.53
Self-esteem	−0.38	.002

Adjusted R^2 = .14, $F_{3,117}$ = 7.17, $p < .01$

10. Which of the following is *not* true?
   a) As self-esteem increases by one standard deviation, satisfaction with genital appearance increases by .38 of a standard deviation
   b) As self-esteem increases by one standard deviation, satisfaction with genital appearance decreases by .38 of a standard deviation
   c) Appearance schemas is the weakest predictor of satisfaction with genital appearance
   d) The relationship between body satisfaction and satisfaction with genital appearance is almost zero and is probably due to sampling error

11. Which of the following is true?
   a) The weakest predictor is body satisfaction
   b) The overall model is statistically non-significant
   c) This study did not have enough participants in it, and therefore the results cannot be relied upon
   d) Together the predictor variables account for 14% of the variation in GAS

Questions 12–15 relate to a study by van der Colff and Rothmann (2009) who assessed whether or not occupational stress, sense of coherence and coping strategies predict burnout and the work engagement of registered nurses. The table below shows a multiple regression analysis with emotional exhaustion as the criterion variable and three types of stress as the explanatory (predictor variables).

Multiple regression analysis: emotional exhaustion predicted by three types of stress

	Unstandardised coefficients	Standardised coefficients	t	P
Constant	7.110		5.10	0.00
Lack of organisational support	0.060	0.19	3.89	0.00
Stress job demands	0.120	0.27	6.14	0.00
Nursing-specific demands	−0.030	−0.06	−1.45	0.15

$R = 0.37, R^2 = 0.14$

12. Emotional exhaustion is predicted by the following regression equation:
    a) $y = (0.060 \times$ lack of organisational support$) + (0.120 \times$ stress job demands$) - (.03 \times$ nursing-specific demands$) + 7.110$
    b) $y = (0.19 \times$ lack of organisational support$) + (0.120 \times$ stress job demands$) - (.03 \times$ nursing-specific demands$) + 7.110$
    c) $y = (0.60 \times$ lack of organisational support$) + (0.120 \times$ stress job demands$) - (.03 \times$ nursing-specific demands$) - 7.110$
    d) $y = (0.19 \times$ lack of organisational support$) + (0.120 \times$ stress job demands$) - (.03 \times$ nursing-specific demands$) + 7.110$

13. Which is the strongest predictor of emotional exhaustion?
    a) Lack of organisation support
    b) Stress job demands
    c) Nursing-specific demands
    d) None of them predict very well

14. The researchers have reported some of their p-values as 0.00. It would have been better to have reported these values as:
    a) $p < .05$
    b) $p < .01$
    c) $p < .001$
    d) $p = .01$

15. Which of the following is true?
    a) The three predictor variables together account for 14% of the variation in scores on emotional exhaustion
    b) The lack of organisational support does not predict emotional exhaustion
    c) Nursing-specific demands are very important in the prediction
    d) As the stress of job demands increase by one standard deviation (SD), emotional exhaustion increases by .27 of a SD

Notes

1 Note that SPSS scatterplots often don't have the edge of the graph positioned on the y-axis (as we have done).

2 Note that when you see the probability reported as $p = .000$ in SPSS, the reported value should really be $p < .001$.

3 This is a conceptual explanation rather than a material one. The mathematical accuracy is lost in the interests of conceptual understanding.

4 This diagram is illustrative only; it does not relate to Hanna et al.

5 These advanced techniques, including statistical or stepwise regression, are beyond the scope of an introductory textbook. Students who wish to learn more about these techniques are referred to either Todman and Dugard (2007) or Tabachnick and Fidell (2007).

Logistic Regression

13

Overview

Logistic regression can be thought of as an extension of linear regression and multiple regression. So far you have seen regression models where a continuous outcome (*y*) is associated with one or more predictor (*x*) variables (in Chapters 11 and 12). Logistic regression shares many similarities but a key difference is that the outcome variable must be dichotomous rather than continuous. A dichotomous variable means each observation can take on only one of two values. For example, blood pressure scored as high (above 140/90 mmHg) or normal (lower than 140/90 mmHg) would be a suitable outcome for logistic regression. Blood pressure measured on a continuous scale should be analysed using linear regression. The questions asked by logistic regression are similar to those posed by linear regression: You may assess the strength of the relationship between a dichotomous outcome variable and one or more predictor variables. You can also predict the probability that an observation will have a particular value on the outcome variable, given knowledge of their predictor variable scores.

In this chapter you will learn how to:

- Assess the relationship between a set of *x* variables and a dichotomous *y* variable

(Continued)

(Continued)

- Interpret logistic regression models with continuous and categorical predictor variables
- Read and understand research papers using logistic regression models

INTRODUCTION

Logistic regression extends linear regression to situations where the outcome variable is dichotomous. Dichotomous variables are categorical variables with only two possible values. For example, sex is dichotomous. It is a single variable that can take on the values of male or female. As we have seen in previous chapters, dichotomous variables are very common in the health sciences. Consequently, logistic regression has often been used in the epidemiological studies discussed in Chapter 5. For example, dichotomous variables could be used to code whether participants:

1. Are suffering from a disease or are well
2. Are obese or normal weight
3. Are smokers or non-smokers

Dichotomous variables are usually coded as 0s and 1s in the dataset. A code of 1 often means that the risk factor or outcome of interest is present (e.g. the participant is ill/obese/smokes) and 0 means the outcome is absent. Whenever you analyse data, it is always crucial to check how your variables have been coded and ensure value labels have been created. Three example studies that employed logistic regression are listed below:

- Hibbeln et al. (2007) used logistic regression to study the effects of varying levels of seafood intake during pregnancy on children's neurodevelopment up to age eight. Measures of poor neurodevelopment included being in the lowest 25% for verbal intelligence and fine motor control
- Cohen et al. (2000) tested the effect of fruit and vegetable consumption on risk of prostate cancer
- Yusuf et al. (2004) computed logistic regression analyses to estimate the contribution of modifiable risk factors to myocardial infarction across 52 countries

THE CONCEPTUAL BASIS OF LOGISTIC REGRESSION

As with other techniques covered in this book, SPSS will do all the calculations for you. We will discuss some of the conceptual features of logistic regression to help you understand,

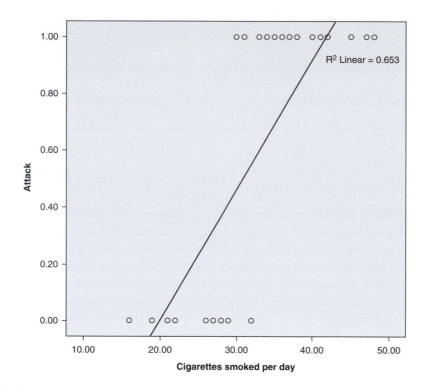

Figure 13.1

interpret and use logistic regression. Inspired by the Yusuf et al. (2004) paper cited above, we will illustrate the use of logistic regression in assessing the association between a history of heart attack and frequency of smoking in a fictional study of 1000 male smokers. Initially for the purposes of illustration, we will work with a sample of just 30 participants as shown in Figure 13.1.

This looks like the scatterplots you have seen in previous chapters except that the dichotomous heart attack variable (on the y-axis) can only take on the values 0 (has not had a heart attack) or 1 (has had a heart attack). We can see that heart attacks are not very common when participants do not smoke very many cigarettes per day. Towards the left of the graph the data points tend to be on the 0 line of the y-axis. As we look towards the right of the graph where participants are smoking more, it becomes more likely that they will have had a heart attack (scoring 1 on the y-axis). So from this graph it looks like smoking more cigarettes increases the risk of heart attack. As in all analyses, however, it is crucial to run an inferential statistical test to see whether the relationship is likely to exist within the population rather than resulting from sampling error. As we will see, the correct test is logistic regression here. However, before we see logistic regression in action, we will spend a little time thinking about the problems of analysing these data using linear regression.

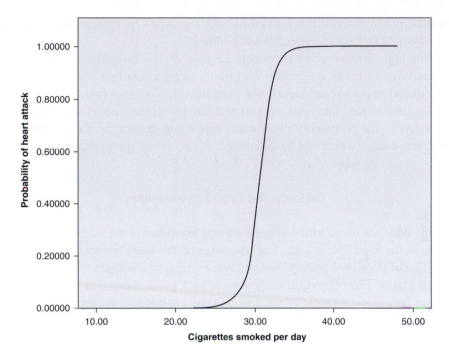

Figure 13.2

A linear regression line has been fitted to the data points on the scatter plot in Figure 13.1. For some values of daily smoking the regression line predicts values of heart attack between 0 and 1. The fitted value may be interpreted as the predicted probability of heart attack given the level of smoking. Participants are predicted to have a heart attack probability of less than 0 if they smoke less than 20 cigarettes per day, or greater than 1 if they smoke more than 45 per day. Probability values must fall between 0 and 1, so this is a problem. Fitting the linear model also violates some of the assumptions of linear regression. In short, it is not a good idea to use linear models with dichotomous outcomes, and that is why we need logistic regression.

Rather than fitting a straight regression line to the data shown in Figure 13.1, it would be ideal to fit one shaped like an s, as shown in Figure 13.2. This does not predict any probabilities above 1 or below 0. In regression analyses, however, we much prefer straight lines that can be described with equations such as:

$$\hat{y} = a + bx$$

This was the form of relationship seen in linear regression (Chapter 11). So really what we want is the best of both worlds. We want to be able to have an s-shaped line of predicted probabilities, but to describe this curvy line with regression coefficients for a straight line. Surely this would be having one's cake and eating it?

Well, with logistic regression it is possible. Logistic regression achieves it by transforming the s-shaped line of predicted probabilities into a straight line that can be described with intercept (*a*) and slope (*b*) coefficients. The transformation involves two steps. First the probabilities are transformed into odds. As you will (no doubt) remember from Chapter 5, odds are calculated as the probability of an event happening divided by the probability of the event not happening (which can be calculated as one minus the probability of the event). Formally this can be written as:

$$Odds = probability/(1 - probability)$$

Second, the odds are transformed into the natural logarithm of the odds.[1] The result can be referred to as the log-odds, or logit. The advantage of this transformation is that it turns the s-shaped line of predicted probabilities in Figure 13.2 into a straight line of predicted log-odds, as in Figure 13.3. The equation generated by logistic regression specifies this linear relationship between the predictor variable and the log-odds of the event occurring in the same format you are familiar with from linear regression (Chapter 11).

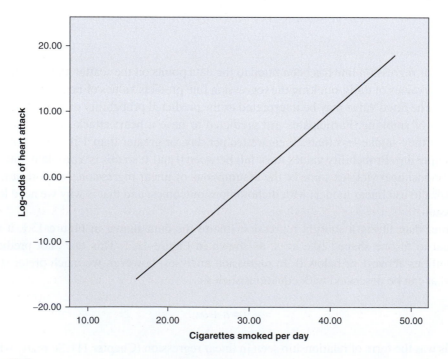

Figure 13.3

The general formula for logistic regression (with a single predictor) is

$$\text{logit } (\hat{y}) = a + bx$$

logit $(\hat{y})$ = the predicted log-odds of the outcome (heart attack in the example)
b = a value representing the slope of the line
a = the constant – the predicted log-odds when the predictor is 0
x = value of predictor variable

As in linear regression, a represents the predicted log-odds of the event when the predictor is 0. b is the slope of the regression line and represents the change in log-odds for a one unit increase in the x variable. Log-odds can take on any value, positive or negative. A value above 0 means the relationship is positive; increasing the predictor variable is associated with an increased chance of the outcome. A value below 0 means that as the predictor variable increases the chance of the outcome decreases. A value of 0 indicates no relationship.

The computer identifies the values of a and b for us. This involves a process called *maximum-likelihood estimation* which generates the values for a and b. Values are selected as the most likely ones to be present in the population to have generated the observed sample data.

In the heart attack example SPSS reports the equation as

$$\text{log-odds (heart attack}') = -32.89 + 1.07*\text{cigarettes}$$

As with linear regression this equation could be used to predict the log-odds that people have a history of heart attack on the basis of the number of cigarettes they smoke daily. This could then be transformed into a probability. We will demonstrate this process later in the chapter. Usually though, health science researchers use this information to illustrate the strength of the relationship between variables. As with linear regression, the slope of the regression line is the key statistic here. In our example the b coefficient is positive, showing that increased smoking is associated with a greater chance of heart attack. The log-odds of heart attack increase by 1.07 for each unit increase in the predictor (number of cigarettes smoked per day).

You probably do not have much of a feel for what an increase in log-odds of 1.07 really means in terms of how big the increase is. Neither do we – log-odds is not an intuitive metric to work with. Fortunately, we can convert log-odds to a more familiar metric very easily. Log-odds can easily be transformed into odds-ratios, and SPSS does this automatically in the logistic regression output. We discussed odds-ratios in Chapter 5. Odds-ratios can never be less than 0. A value between 0 and 1 means that increasing scores on the predictor are associated with less risk of the outcome happening. A value greater than 1 indicates that higher predictor scores are associated with a greater chance of the outcome. An odds-ratio of 1 means there is no relationship between the predictor variable and the outcome. In our example the odds-ratio is 2.93. When comparing odds in terms of ratios we are saying that the odds of heart attack are 2.93 times bigger after a one-unit increase in the predictor. This means that the odds of heart attack are *multiplied* by 2.93 for each extra cigarette smoked per day. Don't forget this is a fictional dataset!

We will see more of the features available in logistic regression as we work through the full dataset from the fictional smoking and heart attack study using SPSS.

Activity 13.1

You can work through the logistic regression with us, using the data set cardiac.sav which is available on our website.

1) To run a logistic regression analysis choose *Analyze*, *Regression*, *Binary Logistic* (Screenshot 13.1).

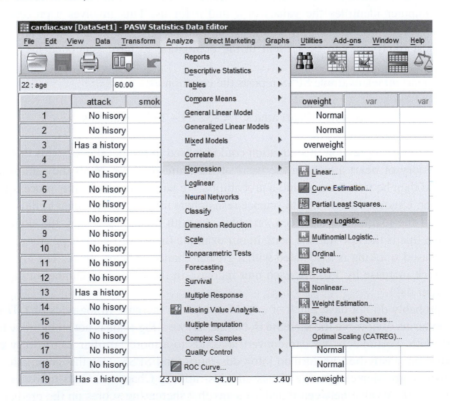

Screenshot 13.1

Next you will see a dialogue box (Screenshot 13.2).

2) The outcome variable, *attacks*, is coded 1 for those who have had a heart attack and 0 for those who have not. It is always important to check the coding of your variables.

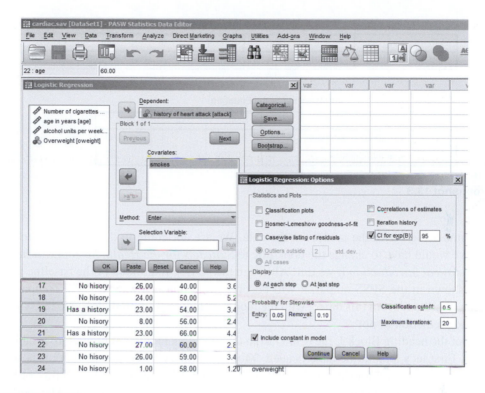

Screenshot 13.2

In SPSS, the logistic regression model will predict the probability of the outcome equalling 1. Move this variable to the *Dependent* box. Move the predictor variable, *smokes* (not *smokes10*), to the covariates box. It is also a good idea to click the *Options* button, as shown, and tick the box to generate confidence intervals on the exp(B) statistic (exp(B) is the odds-ratio). The default setting is for 95% confidence intervals, and this will be what you want for most purposes.

3) Click *Continue* and *OK*. The initial SPSS output (not shown) gives descriptive details including the number of cases, missing values, and the coding of the outcome variable.

Under the heading Block 0, SPSS produces the output shown in Screenshot 13.3.

This model reported here contains no predictor variables. You can see that only the 'Constant' is included in the equation and the *smokes* variable is listed under the heading 'Variables not in the equation'. You may wonder why SPSS produces this output and you will not often want to look at it. However, it is an important component of the calculation so it is worth us spending a few minutes thinking about it.

The model reported in the Block 0 output is a baseline model. This tests how well we can predict the observed outcome without any predictor variables. How well the model prediction fits the observed data is summarised in a statistic called '–2 Log likelihood'. The lower

Variables in the Equation

		B	S.E.	Wald	df	Sig.	Exp(B)
Step 0	Constant	-1.386	.079	307.490	1	.000	.250

Variables not in the Equation

			Score	df	Sig.
Step 0	Variables	smokes	60.360	1	.000
	Overall Statistics		60.360	1	.000

Screenshot 13.3

this number the better the model fits the data. We are not going to discuss the calculation here; we would have to change the book title to *Statistics for the Health Sciences: A heavily mathematical introduction* if we did! Although the −2 Log likelihood of the baseline model is not shown in the SPSS output, it will become important below. SPSS will compare the −2 Log likelihood from this model with the model including your predictor(s) to tell whether they aid prediction or not.

Under the heading Block 1, the results from the model including our predictor variable are shown. First let's look at the table headed 'Model Summary' (Screenshot 13.4); this shows the −2 Log likelihood for this model as 937.78. The model predicts the probability of heart attack (in the form of logit(heart attack′)) for each observation in the analysis. The model fit is based on how well this prediction fits observed heart attack status.

Next look at the Omnibus Tests of Model Coefficients (Screenshot 13.5).

Model Summary

Step	-2 Log likelihood	Cox & Snell R Square	Nagelkerke R Square
1	937.777[a]	.061	.097

a. Estimation terminated at iteration number 5 because parameter estimates changed by less than .001.

Screenshot 13.4

Omnibus Tests of Model Coefficients

		Chi-square	df	Sig.
Step 1	Step	63.028	1	.000
	Block	63.028	1	.000
	Model	63.028	1	.000

Screenshot 13.5

This table compares the −2 Log likelihood of the current model with the baseline model. The reported chi-square statistic is calculated from the difference between the −2 Log likelihoods of the two models. Incidentally we can infer the −2 Log likelihood of the baseline model by adding the −2 Log likelihood of the current model to the difference between the two models (you won't usually want to do this, however):

$$937.78 + 63.03 = 1000.81$$

The larger the difference the better the model with predictors is doing at predicting the outcome variable relative to the baseline. In this case the improvement in fit is significant (chi-square(1) = 63.03, $p < .001$). This tells us that adding the smoking predictor gives a significantly better prediction of heart attack compared to the baseline model. If this test was non-significant then there would not be any evidence that the predictor variable was helpful in predicting the outcome. The degrees of freedom for this test are calculated as the number of extra parameters estimated in the new model. We have one extra parameter here: the b coefficient for cigarettes smoked (both models estimate the constant). This chi-square test of significance is analogous to the ANOVA test of the overall fit of a linear regression model as described in Chapter 11.

In Chapter 11 you also saw that a linear regression model provides you with an R^2 measure of how much variation in the outcome variable is explained by the predictor(s). In logistic regression, calculation of an analogous statistic is not so straightforward and several different methods have been put forward. SPSS provides the results from two approaches; the Cox and Snell and the Nagelkerke R^2 measures. The Nagelkerke approach seems to be the one that is most often reported, so we suggest you focus on this one. These are shown in the Model Summary table (Screenshot 13.6).

Logit(heart attack′) may easily be converted into predicted probability of heart attack. The SPSS output shows a classification table (Screenshot 13.7) which tells us how well the model does in terms of predicting who has had a heart attack and who has not. If the predicted probability for a case is above .5 then it is classified as a predicted heart attack. If it is below .5 then the prediction is classified as no heart attack. Overall, this model is classifying 80.5% of the sample correctly. This may sound impressive, but it is little improvement on the baseline model accuracy shown in Block 0 of the SPSS output (80% accuracy).

The next part of the SPSS output (Screenshot 13.8) shows how the predictor variable relates to the outcome.

Model Summary

Step	-2 Log likelihood	Cox & Snell R Square	Nagelkerke R Square
1	937.777[a]	.061	.097

a. Estimation terminated at iteration number 5 because parameter estimates changed by less than .001

Screenshot 13.6

Classification Table[a]

Observed			Predicted		
			history of heart attack		
			No hisory	Has a history	Percentage Correct
Step 1	history of heart attack	No hisory	798	2	99.8
		Has a history	193	7	3.5
	Overall Percentage				80.5

a. The cut value is .500

Screenshot 13.7

Variables in the Equation

		B	S.E.	Wald	df	Sig.	Exp(B)	95% C.I.for EXP(B)	
								Lower	Upper
Step 1[a]	smokes	.094	.013	56.255	1	.000	1.098	1.072	1.126
	Constant	-3.370	.291	134.133	1	.000	.034		

a. Variable(s) entered on step 1: smokes.

Screenshot 13.8

As noted above, the logistic regression model has the form

$$\text{logit } (\hat{y}) = a + bx$$

We can flesh out the equation from Screenshot 13.8, looking in the column headed B. The constant is a in the equation (−3.37). The *smokes* line shows the b coefficient which is the predicted increase in log-odds of heart attack for a one cigarette increase in daily smoking (.09). As the log-odds coefficient is positive, we know that more smoking is associated with increased chance of heart attack. We can calculate the logit(heart attack´) for each participant using this equation. For example, for a participant who smokes 11 cigarettes per day the equation would be:

$$\text{logit } (\text{heart attack}´) = -3.37 + (.09 \times 11) = -2.38$$

We can convert the logit back to the odds and then to the probability with a simple sum that has been confined to a footnote.[2] This gives an individual smoking 11 cigarettes per day a .08 probability of having had a heart attack (based on this fictional data).

Activity 13.2

If someone smokes 42 cigarettes per day, what is their logit(heart attack´)?

As with linear regression SPSS also produces a significance test for each predictor in the model. In the case of logistic regression this is a Wald test rather than a *t*-test. The Wald statistic is calculated by dividing the log-odds by the estimated standard error (shown in the S.E. column of the SPSS output) and squaring the result. The significance of the Wald statistic is tested using the chi-square distribution. It is highly significant here ($p < .001$), confirming that higher levels of smoking are significantly associated with a greater chance of heart attack.

As noted above, log-odds is not a convenient metric to work in, whereas the odds-ratio is more intuitive. SPSS provides the odds-ratio for a one cigarette increase in smoking in the exp(B) column (1.10) also shown in Screenshot 13.8. The odds-ratio may be interpreted as the odds of heart attack being multiplied by 1.10 for each extra cigarette smoked per day. The 95% confidence intervals on the odds-ratio are also provided here as we asked for these in the options when setting up the analysis. We can interpret these as showing that we are 95% confident that the odds-ratio in the population lies somewhere between 1.07 and 1.13. As odds-ratios are easier to interpret than log-odds we shall focus on them for interpretation.

It is important to note that *both* the log-odds and the odds-ratio are unstandardised. There is nothing analogous to the beta coefficient in linear regression presented here. If you change the scale that cigarette smoking is measured on, then you will change both the log-odds and the odds-ratio. We chose to scale the predictor so that one unit equates to one cigarette per day. We might want to rescale the smoking predictor so that one unit equates to 10 cigarettes. To do this we could simply divide the smoking variable by 10 before running the analysis. If we do this, the log-odds coefficient is .938 and the odds-ratio is 2.56 (95% confidence interval 2.00, 3.27). The significance of the predictor and fit of the model does not alter at all, however. We have included smoke divided by 10 in the cardiac.sav data file on the companion website in case you would like to check this yourself.

WRITING UP THE RESULT

You might have felt that logistic regression produces a lot of complex information which is tricky to interpret. However, when you write up your results you usually don't need to include much detail. In particular it is best to focus on the odds-ratio as the log-odds are not intuitive to understand. With reference to the present example you might say:

> *A logistic regression model was conducted to test whether frequency of smoking predicted a history of heart attack. The analysis showed that more frequent smoking was significantly associated with heart attack (chi-square(1) = 63.03, p < .001). The odds-ratio for an increase of 10 cigarettes per day was 2.56 (95% confidence interval: 2.00, 3.27).*

LOGISTIC REGRESSION WITH MULTIPLE PREDICTOR VARIABLES

So far we have only seen logistic regression with one predictor variable. Logistic regression can also accommodate multiple predictors. As such, it works much like the multiple regression models that you saw in Chapter 12 except that the outcome variable is binary. The logistic regression equation with multiple predictors has the following form:

$$\text{logit (outcome}') = a + (b_1 x_1) + (b_2 x_2) + (b_3 x_3) \cdots$$

To illustrate logistic regression with multiple predictors we will add more predictors to our fictional data set predicting history of heart attack in a sample of smokers. The variables we will add are

- Age (measured in years)
- Alcohol consumption (measured on a scale where one unit equals five units of alcohol per week)

Activity 13.3

Let's run the analysis in SPSS from the cardiac.sav dataset. We need to find the logistic regression dialogue box in the same way that we saw above. You should set up the dialogue box so it looks like Screenshot 13.9.

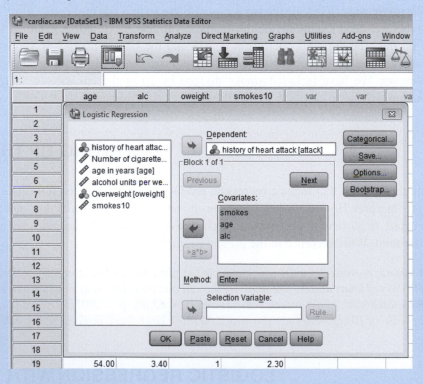

Screenshot 13.9

Don't forget to ask for 95% confidence intervals on the odds-ratio (exp(B)) from the *Options* dialogue box.

In Block 0 of the output we again find a baseline model without any predictors, only the constant. This is exactly the same output that we saw above, so we will not dwell on it again here. Our model with three predictors will be compared against this baseline.

In Block 1 we see the results regarding the model with all three predictor variables included. The Omnibus Tests of Model Coefficients (Screenshot 13.10) compares the overall model fit to the baseline model. The chi-square value is the difference between the -2 Log likelihood of the two models. There are three degrees of freedom because there are three more parameters in this model than in the baseline model: one each for the smoking, alcohol and age b coefficients. This test is significant (chi-square$(3) = 153.03$, $p < .001$), showing that the overall model is a significantly better fit to the data than the baseline model.

Omnibus Tests of Model Coefficients

		Chi-square	df	Sig.
Step 1	Step	153.027	3	.000
	Block	153.027	3	.000
	Model	153.027	3	.000

Screenshot 13.10

The Model Summary (Screenshot 13.11) contains the R^2 measures that provide a more interpretable assessment of how well the overall model fits the data.

Model Summary

Step	-2 Log likelihood	Cox & Snell R Square	Nagelkerke R Square
1	847.778[a]	.142	.224

a. Estimation terminated at iteration number 5 because parameter estimates changed by less than .001

Screenshot 13.11

Information on the individual predictors is presented in the Variables in the Equation table (Screenshot 13.12).

Variables in the Equation

		B	S.E.	Wald	df	Sig.	Exp(B)	95% C.I.for EXP(B) Lower	Upper
Step 1[a]	smokes	.053	.015	12.601	1	.000	1.055	1.024	1.086
	age	.060	.009	45.422	1	.000	1.061	1.043	1.080
	alc	.619	.106	33.768	1	.000	1.857	1.507	2.288
	Constant	-7.880	.660	142.636	1	.000	.000		

a. Variable(s) entered on step 1: smokes, age, alc.

Screenshot 13.12

Let's start by looking at the *smokes* line. This was the variable we used when predicting heart attack with a single variable in the previous analysis. When there was only one predictor we found an odds-ratio of 1.10. In this model we have exactly the same heart attack and smoking scores but we have added extra predictors as well. After adding the new predictors, smoking now has an odds-ratio of 1.06. The Wald test shows this effect is significant ($p < .001$).

So smoking has a lower odds-ratio in this model including other predictors than when it was the only predictor. Why has this happened? The answer is that when there are multiple predictors in the model, only the *independent* contribution of each predictor is represented in these figures. Only the contribution of smoking that is not associated with alcohol use and age is represented here. The interpretation of the odds-ratio for smoking from this model are similar to those from the single predictor model with a small addition. We can say that a one cigarette increase multiplies the odds of heart attack by 1.06 *holding the other predictors constant*.

The other predictors in the model may be interpreted in a similar way. For example, on the weekly alcohol scale a one-point increase in alcohol consumption (which actually represents five alcohol units) has an odds-ratio of 1.9. So does this imply alcohol consumption is a more important predictor of heart attack than smoking? No. Remember the log-odds and odds-ratios are dependent upon the scale of measurement. As we saw above, the size of the odds-ratio for smoking varied depending on whether one unit represents a one cigarette increase or a 10 cigarette increase in daily use. To make the predictors more comparable you could standardise them (as described in Chapter 4) prior to analysis. This puts all the predictors onto the same scale, which has a mean of 0 and a standard deviation of 1. Creating *z*-scores of this sort is easy to do in SPSS:

Select Analyze, Descriptive Statistics, Descriptives (Screenshot 13.13)

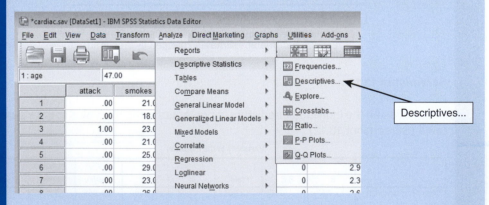

Screenshot 13.13

In the dialogue box, move the variables to be standardised into the *Variables* list. For our current purposes the most important thing to do is to tick the box for *Save standardized values as variables* as shown in Screenshot 13.14. Then click *OK*.

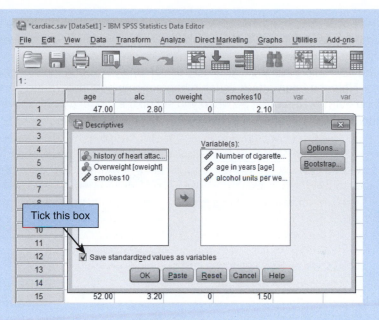

Screenshot 13.14

When you do this, the output will show the descriptive statistics (mean, standard deviation, etc.) for the variables you selected. However, we are not particularly interested in this output for our current purposes. If you look at the dataset (in the *Data View*) you will see extra columns have been added with a Z in front of the variables names (Screenshot 13.15).

Zsmokes	Zage	Zalc
.16801	-.81885	-.15640
-.25343	1.35055	-2.32581
.44897	1.44916	1.02692
.16801	-2.49521	.43526
.72993	-1.01607	1.42136
1.29186	1.15333	-.74805
.44897	-.02998	-.94527
.87041	.75890	-.55083
-1.65823	1.74499	.04082
-.95583	-.42441	.04082
-.53439	1.05473	-.35361
1.29186	-1.01607	.43526
.02753	1.05473	.43526
.30849	.06863	-.15640

Screenshot 13.15

(sidebar) **Activity 13.3 Cont'd**

These are the standardised versions of the predictors with means of 0 and standard deviations of 1. You can check this using the *Descriptives* command if you don't believe us!

Now we will re-run the logistic regression analysis using the standardised predictors. Note the heart attack variable has not changed, but we are going to predict it using our new *z*-scores. So when you set up the model (check above if you need a reminder) it should look like Screenshot 13.16.

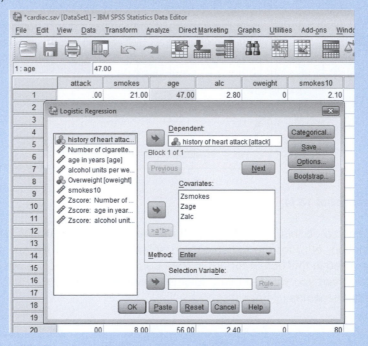

Screenshot 13.16

Most of the results will look exactly as they did when we used the unstandardised predictors. This includes the Wald statistics and associated *p*-values for the predictors. Standardising the predictors does not change their fundamental association with the outcome. The odds-ratios (and log-odds) coefficients for the predictors should look different, however, as shown in Screenshot 13.17.

								95% C.I.for EXP(B)	
		B	S.E.	Wald	df	Sig.	Exp(B)	Lower	Upper
Step 1[a]	Zsmokes	.379	.107	12.601	1	.000	1.461	1.185	1.802
	Zage	.604	.090	45.422	1	.000	1.829	1.534	2.180
	Zalc	.628	.108	33.768	1	.000	1.873	1.516	2.314
	Constant	-1.702	.100	288.148	1	.000	.182		

Variables in the Equation

a. Variable(s) entered on step 1: Zsmokes, Zage, Zalc.

Screenshot 13.17

In the standardised scores, a single unit represents 1 standard deviation. Therefore the exp(B) column shows the odds-ratios associated with a 1 standard deviation increase in each predictor. For example, a 1 standard deviation increase in smoking multiplies the odds of heart attack by 1.46 (95% confidence interval 1.19, 1.80). A 1 standard deviation increase in age multiplies the odds by 1.80 (95% confidence interval 1.53, 2.18). As all the predictors are now scored on the same scales, comparisons now make more sense.

Answering questions about which predictors are more important though, is not necessarily straightforward. Comparison between predictors may be made more difficult by patterns of inter-correlation between predictors. 'Importance' may also mean different things in different contexts.

LOGISTIC REGRESSION WITH CATEGORICAL PREDICTORS

As well as handling continuous predictor variables, logistic regression can also include categorical predictors (as can linear regression). We will extend the heart attack example by adding a categorical predictor which can take on one of two values (note predictor values taking on any number of values can be included); participants are coded as either overweight or normal weight, depending on whether their body-mass index is above 25. This variable is called *oweight* in the cardiac.sav dataset.

Access the logistic regression dialogue box as described above, and set *attack* as the dependent variable and oweight as a covariate. Then press the *Categorical* button and move *oweight* from the covariates list to the *Categorical Covariates* list as shown in Screenshot 13.18. The reference category setting is very important to the interpretation, as we will show you. In this first run, click the Radio button for *First* as shown in Screenshot 13.18 and then click the *Change* button immediately above it.

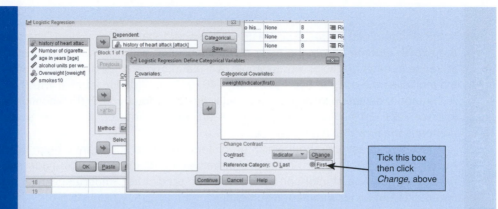

Tick this box then click *Change*, above

Screenshot 13.18

Then press *Continue* and *OK* to run the model. In most ways the model runs as the previous logistic regression models we have seen. The Variables in the Equation box is shown in Screenshot 13.19.

Variables in the Equation

| | | B | S.E. | Wald | df | Sig. | Exp(B) | 95% C.I.for EXP(B) | |
								Lower	Upper
Step 1[a]	oweight(1)	1.211	.165	54.090	1	.000	3.358	2.432	4.638
	Constant	-1.977	.125	250.543	1	.000	.139		

a. Variable(s) entered on step 1: oweight.

Screenshot 13.19

As this is a categorical variable predictor with two levels, the coefficients refer to comparisons of the odds at the two different levels of the predictor. The dialogue box was setup with the reference category of *First*. The first category is the one with the lowest coding. In our case it is 0 which indicates normal weight. The output compares all the other categories of *oweight* to this one. In this example there is only one other category, overweight, coded as 1. So the output on the *oweight(1)* line compares the people in the overweight category to those in the normal weight category. If we look at the odds-ratio we can see that the odds of heart attack are 3.36 times higher for overweight men than normal weight men. The Wald test shows that this is a significant effect ($p < .001$), and the confidence intervals show us that we are 95% confident that the odds-ratio in the population falls between 2.43 and 4.64.

To become more familiar with categorical predictors, re-run the analysis but select *Last* as the referent category when setting up the model, as shown in Screenshot 13.20.

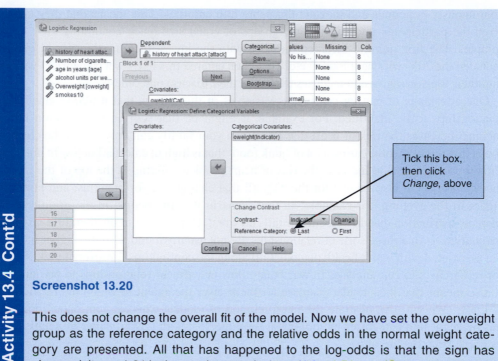

Screenshot 13.20

This does not change the overall fit of the model. Now we have set the overweight group as the reference category and the relative odds in the normal weight category are presented. All that has happened to the log-odds is that the sign has changed: it was 1.21 in the previous analysis and it is –1.21 now (Screenshot 13.21). The odds-ratio looks a lot different now though, at .30. Remember, an odds-ratio less than 0 is not possible. This result shows that the odds decrease by a factor of .30 when comparing normal weight people to overweight people. Thus, there is a lower probability of having a heart attack for men of normal weight.

Variables in the Equation

		B	S.E.	Wald	df	Sig.	Exp(B)	95% C.I.for EXP(B) Lower	Upper
Step 1[a]	oweight(1)	-1.211	.165	54.090	1	.000	.298	.216	.411
	Constant	-.765	.107	50.764	1	.000	.465		

a. Variable(s) entered on step 1: oweight.

Screenshot 13.21

CATEGORICAL PREDICTORS WITH THREE OR MORE LEVELS

Many researchers will decide to cut continuous predictors into discrete categories. For example, as we will see below, Emerson et al. (2006) were predicting the presence of a range of health outcomes with family income using logistic regression. Income was measured continuously in pounds and they cut this score into quintiles. This means that they catego-rized the participants into five income groups of equal size (each containing 20% of the sample). The first quintile included the 20% with the lowest income, the second quintile included the 20% with next lowest, etc. They then entered this five-level categorical variable into their logistic regression analyses to predict their disease outcomes.

One advantage of cutting continuous variables in this way is that it allows curvilinear relationships to be identified. For example, it might be that scoring very low on family income increases the risk of heart disease. When your family can only afford the cheapest foods this might involve eating a lot of 'junk food' that is high in calories but low in nutrition. This type of diet could increase the risk of heart problems. Being at the top of the income distribution could also be bad for the diet: all that champagne for breakfast and port with cigars in the evening, for example! In this scenario it is the people in the middle of the income distribution that do best and the tails do worst. Our reading of the literature on health inequalities is that these sorts of relationships are not usually found. Usually higher incomes are associated with better health outcomes all along the continuum. However, it makes sense for researchers to run analyses in ways that allow curvilinear relationships to be detected. It also means that their readers can see for themselves the extent to which the relationship is linear. We will demonstrate the interpretation of models where a continuous predictor has been cut into categories by looking at the Emerson et al. (2006) paper in detail in our example from the literature.

Example from the Literature

Emerson et al. (2006) used the British Child and Adolescent Mental Health Survey to examine whether social inequalities in a range of health outcomes were present in childhood and adolescence. The survey included 10,438 young people from across the UK. The health outcomes studied were all constructed as binary mea-sures and analysed using logistic regression. Some of these were naturally binary, such as eczema, asthma and psychiatric disorder (all coded as present or absent). They also studied the answer to a general question about health status which was coded on a five-point scale (very good, good, fair, bad and very bad). To make this variable into a binary outcome suitable for logistic regression they collapsed (i.e. combined) the very good and good categories to form a 'good' category and the fair, bad and very bad categories to form a 'fair to very bad' category.

These outcome variables were predicted from household income using logistic regression. Income quintile (described above) was entered into logistic regression models as a categorical variable to predict the health outcomes. The authors exam-ined whether the effect of income differed for boys and girls and for younger (5–10-years-old) and older (11–15-years-old) children. We report the analyses for younger children in Table 13.1. Note that each line of the table reports a separate logistic regression model.

Table 13.1

Outcome	Prevalence	Income quintile					Nagalkerke R^2	p-value
		1 (low)	2	3	4	5 (high)		
Fair–very bad health (boys)	7%	3.4*	2.4*	2.0*	1.3	1	.03	<.001
Asthma (boys)	18%	1.8*	1.6*	1.4*	1.4	1	.01	<.01
Eczema (boys)	14%	1.1	.9	.8	.9	1	.00	n.s.
Eczema (girls)	15%	.6*	.8	1.0	.8	1	.01	<.05
Psychiatric disorder (boys)	10%	3.0*	2.1*	1.2	1.1	1	.04	<.001

*p <.05

There are a number of interesting features in these results. First, we will look at the statistics for overall model fit, starting with the p-values. This is the significance test on the differences between the fit for the models including income as a predictor and the baseline models including no predictors. These are significant in all cases except eczema in boys; there is no evidence that income predicts eczema in boys. In all other cases knowing about income improves the prediction of whether a child has the outcomes studied. Next we will look at the Nagalkerke R^2 estimates, which provide an indication of how well knowing income improves prediction of disorder. In all cases these look quite low. Even very small effects will be significant in large datasets. However, statistically small effects may be very important in terms of public health policy.

Next, look at the odds-ratios. Remember income was entered as a five-category predictor. Quintile 5, containing the highest income families, has been chosen as the reference category. All other quintiles are separately compared to this reference category. The odds-ratios shown are the odds of disorder in each quintile relative to the odds in the reference category. Therefore the odds-ratios shown in the reference category column are 1. Where odds-ratios are significantly different from 1 (p < .05) they have been marked with an *. For example, the odds of having fair–very bad health in the poorest quintile is significantly different from those in the richest quintile. The odds-ratio is quoted as 3.4. This means the odds of poor health are 3.4 times greater in the poorest quintile relative to the richest quintile. The odds in the second quintile of income is also significantly different from the reference category; the odds-ratio is quoted as 2.4. Are the odds in quintile 1 different from quintile 2 (the two most affluent quintiles)? This is not clear from the results as presented here. The question could be answered by re-running the model specifying a different reference category in the predictor variable.

For most of the health outcomes studied here we see the expected social gradient in health; those who are better off have less risk of disease. This is not true for eczema in girls though. Income is a significant predictor of the outcome, but the odds-ratios in lower income quintiles are less than 1. This indicates that the chance of eczema is lower in the lower income quintiles relative to the highest. The only significant comparison is between the lowest and highest income quintiles, however.

Summary

Binary logistic regression is used to analyse outcome variables which can take on one of two values. It shares many similarities with the regression models for continuous outcome variables covered in Chapters 10 and 11. In particular, it may include one or more predictor variables and these may be continuous and/or categorical. As we have seen in the Example from the Literature it is common for health science researchers to cut up continuous variables into groups and use the groups as categorical predictors.

As in other types of regression, logistic regression provides a significance test of the overall model and indices of how well the model fits the data. The relationship between the predictors and the outcome are most usefully expressed as odds-ratios. Binary logistic regression is widely used by health scientists and forms the basis of many more advanced models as well. Therefore it is a key technique for you to become familiar with.

MULTIPLE CHOICE QUESTIONS

1. Binary logistic regression may be used with the following types of outcome variables:
   a) Variables that take on one of two possible values
   b) Continuous variables scored on an interval scale
   c) Variables that take on one of many possible values
   d) Continuous variables scored on an interval-ratio scale

2. Logistic regression can include which type of predictor variables?
   a) Continuous
   b) Categorical with only two possible values
   c) Categorical with three or more possible values
   d) a), b) and c) are all correct

3. If a continuous predictor variable has an odds-ratio of 1.4 in a logistic regression model, this implies that for every unit increase in the predictor:
   a) The probability of the outcome increases by 1.4
   b) The probability of the outcome is multiplied by 1.4
   c) The odds of the outcome increase by 1.4
   d) The odds of the outcome are multiplied by 1.4

4. In logistic regression the baseline model contains:
   a) A white line which you must stand behind when serving
   b) All your predictor variables and a constant term
   c) A constant but no predictor variables
   d) All the predictor variables but no constant

5. Log-odds can take on values between:
   a) – infinity and infinity
   b) 0 and 1
   c) 0 and infinity
   d) −1 and 1

6. In logistic regression, −2 Log likelihood measures:
   a) Model fit: the higher the value, the better the fit
   b) Model fit: the lower the value the better the fit
   c) The probability of a Type 1 error
   d) The chances of tripping over a log when running (multiplied by −2)

7. Which of the following would be suitable predictor variables in a logistic regression model?
   a) Heart rate (measured in beats per minute)
   b) Waist/hip ratio (cut into quintiles)
   c) Gender (male or female)
   d) All of the above

The next questions refer to a study predicting the presence of depression from severity of life events over the previous six months (measured on a continuous scale, with higher scores indicating greater severity) and gender (coded $0 =$ female, $1 =$ male).

The model summary output showed:

Omnibus Tests of Model Coefficients

		Chi-square	df	Sig.
Step 1	Step	24.664	2	.000
	Block	24.664	2	.000
	Model	24.664	2	.000

Model Summary

Step	-2 Log likelihood	Cox & Snell R Square	Nagelkerke R Square
1	20.323[a]	.460	.682

a. Estimation terminated at iteration number 7 because parameter estimates changed by less than .001.

8. Why are there two degrees of freedom in the Omnibus Tests of Model Coefficients?
   a) Because depression can take on two possible values
   b) Because the baseline model contains two additional parameters
   c) Because the model including predictors contains two additional parameters
   d) Because gender can take on two possible values

9. Does the model as a whole significantly improve prediction of depression relative to the baseline model?
   a) No
   b) Yes, because the chi-square test is significant
   c) Yes, because the Nagalkerke R^2 is above 0
   d) Yes because the -2 Log likelihood is positive

The Variables in the Equation output from the model predicting depression is shown below:

Variables in the Equation

	B	S.E.	Wald	df	Sig.	Exp(B)	95% C.I.for EXP(B) Lower	Upper
Step 1[a] lifeevents	.928	.300	9.575	1	.002	2.529	1.405	4.552
gender(1)	.403	1.278	.099	1	.752	1.497	.122	18.332
Constant	-10.084	3.086	10.679	1	.001	.000		

a. Variable(s) entered on step 1: lifeevents, gender.

10. How are the Wald statistics calculated?
    a) The log-odds^2/standard error
    b) The log-odds/standard error^2
    c) The (log-odds/standard error)^2
    d) By thinking of a number and then doubling it

11. According to the Wald tests, which predictor(s) make a significant contribution to the model?
    a) Life events
    b) Gender
    c) a) and b)
    d) None of the predictors are significant

12. We can be 95% confident that the population odds-ratio for life events falls between:
    a) We have no idea of the 95% confidence intervals from this output
    b) 1.41 and 4.55
    c) .12 and 18.33
    d) .30 and 9.58

13. If the life events variable was standardised before running the analysis the effect would be:
    a) The overall model fit would change
    b) The Wald significance test of the life events effect would change
    c) The odds-ratio for life events would change
    d) The odds-ratio for gender would change

14. Which of the following are different approaches to calculating R^2 type statistics for logistic regression:
    a) Wald test
    b) Nagelkerke
    c) Cox and Snell
    d) Both b) and c) above

15. If you had an exp(B) of −1.4 what would this mean?
    a) If you increase your predictor variable by one unit the odds of being in the condition coded as 1 would be 1.4 times lower
    b) If you increase your predictor variable by one unit the odds of being in the condition coded as 1 would be 1.4 times higher
    c) You have made a mistake as you cannot have a negative exp(B)
    d) None of the above

Notes

1 We are not going to go into the process of log transformation as we are trying to avoid mathematical detail in this book. If you are interested though, then you can easily find out more with a quick internet search.
2 Converting the log-odds to the odds involves taking the inverse of the natural logarithm of −2.38 which gives .09. The odds can be converted by to a probability by dividing the odds by 1 + odds. This rounds to .08. Odds and probabilities are very similar when the probability is low.

Interventions and Analysis of Change

14

Overview

In this chapter we will focus on measuring and analysing change. We will be explaining how to design research that can measure change in an outcome variable and how to analyse the data from such research designs. We will also explain the importance of proper reporting of intervention and change research. We aim to cover randomised control trials as well as single-case designs and will we also explain how to carry out the analyses we cover in SPSS.

   Thus in this chapter you will learn about:

- Interventions
- Randomised Control Trials (RCTs)
- CONSORT guidelines for reporting RCTs
- Analysis of RCTs
- Single-case designs
- Visual analysis of single-case designs
- Running the analyses using SPSS

(Continued)

(Continued)

In order to best understand our discussions in this chapter you should make sure that you have read the chapter on measuring associations (Chapter 9), differences between two groups (Chapter 7) and differences between three groups (Chapter 8).

INTERVENTIONS

Much medical and health science research is designed to measure the effectiveness of one treatment or another. Such treatments can be pharmaceutical in nature or they might be physical, surgical or even psychological. We often call these treatments 'interventions'. An intervention is simply some means of researchers (or practitioners for that matter) intervening to alter some variable of interest. Usually, in the health sciences the variables of interest are disease or health relevant variables and so an intervention is often some procedure designed to reduce disease or increase healthy behaviours (e.g. exercising more or using dental floss). If you think about it, interventions are quite similar to independent variables in the typical experiment that we described in Chapter 1. In the typical experiment we have a variable that we are interested in (the dependent variable) and we manipulate another variable (the independent variable) to see if it has an effect on the dependent variable. We suggested in Chapter 1 that an experimental design consists of an independent variable where participants are randomly allocated to the different conditions of this variable, and then we do something different to each group (e.g. give them different treatments) to see what effect this has on the dependent variable. The treatments that we introduce as conditions of the independent variable could, within the context of clinical research, be regarded as interventions.

HOW DO WE KNOW WHETHER INTERVENTIONS ARE EFFECTIVE?

Let us imagine a scenario. You are a clinician and you think you have a fantastic new way of treating people with halitosis. You therefore invite people with halitosis to take part in a trial for your new intervention. You find that most of the people who take part improve in terms of their symptoms of halitosis. On the face of it your treatment seems to have worked as most people see an improvement. But a moment's thought (or rereading Chapter 1) would bring to mind a number of problems with trying to draw conclusions from this trial. First of all, how do we know that your treatment has improved symptoms; it might be that the participants in your study had spontaneous improvements in their breath, or perhaps taking part in your study led them to be more mindful of their condition, and they took additional measures to improve their symptoms beyond those that you included in your intervention. Also, if you were the person assessing symptoms before and after the intervention you might have subconsciously biased your assessment of symptoms in line with your expectations. And of course, the difference in halitosis symptoms that you observe before and after your intervention might simply be due to sampling error. These are all problems associated with trying to determine whether or not an intervention has been effective.

Example from the Literature

Porter and Scully (2006) present a brief paper on the causes and treatment of halitosis (or oral malodour). Although this is not a research paper it does provide a nice overview of the treatment of halitosis and suggests that gentle tongue cleaning and a mouthwash of chlorhexidine gluconate are effective, at least in the short term. It is interesting to note, however, that the evidence that they cite for the benefits of chlorhexidine gluconate is only a pilot study (Quirynen et al., 1998).

What Then Do We Need?

A first important improvement to the design would be to introduce a no intervention condition so that we would have a comparison group to act as a 'control'. If we get more improvement in the intervention group then we have better evidence for the efficacy of the new intervention. One problem with such a design relates to how you allocate people to conditions. For example, you might allocate the first 20 people to the new intervention group and the next 20 people to the control group. The problem with such a method of allocation is that there might be some characteristic that distinguishes the first 20 people who volunteer for your study from the last 20 people. Perhaps the first volunteers are much keener to improve their symptoms and it is this that accounts for the later improvements rather than your intervention. We therefore need to have a less systematic way of allocating participants to groups. We should ideally use random allocation (we touched on this in Chapter 1, see page 12). If we randomly allocate participants to the two groups (e.g. through the flip of a coin or using random number lists) then any differences between the two groups (e.g. in terms of motivation, etc.) are likely to be minimised and be random in nature. With such a method of allocating participants we can be much more confident that it is our new intervention that has led to an improvement in symptoms rather than some other extraneous variable that we have failed to control for.

Blinding

A control group and random allocation of participants to conditions are ways of making sure that our assessment of the intervention is reliable. However, on their own they do not make for a perfect research design. We alluded to one of the reasons for this earlier. If you have devised the new intervention and then you yourself decide to assess both the control and intervention groups for their symptoms of halitosis before and after the intervention then you might be unwittingly biased in your assessment of the symptoms. This is often inescapable no matter how hard we try as researchers. Also, even if you have been completely unbiased in your assessments you are still open to this criticism from doubters of your new intervention. They might reasonably say 'ah but you knew which group each participant was in and therefore you may have been biased in your recording of symptoms'. This is a difficult charge to allay in such a study, and so how do we get around this?

We get around it through *blinding*. Blinding is where you as a researcher do not know which condition each participant has been allocated to. If you are kept blind to each participant's trial condition your assessments of symptoms cannot be influenced by the condition they were in, nor by your prior expectations. Blinding is a crucial part of a clinical trial. At the very least you need to have the researchers blind to the condition that each participant is allocated to. Such a procedure would be known as *single blinding*.

We are now creating a good research design which will enable us to determine the effectiveness of the new intervention. Are there any other problems that we need to overcome? Well, yes there are. We have looked at the problem of researcher bias influencing the outcome, but what about participant bias? Quite often participants are very keen to do what the researcher wants them to do, and they modify their behaviour to please the researcher. This means that it might not be the intervention that is effective but other behaviour changes in the participants. Such subtle changes from the participants are often called *demand effect*. Another problem has to do with the *placebo effect*. The placebo effect arises when the intervention that a participant receives has no active ingredient, but still leads to an improvement of symptoms. For example, when trying to establish whether or not a new drug is effective we would give some of our participants a pill that looks like the new drug but which has no active ingredient (e.g. a sugar pill). The participant would then not know whether they are getting the new treatment or the placebo, and thus we could see how strong the placebo effect is for the trials being carried out. In order for this to work, participants have to be randomly allocated to the placebo and intervention conditions and they must be naïve (or blind) to the condition that they are in. That is, they must either all believe that they getting a sugar pill, all believe that they are getting the intervention or not know whether they are getting the placebo or the actual intervention. In such a study the participants are said to be blind to the intervention. When we combine blinding of the researchers with blinding of the participants then we have what is known as a *double blind* study. And such procedures make our findings much more reliable and much less open to question by other researchers and clinicians.

The Placebo Effect

There is considerable evidence that the placebo effect has a strong influence on participants' responses (e.g. Price et al., 2008). A placebo effect occurs when a participant in a study receives an intervention which has no obvious meaningful 'active ingredient'.

(Continued)

An example would be participants in a study of the effects of paracetemol on migraine headaches being given a sugar pill rather than a paracetemol tablet. The sugar pill contains no obvious active analgesic ingredient, and so on the face of it should have no beneficial effects on the relief of migraine pain. If the sugar pill is acting as a placebo we would see an improvement in the migraine symptoms of those participants who were given these as a treatment. Although there is considerable evidence for the existence of placebo effects there is also research which suggests that these effects might not be reliable. For example, Hrobjartsson and Gotzsche (2001) found that the strength of the placebo effect appears to be related to the size of the sample, and thus they suggested that such effects were unreliable. This was a finding that they replicated three years later (Hrobjartsson and Gotzsche, 2004).

Although there is still a little controversy surrounding the placebo effect we still need to take account of these effects in our trials. For this reason we need to be sure to include blinding in studies where possible and appropriate.

Activity 14.1

Think about our halitosis example. Write down how you would be able to discount a placebo effect explanation for the improvements that we might observe in our new intervention condition (you can find some suggestions from us about this at the back of the book).

RANDOMISED CONTROL TRIALS (RCTs)

We have now outlined all the major elements of perhaps the most robust way of researching the effectiveness of an intervention, the randomised control trial (RCT). The RCT has the following key features:

- Intervention and one or more control conditions
- Random allocation of participants to conditions
- Blinding (usually at least double blinding)

Because of these features, such research is held to be the 'gold standard' for clinical trials. Some authors have suggested that there is a hierarchy of research methods in terms of the reliability of the evidence provided by them. An example 'evidence ladder' (taken from Sutherland, 2001) is presented in Figure 14.1.

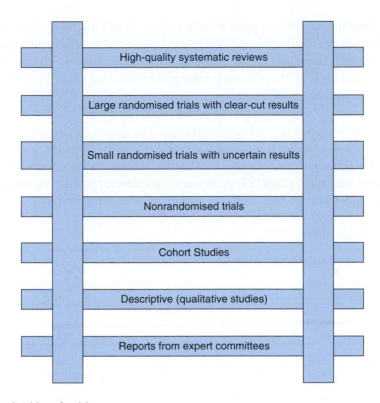

Figure 14.1 Ladder of evidence

You can see that at the top of the ladder are systematic reviews of published research, but on the next rung down sit RCTs. Given that systematic reviews are only as good as the studies on which they are based, then it can be reasonably be argued that RCTs are the most important rung in this ladder. Without RCTs we would not have good quality research on which to base the systematic reviews.

DESIGNING AN RCT: CONSORT

How would you go about designing an RCT? There are a number of critical things that we have to consider in order to run a high quality RCT. In the past, published RCTs have been extremely variable in quality, and because of this researchers and journal editors got together to generate some guidelines for running and reporting RCTs. These guidelines are called CONSORT which stands for Consolidated Standard of Reporting Trials and were originally published by Begg et al. in 1996. The latest version of CONSORT (Moher et al., 2010) contains a 25-item checklist and a flow diagram that researchers can use to help them design and report their RCTs. The 25-item checklist is focussed on the features of the RCT that should be reported when the researchers publish their findings (see Table 14.1). If you have a look at the checklist you can see that it is divided into the sections typically included in a research report (i.e. Abstract, Introduction, Method, Results and Discussion). Within each of these sections is an indication of the minimum information required about the RCT. If you are designing and reporting an RCT then you should consult this CONSORT table and you should also consult the original paper by Moher et al. (2010) which can be found on the CONSORT website (www.consort-statement.org). The paper by Moher et al. contains detailed explanations of what is required for each item in the checklist, and very usefully contains good examples of how to report information about each item in a research report. It should be noted that the CONSORT guidelines were developed with two-group RCTs in mind, but the guidelines can be extended with care to other forms of RCT.

Table 14.1 CONSORT checklist

Section /topic	Item no.	Checklist item	Reported on page no.
Title and Abstract			
	1a	Reported as an RCT in the title	
	1b	Abstract to contain structured summary of research	
Introduction			
Background and objectives	2a	Scientific background and explanation of rationale for the study	
	2b	Identify the specific objectives and hypotheses	
Methods			
Trial designs	3a	Description of trial design including allocation ratio	
	3b	Important changes to methods after trial commencement with reasons	
Participants	4a	Eligibility criteria	
	4b	Settings and locations where the data were collected	
Interventions	5	The interventions for each group with sufficient details to allow replication, including how and when they were administered	
Outcomes	6a	Completely defined pre-specified primary and secondary outcome measures, including how and when they are assessed	
	6b	Changes to trial outcomes after the trial commenced with reasons	
Sample size	7a	Sample size determination	
	7b	Explanation of interim analyses and stopping guidelines	

Table 14.1 Cont'd

Section /topic	Item no.	Checklist item	Reported on page no.
Randomisation:			
Sequence generation	8a	Method used to generate the random allocation sequence	
	8b	Type of randomisation used	
Allocation concealment mechanism	9	Mechanism used to implement the random allocation sequence, including details of steps taken to conceal the sequence until interventions were assigned.	
Implementation	10	Who generated the random allocation sequence, who enrolled participants and who assigned participants to interventions?	
Blinding	11a	If done, who was blinded after assignment to interventions and how?	
	11b	If relevant, description of the similarity of interventions	
Statistical methods	12a	Statistical method used to compare groups for primary and secondary outcomes	
	12b	Methods for additional analyses, such as subgroup analyses	
Results			
Participant flow diagram	13a	For each group the no. of participants who were randomly assigned, received intended treatment and were analysed for primary outcome	
	13b	For each group, losses and exclusions after randomisation, with reasons	
Recruitment	14a	Dates defining periods of recruitment and follow-up	
	14b	Why the trial ended or was stopped	
Baseline data	15	A table showing baseline demographic and clinical characteristics for each group	
Numbers analysed	16	For each group, the number of participants included in each analysis and whether the analysis was by original assigned groups	
Outcomes and estimation	17a	For each primary and secondary outcome, results for each group and the estimated effect size with confidence intervals	
	17b	For binary outcomes, presentation of both absolute and relative effect sizes	

(Continued)

Table 14.1   Cont'd

Section /topic	Item no.	Checklist item	Reported on page no.
Ancillary analyses	18a	Results of any other analysis performed, including subgroup analysis, distinguishing pre-specified from exploratory	
Harms	19	All important harms or unintended effects in each group	
Discussion			
Limitations	20	Limitations addressing sources of potential bias and imprecision	
Generalisability	21	Generalisability or applicability of the trial findings	
Interpretation	22	Interpretation consistent with results, balancing benefits and harms and considering other relevant evidence	
Other information			
Registration	23	Registration number and name of trial registry	
Protocol	24	Where the full trial protocol can be accessed if available	
Funding	25	Sources of funding and other support	

You will notice from the table that there is a column that is headed 'Reported on page no.'. This is for the authors of research papers to indicate on which page of their manuscripts each item in the checklist has been addressed. This checklist ensures not only consistency in reporting of RCTs but also better consistency in their design.

An additional safeguard for the correct reporting and interpretation of RCTs is a requirement to register them before the research is undertaken. Registration of such trials can be made on the International Standard Randomised Control Trial Number Register which can be found at: http://www.controlled-trials.com/isrctn/search.html

When registering a trial we have to supply certain basic information relating to the design and the specific hypotheses being tested. Such registration acts as a safeguard against researchers changing their hypotheses to fit their findings, and ensures that the researchers adhere to the procedures that they have outlined in advance.

THE CONSORT FLOW CHART

The other important component of CONSORT is the encouragement to visually present information about the flow of participants through each phase of the trial with a flow chart.

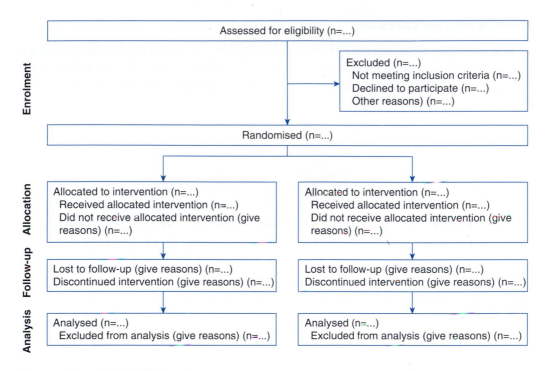

Figure 14.2   CONSORT flow chart

The recommended format of these flow charts is presented in Figure 14.2. This flow chart was developed for the typical two-group RCT but can be modified to represent the same information for more complex designs. If you look at the flow diagram you can see that authors are encouraged to give information about the numbers of participants who were originally assessed for eligibility, then the next stage down contains details of how many were excluded from the study and the reasons for exclusion. This is followed by the randomisation information, in which you are expected to give details of the total number of participants allocated to conditions, as well as how many actually received the interventions in each condition and the reasons why some participants did not receive the intervention. The next level provides information about how many participants were assessed at follow-up, how many were lost to follow-up and how many discontinued the intervention (along with reasons for such discontinuation). Finally, you should provide details of how many participants were included in the analysis from each condition, how many were excluded from analysis, and what reasons there were for such exclusion. Presenting information in such a way provides a clear and concise overview of the numbers of participants involved in the study and allows for appropriate comparison across studies. This also allows other researchers to assess the quality of the RCT that you are reporting.

Example from the Literature

A nice example of a CONSORT flow chart is that presented by Williamson et al. (2009) when presenting their research investigating the impact of a weight management intervention on the quality of life of type 2 diabetes patients. The flow chart that they present is as in Figure 14.3.

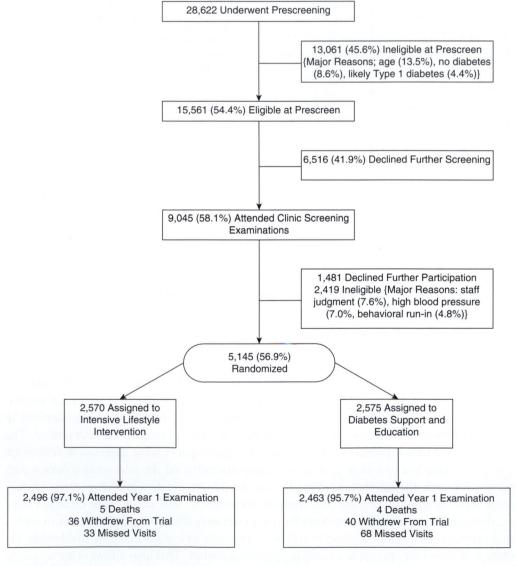

Figure 14.3

You can see from the chart that over 28,000 people underwent the prescreening process, and 54.5% of these were deemed eligible for the study. Of those deemed not eligible, the majority of these were because of their age, because they didn't have diabetes or because they had type 1 diabetes. We can see that of those deemed eligible, 41.9% declined to take part in the study. Of the remaining 9000 or so who attended the clinic for examination, 1481 declined to take part and 2419 were ineligible. This means that just over 5000 participants were randomised. 2570 were allocated to the intensive lifestyle intervention and 2575 were allocated to the diabetes support and education condition. These participants were then tested after a year, and of the intensive lifestyle participants 2496 attended this assessment session and 2463 of the diabetes support and education participants attended also. The flow chart doesn't say how many from each condition were included in the analysis of the outcome measures and this is a weakness in the reporting here. Also, it doesn't contain this information in the actual reporting of the statistical analyses. We have to presume that all of the participants who were assessed at one year follow-up were included in the analyses (but we don't know for sure).

IMPORTANT FEATURES OF AN RCT

You will notice that in Table 14.1 we have highlighted some of the items. We have done this because these items specifically relate to features of RCT design. We stated previously (see pages 430–431) that a control condition, random allocation of participants to conditions and blinding were important features of high quality research. These are the features that are included in the CONSORT statements above but there are factors that we need to take into account when implementing such design features.

Random Allocation

Random allocation of participants to conditions is not necessarily as straightforward as you would think. For our halitosis study let us imagine that we have an intervention condition and a control condition. How should we go about randomly allocating participants to each of these two conditions?

Activity 14.2

Before you read any further think about how you might randomly allocate participants to the two conditions of our halitosis study.

One way would be to toss a coin. This is a random process, where there are two possible outcomes where one (say 'heads') could be equated with allocation to the intervention condition and the other (tails) could be equated to allocation to the control condition. When a participant is included in the study the researcher could toss a coin to see which condition they are allocated to, and this would provide us with random allocation. The CONSORT guidelines though do not recommend this approach to random allocation. Why do you think that they wouldn't? The answer is that there is potential for bias to creep into to such a system of random allocation. If it is left up to the researcher to allocate each participant on the toss of a coin then there is scope for the researcher to decide that certain coin tosses were not valid (for example they might drop the coin, decide that they didn't toss the coin high enough, that they forgot to use their lucky penny, etc.). Such an approach potentially introduces bias in the allocation of participants to conditions which randomness is meant to avoid. How should we randomly allocate participants? A better way would be to decide on the allocation of participants to conditions before they are even recruited. For example, we would decide on the allocation of each participant before we even knew which participants were going to be taking part in the study. We could use coin tossing for this. Thus if we knew we were going to need 20 participants in the study we would toss a coin 20 times and the order of allocation to conditions would be determined by the 20 coin tosses. Our allocation table would look like that presented in Table 14.2.

Table 14.2   Random allocation sequence generated through tossing a coin

Participant	Outcome of coin toss	Allocated condition
1	Heads	Intervention
2	Heads	Intervention
3	Tails	Control
4	Tails	Control
5	Tails	Control
6	Heads	Intervention
7	Tails	Control
8	Heads	Intervention
9	Heads	Intervention
10	Heads	Intervention
11	Heads	Intervention
12	Tails	Control
13	Heads	Intervention

Table 14.2   Cont'd

Participant	Outcome of coin toss	Allocated condition
14	Tails	Control
15	Tails	Control
16	Tails	Control
17	Heads	Intervention
18	Heads	Intervention
19	Tails	Control
20	Heads	Intervention

You can see that the first two people who were recruited would be allocated to the intervention group and then the third, fourth and fifth people would be allocated to the control group, and so on. This is better than tossing a coin at the point the participant is recruited, as the researcher is not biased in allocation as a result of them knowing details about the participants. There are though better ways of ensuring the allocation sequence is truly random. Tossing a coin is open to potential bias, and so we can generate random allocation sequences through other means, for example through the use of random number tables or a random number generator feature of a program like Microsoft© Excel or SPSS. We have produced a document to show you how to generate a random allocation sequence in SPSS, and this is available on the companion website for this book. The random allocation sequence that we have generated using SPSS is presented below in Screenshot 14.1.

Restricted Randomisation

Both of the methods of generating randomisation sequences that we have described above and on the companion website (coin tossing and using SPSS) are examples of simple (unrestricted) randomisation. Take a look back at these allocations, what do you notice? You should notice that they have both led to unequal numbers of participants being allocated to each condition of the RCT. In the coin tossing sequence we would allocate 11 participants to the intervention condition and 9 to the control, whereas in the SPSS sequence we would allocate 12 participants to the intervention condition and 8 to the control. Quite often in research it is desirable to have equal numbers of participants in each condition. This often results in our data analyses being more robust to violations of assumptions and more reliable. With simple random allocation we often get unequal sample sizes across our conditions, and the smaller the samples the more likely this is to happen. There is a really good paper published in *The Lancet* by Schulz and Grimes in 2002 which discusses random allocation of participants and ways of overcoming this problem with unequal sample sizes. We suggest that you have a look at the paper for more information on randomisation.

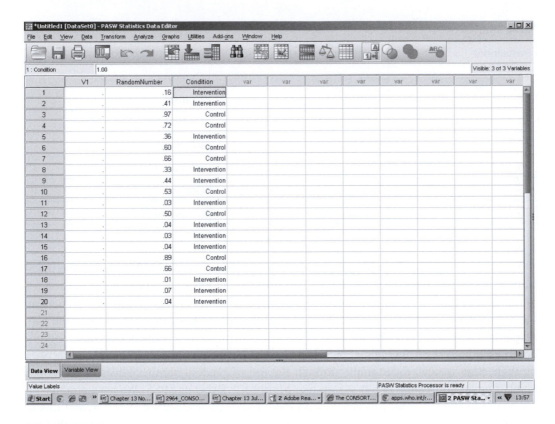

Screenshot 14.1

However, we will illustrate here one way of ensuring that there is not a large disparity between your conditions in the sample sizes. The approach we will describe here is called *replacement randomisation*.

Replacement Randomisation

In replacement randomisation you have to decide before you generate your randomisation sequence how much disparity between groups you are willing to tolerate. So, for example, we might decide for our halitosis study that we can tolerate a sequence that has 11 in one condition and 9 in the other, but that is the maximum disparity that we will allow. Let us assume that the first sequence we generate with SPSS is the one that we have illustrated above. In this sequence we have 12 in the intervention condition and 8 in the control condition. The disparity between the two groups is greater than we have said that we want to tolerate, and so what we would do is to get SPSS to generate another random sequence. We have done this in Screenshot 14.2.

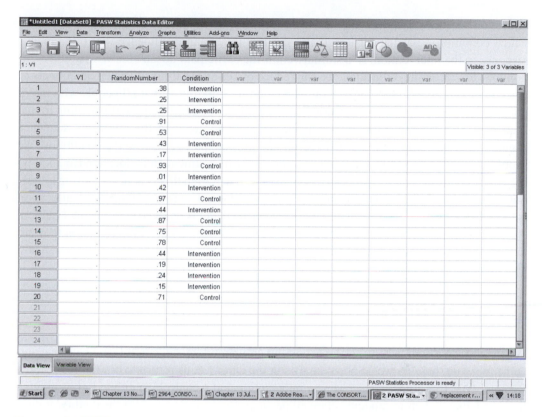

Screenshot 14.2

Here there are again 12 participants in the intervention condition and 8 in the control condition. We would thus get SPSS to generate another random sequence for us, and keep doing so until we get the first sequence that falls within the disparity limits that we specified before we started generating randomisation sequences (i.e. the first sequence where there are 11 or 10 participants in either the intervention condition or the control condition). Schulz and Grimes (2002) suggest that this is an adequate means of ensuring equivalent sample sizes across conditions as long as it is carried out before the RCT begins.

BLINDING

Not surprisingly, randomisation is a critical feature of RCTs ('it does what it says on the tin') but on its own it is not enough to guard against bias creeping into studies. We suggested above that researchers and participants can bias findings if they know which conditions the participant is in. We suggested that the best way to ensure that such biasing does not occur is through blinding. Blinding is where the important people in a study do not know the allocation sequence. If the people who are allocating participants to conditions do not know which condition a participant is actually in, then they cannot influence that participant's response to the intervention. In a similar vein if the participant doesn't know what intervention they are receiving, then again we can reduce biases due to things like demand effects or placebo effects. The CONSORT recommendation for blinding is that all people who might potentially bias the findings by knowledge of the allocation sequence should be blind to that sequence. The recommendation is that the people who generate the allocation sequence should not be the ones who actually recruit and allocate participants to the conditions. We should also, where possible, prevent those who do the recruitment and allocation from knowing which conditions participants are being allocated to. Often this is done by putting allocation information for each participant in a blank envelope. The information about allocation is then accessed once the participant has been recruited and is ready to start the intervention. All baseline data should be collected prior to any knowledge about which condition they are in. Finally, when the intervention is completed, the people doing the data analyses should also be blind to the conditions.

ANALYSIS OF RCTs

When we have a comparatively simple parallel group randomised control trial with one outcome measure, how do we go about analysing the data? Let us return to our halitosis study. Remember in this study we have a new intervention and a control condition. Let us assume that immediately before randomisation all participants were assessed for the quality of their breath by an independent rater who was blind to the condition that each participant was to be allocated to. This rating constitutes our baseline data and is made on a seven-point scale where 1 equals 'smells like a sewer' and 7 equals 'smells like a rose'. The same rater then assesses breath quality again one month later, and this is our follow-up data. In the literature such a design is often called a pretest/posttest design because we have repeated testing before and after an intervention. What would be the best way of analysing these data? One approach would be to calculate gain or change scores. This would be done by subtracting the breath ratings at time 1 from the ratings at time 2 for each group. We could then run an independent *t*-test (or equivalently a between-participants ANOVA) comparing the two conditions on their gain scores. If there is no effect of the new intervention in quality of breath, then we would expect the change from time 1 to time 2 to be about the same for both groups. If the intervention is having an effect, however, we would expect a significant difference to be seen between the two gain scores that we calculated. There is though some criticism of the analysis of gain scores in such designs (e.g. Rausch et al., 2003; but also see Dimitrov and Rumrill, 2003).[1]

Perhaps the best way of analysing data from the simple parallel-group RCT is to use *Analysis of Covariance (ANCOVA)*. We won't be going into too much detail about ANCOVA here, but we want to give you an overview of what this statistical technique does. ANCOVA is like a cross between multiple regression and ANOVA. In such an analysis the dependent variable would be the posttest scores (e.g. posttest breath ratings) and the independent variable would be the conditions that participants were allocated to (intervention versus control). However, before we ran the analysis we would try to take account of participants' pretest breath ratings scores, and these would be included in the analysis as a *covariate*. If you think back to Chapter 12 where we introduced hierarchical regression, then ANCOVA is a bit like that. In the first stage we would look at the relationship between posttest scores and the pretest scores, we would then look to see if condition that participants were allocated to could account for any of the variation in posttest scores once pretest scores had be controlled (or partialled out – see Figure 14.4). You should refer back to Chapter 12 for an explanation of this.

Referring to Figure 14.4, the difference between the conditions (intervention versus control) in posttests scores after we have controlled for pretest scores is represented by the area labelled c. The areas a and b represent the variance in posttest scores which are partialled out of the analysis. Why would we need to take account of pretest scores? One of the best reasons for doing this is that it tends to make your analyses more powerful. Also, some authors have argued that analysing change scores has a number of problems associated with it, and thus they recommend ANCOVA (e.g. Rausch et al., 2003).

You should bear in mind that ANCOVA has similar assumptions to ANOVA, but has an additional assumption which is called the *assumption of homogeneity of regression slopes*. Essentially, this assumption stipulates that the correlation between the pretest and posttest scores for the intervention condition should be the same as for that for the control condition. We don't feel that it is appropriate to include an in-depth discussion of this here, and so we would refer you to other texts (e.g. Dancey and Reidy, 2011).

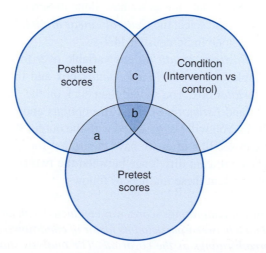

Figure 14.4 Illustration of the partialling out of variance in the posttest scores due to pretest scores in ANCOVA

RUNNING AN ANCOVA IN SPSS

We are going to illustrate the analysis of the data from the halitosis study presented in Table 14.3.

Table 14.3 Pretest and posttest breath ratings for the new intervention and control conditions

New intervention group		Control group	
Pretest	Posttest	Pretest	Posttest
1.00	2.00	2.00	2.00
1.00	4.00	2.00	2.00
2.00	6.00	1.00	0.00
3.00	4.00	3.00	2.00
2.00	3.00	2.00	1.00
2.00	5.00	2.00	0.00
1.00	4.00	2.00	1.00
0.00	5.00	1.00	2.00
1.00	3.00	1.00	2.00
2.00	5.00	1.00	2.00

You should set up your SPSS data file as we have done in Screenshot 14.3.

To run the analysis you should select the *General Linear Model*, *Univariate* option and set up the dialogue as we have done in Screenshot 14.4.

You should move the *Posttests breath ratings* variable over to the *Dependent Variable* box, the *Condition* variable over to the *Fixed Factors* box and the *Pretest breath ratings* variable over to the *Covariates* box. You should then click on the *Options* button and select the *Descriptive statistics* and *Estimates of effect size* options and finally click on *Continue* and *OK* to run the analysis. You will be presented with the output shown in Screenshot 14.5.

From the output we can see that after we have controlled for (partialled out) the pretest breath ratings we have a significant difference between the two conditions in their posttest breath ratings. We might present these findings as follows:

Analysis of the posttest breath ratings scores was conducted with an analysis of covariance (ANCOVA) which had a between-participants factor of condition (intervention versus control) and pretest breath ratings as the covariate. The analysis showed that there was no relationship between the pretest and posttest breath ratings ($F_{1,17} = 0.24$, p = .628, partial eta-square = 0.01). There was, though, a significant difference between the conditions in

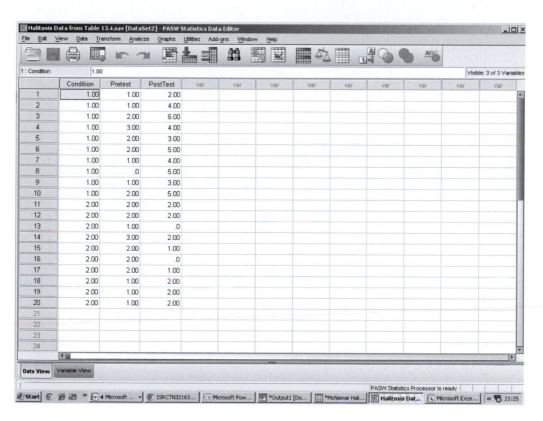

Screenshot 14.3

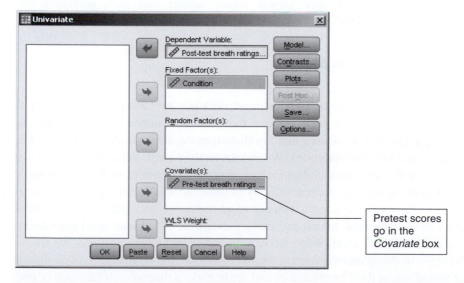

Screenshot 14.4

Descriptive Statistics

Dependent Variable:Post-test breath ratings

Condition	Mean	Std. Deviation	N
Intervention group	4.1000	1.19722	10
Control group	1.4000	.84327	10
Total	2.75000	1.71295	10

Tests of Betwees-Subjects Effects

Dependent Variable:Post-test breath ratings

Source	Type III Sum of Squares	df	Mean Square	F	Sig.	Partial Eta Squared
Corrected Model	36.723[a]	2	18.361	16.405	.000	.659
Intercept	21.327	1	21.327	19.055	.000	.528
Pretest	.273	1	.273	.244	.628	.014
Condition	36.630	1	36.630	32.727	.000	.658
Error	19.027	17	1.119			
Total	207.000	20				
Corrected Total	55.750	19				

a. R Squared = .659 (Adjusted R Squared = .619)

> This shows whether there is a significant relationship between pretest and posttest scores

> This row tells us if we have a significant effect of condition after controlling for pretest scores

Screenshot 14.5

their posttest breath ratings once pretest breath ratings had been partialled out $(F_{1,17} = 32.73, p < .001, partial eta-square = 0.66)$.

McNEMAR'S TEST OF CHANGE

The above suggestion for analysis would be appropriate when we have pretest and posttest scores measured on a continuous scale (or one that can be assumed to be continuous). Sometimes we have outcome measures that are dichotomous, for example whether or not someone has a disease (e.g. has halitosis). We cannot analyse such dichotomous variables using ANCOVA, ANOVA or *t*-tests, and so we have to use an alternative such as McNemar's test of change. Let us change the example slightly to illustrate McNemar's test. Let us suppose that we have randomly selected a number of participants, and then we use trained judges to assess the participants' breath and make a diagnosis of halitosis (oral malodour). Obviously, some of the participants will receive a diagnosis and others will not. We would then give all the participants an intervention consisting of our new treatment. At one-month follow-up we would assess their breath again, and again make a diagnosis of halitosis or not. You should be able to see that in this example we have a dichotomous outcome variable

Table 14.4 Contingency table showing frequency of diagnosis of halitosis pre- and post-intervention

	Posttest halitosis	Posttest no halitosis	Total
Pretest halitosis	50	███████████	56
Pretest no halitosis	███████████	133	144
Total	61	139	200

which is whether or not participants receive a halitosis diagnosis. We also have a repeated measures element to the study, as each participants is tested at two time points (pretest and posttest). For illustration's sake let us say that we recruited 200 participants and at the initial assessment (pretest) 56 received a halitosis diagnosis. At posttest we find that of the original 56 who had halitosis only 50 now have it, and of the original 144 who didn't have halitosis 11 now have it. We want to know whether or not these differences in diagnoses are statistically significant, or whether it could merely represent chance changes. We can present the halitosis numbers in a contingency table format (similar to that seen earlier for chi-square) (Table 14.4).

McNemar's test works by looking at those participants who change diagnosis from pretest to posttest. This makes some intuitive sense, because there will only be evidence of the effectiveness of the intervention if some of the participants change their diagnosis from having halitosis to not having halitosis. If no participants change, then the intervention has made no impact. Thus McNemar's test focusses on the cells in the above table that indicate a change of diagnosis (the cells in the table that are shaded). We would use these change values to calculate a chi-square value, and then use this to discover whether the values in the shaded cells represent a significant difference from what we would expect by chance. We do not intend explaining the calculation of the McNemar chi-square, but we will demonstrate how to get this using SPSS.

RUNNING McNEMAR'S TEST IN SPSS

In order to run the McNemar's test you need to set up three variables so that you can represent the columns and rows in the above table (much like you had to do for chi-square). The first variable (we have called it 'pretest') represents the rows in the table and the second variable (we have called it 'posttest') represents the columns. The third variable contains the frequency counts that are in the actual cells (we have called this 'Counts'). The data file should look like Screenshot 14.6.

You will notice that we type condition numbers into the pretest and posttest variables. To make the data table more meaningful you should go to the *Variable View* table and use the *Values* characteristic for the pretest and posttest variables to indicate what each number means. We have set it up so that a 1 represents halitosis and a 2 represents no halitosis for

Screenshot 14.6

both the pretest and posttest variables. When you click on the road sign icon you will see Screenshot 14.7 in your *Data View* screen.

To run the analysis you need to first weight the cases. You can do this by clicking on the *Data* and *Weight Cases* options, and then selecting the *Weight Cases by* option and moving the *Counts* variable across to the relevant box. Once you have done this click on *OK*. To run the McNemar test you should click on *Nonparametric Tests*, *Legacy Dialogs* and *2 related samples*, you will be presented with a dialogue box (Screenshot 14.8).

You should select both the *Pretest* and *Posttest* variables together by holding the *Shift* key down on the keyboard and then clicking on the *Posttest* variable. When both are highlighted, click on the arrow to move them across to the *Test Pairs* box. You should then deselect the *Wilcoxon* option and select the *McNemar* option and then click on *OK* (Screenshot 14.9).

The output will look like Screenshot 14.10.

You can see from the output that you are presented with a frequency counts table and a table containing the results of the statistical analysis. You should note that in the test statistics table you are simply given the *p*-value (SPSS doesn't usually give you the chi-square

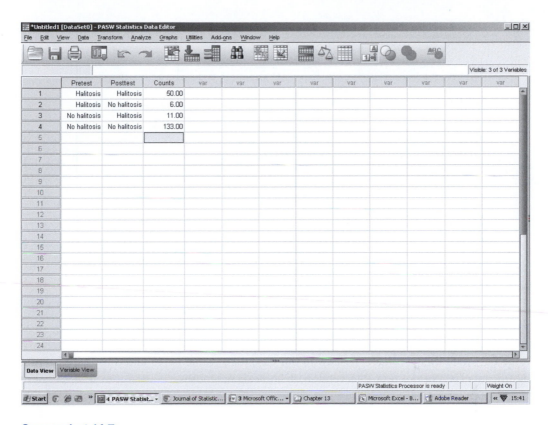

Screenshot 14.7

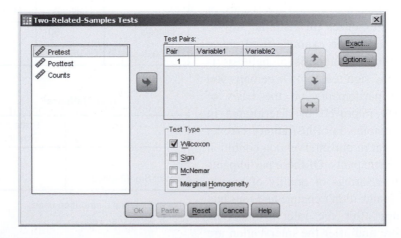

Screenshot 14.8

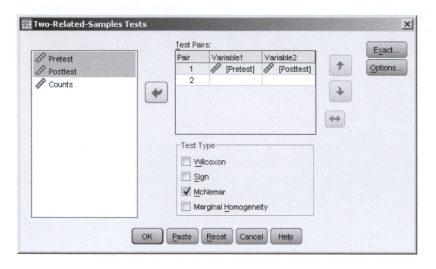

Screenshot 14.9

value on which this *p*-value is based). In our case the *p*-value is .33 and thus there is not a significant effect of our new intervention on halitosis diagnoses.

THE SIGN TEST

A simpler alternative to the McNemar test of change is the *sign test*. The sign test is based upon the binomial distribution and is a test of dichotomous responses (in a similar way to McNemar's test). The example used above about receiving a diagnosis of halitosis is suitable for the sign test too. Or perhaps you could code participants on the basis of whether they improved or deteriorated in terms of symptoms. For illustration's sake let us suppose that in our intervention condition we had 20 participants. Of these participants 13 had higher ratings of quality of breath, three participants didn't change and four had lower ratings after the intervention. The ratings before and after the intervention are presented in Table 14.5.

Pretest & Posttest

Pretest	Posttest	
	Halitosis	No halitosis
Halitosis	50	6
No halitosis	11	133

Test Statistics[b]

	Pretest & Posttest
N	200
Exact Sig. (2-tailed)	.332[a]

a. Binomial distribution used.

b. McNemar Test

Screenshot 14.10   McNemar test, crosstabs

Table 14.5   Ratings of breath quality before and after the intervention

Participant	1	2	3	4	5	6	7	8	9	10	11	12	13	14	15	16	17	18	19	20
Before	3	4	3	3	5	6	6	0	6	1	5	3	2	6	4	3	3	7	2	5
After	5	7	5	3	4	7	6	3	7	2	5	6	5	4	2	4	4	4	3	7

It is clear from these ratings that more participants improved in terms of the rated quality of their breath (13) than did those who deteriorated (4). It would thus appear that the intervention might be effective. However, we don't know whether the difference between these two outcomes could have been a chance finding or whether it will be statistically significant. We can use the sign test to provide this information for us. You should note that the sign test discards all the participants who do not change from before to after intervention. These are called 'ties' and are not used in the calculations for the sign test.

RUNNING THE SIGN TEST USING SPSS

In order to run the sign test using SPSS you need to set up two columns of data, with one containing the data for one condition and the other the data for the other condition. In our example we have the ratings before and after intervention to input and so we have set up the SPSS data file as in Screenshot 14.11.

Once you have entered the data you can run the sign test. To do this you need to click on the *Analyze*, *Nonparametric Tests*, *Legacy Dialogs* and *2 related samples* options. You will be presented with the same dialogue box that we showed you earlier for the McNemar test. You should then select both the *Before* and *After* variables and move them across to the *Test Pairs* table. You should then deselect the *Wilcoxon* option and select the *Sign Test* option. You can then click on *OK* to run the sign test (Screenshot 14.12).

The output will look like Screenshot 14.13.

You can see that the first table in the output gives you the numbers of participants who improved, the numbers who deteriorated and the numbers who didn't change. The second table gives the *p*-value for the sign test, and we can see that in this case there is a significant effect such that there are significantly more improvers than deteriorators.

INTENTION TO TREAT ANALYSIS

Intention to treat analysis is where all participants who were randomised are included in the analyses of the outcome measures. In addition, all participants should be analysed in the groups to which they were originally randomised. For example, suppose we had 20 participants in our halitosis study with 11 in the new intervention group and 9 in the control group, and the outcome measure was breath quality as measured by an independent rater who was

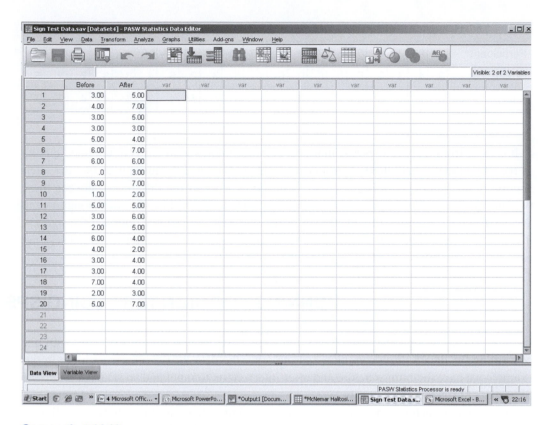

Screenshot 14.11

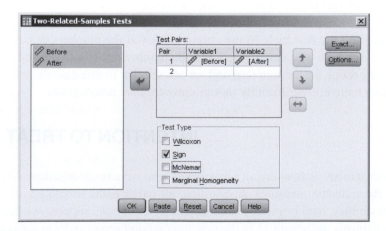

Screenshot 14.12

Frequencies

		N
After - Before	Negative Differences[a]	4
	Positive Differences[b]	13
	Ties[c]	3
	Total	20

a. After < Before

b. After > Before

c. After = Before

Test Statistics[b]

	After - Before
Exact Sig. (2-tailed)	.049[a]

a. Binomial distribution used.

b. Sign Test

Screenshot 14.13 Sign test

blind to condition. In an intention to treat analysis we would compare the two conditions on this measure of breath quality, but we would need to ensure that all 11 from the new intervention condition and all 9 from the control condition were included in this analysis. However, there are often problems with such clinical trials that make intention to treat analyses difficult. For example, participants may drop out of the study before the follow-up assessment. Or some participants may have failed to adhere to the instructions related to the condition they were allocated to. For example, let us suggest that the new intervention was a mouthwash that had to be administered three times per day immediately after meals. It might be that some participants have forgotten to do this and thus have compromised the intervention to some degree. We need to decide what to do about such participants. The most obvious thing to do is not to include them in the final analysis, as they have not properly adhered to the intervention instructions. However, if we do this we may have introduced some bias into the study and undermined the benefits of the random allocation of participants to conditions. If you decide to exclude the participants from the analysis you need to report how many participants have been excluded and the reasons for such exclusion (this information can be included in your flow chart). These would be classified as missing data, and if you remember from Chapter 6 there are a number of alternative ways of dealing with missing data.

CROSSOVER DESIGNS

The traditional RCT design is considered the 'gold standard' in health research and is recommended whenever it is possible (see the ladder of evidence that we presented earlier in Figure 14.1). One of the problems with this, though, is that often it is not economically viable, and thus alternative designs are required. A commonly utilised alternative is the crossover design in which all participants receive the treatment and they act as their own controls. In such a design participants would be randomly assigned to one of two treatment sequences:

1) Control period followed by the intervention period
2) Intervention period followed by a control period

The design would look something like that presented in Figure 14.5.

You can see from the figure why these are called crossover designs. One group of participants will receive the intervention for a set period of time and then the intervention will be withdrawn. The other group of participants will have a period without treatment and they will then crossover to the intervention condition. Such designs can be more ethical than the standard RCT because all of the participants will receive treatment at some time, and this is thus a particular advantage of crossover designs. We would want to take measures of the outcome variable at various timepoints to see what effect introducing the conditions in the different orders has. Thus, we would expect a reduction in symptoms first followed by an increase in symptoms in the 'Intervention–Control' sequence, and in the 'Control–Intervention' sequence we would expect no change in symptoms from baseline followed by a reduction when the intervention was introduced.

One of the limitations of such designs is that we can get carryover effects where the changes brought about by the intervention continue into the following control condition. This means that the increase in symptoms observed when intervention is withdrawn might not be equivalent to the decrease in symptoms when the intervention is introduced in the 'Control–Intervention' sequence. This can be alleviated somewhat by introducing a 'washout' period between one phase and the next.

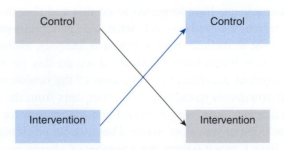

Figure 14.5   Illustration of the order of conditions in a two-period crossover design

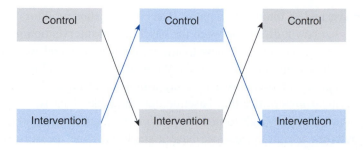

Figure 14.6   Example of a three-period crossover design

The type of crossover design that we have considered thus far is called a two-period design because there are two phases to each of the treatment sequences (Control followed by Intervention, or Intervention followed by Control). We can extend this sort of design to incorporate more periods if we wish. Ebbutt (1984) recommends using three-period designs where, in effect, there are two crossovers. This is illustrated in Figure 14.6.

You can see from Figure 14.6 that one group of participants will start with the Control condition and then they will cross to the Intervention condition and then cross back to the Control condition. The other group starts with the Intervention and then crosses to the Control and finally crosses back to the Intervention condition. According to Ebbutt (1984) the advantage of this extra period in the design is that it allows the researcher to more closely examine any carryover effects from Control to Intervention or from Intervention to Control.

If we wanted to statistically analyse the effects in this sort of design on an outcome mea-sure, we could conduct one-way within-participants ANOVAs on each condition to see how the intervention phases differ from the control phases.[2]

SINGLE-CASE DESIGNS (*N* = 1)

So far in this book we have covered analytical techniques which are based upon samples of participants and using these samples to generalise to underlying populations. We have sug-gested in this chapter that the gold standard for research in the health sciences is the ran-domised control trial, which if appropriately designed allows stronger inferences to be made about causality (e.g. an intervention caused a change in the outcome variable). A form of research which is often neglected and often misunderstood is that involving single partici-pants rather than samples of participants. These types of studies are called *single-case designs* or *single-case experimental designs*.

The typical single-case design is one where a clinician might give a patient a particular intervention and record the effect of this intervention on some particular outcome variable. In many ways conceptually it is quite similar to the pretest/posttest designs that we described earlier in the chapter. In a basic single-case design there are two phases that we are interested in, a baseline phase and an intervention phase. The clinician then monitors a particular outcome variable to see how it differs between the baseline and intervention phase. For example, suppose we were interested in a new treatment for psoriasis and we wanted to test a single patient who had symptoms of psoriasis. We would need a baseline period where we measured the symptoms of psoriasis across say a number of days. According to Kazdin (1978), it is of critical importance that baseline data is stable. That is, we need to have a baseline phase that is long enough to provide us with good consistent and stable measurements of the outcome variable. Once we have a stable baseline measure we would then introduce the new intervention, and measure the symptoms of psoriasis again across a number of days until we had a stable measure in the intervention phase. We could then compare the symptoms in the baseline phase with those from the intervention phase to see if there was a noticeable difference. The most common method of deciding whether there is a difference between baseline and intervention phases is through visual analysis of a graph. In such a graph the symptoms on the baseline and intervention phases would be plotted over time (e.g. see Figure 14.7).

An examination of Figure 14.7 might suggest that there are markedly fewer symptoms of psoriasis in the intervention phase compared to the baseline phase. We might be tempted to conclude that the intervention has been effective for this single patient. However, such a conclusion might not be warranted, and the reason for this highlights one of the potential weaknesses of a single-case design like this one. Because we have one baseline phase and one intervention phase, and we are dealing with real people living their lives alongside being treated, we have no control over potential confounding factors. It might be the case that a factor other than the intervention is responsible for improvement in symptoms, for example perhaps in the intervention phase it was much sunnier than in the baseline phase. It could be

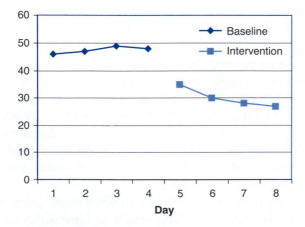

Figure 14.7 Graph showing the difference between symptoms during the baseline and intervention phases for a single-case design

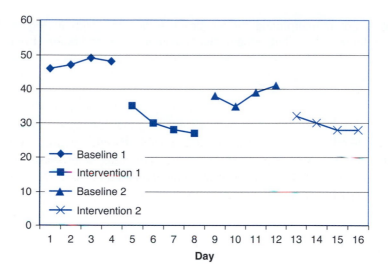

Figure 14.8 Illustration of a single-case design graph with four phases

that the sunshine rather than our intervention is responsible for the improvement in symptoms. To overcome come such problems it is advisable to utilise slightly more complex single-case designs such as one with repeated baseline measures and repeated interventions. A single baseline and intervention design is often called an AB design, where the A is the baseline and the B is the intervention. The recommendation is to have something more like an ABAB design, where there is a baseline phase followed by an intervention phase and then the intervention is withdrawn for a period and then re-introduced. If the intervention is effective we would expect an improvement in symptoms during the first intervention phase and a deterioration when the intervention is withdrawn. Finally, the re-introduction of the intervention should result in an improvement in symptoms again. The addition of the two extra phases allows us to be more confident in the success of the intervention should we see symptom improvements in both the intervention phases. The graph of such a design might look like the one presented in Figure 14.8.

From Figure 14.8 we can see that there was an improvement in symptoms from the baseline phase to the first intervention phase. There was then a slight deterioration in symptoms in the withdrawal phase, followed by another improvement when the intervention was re-introduced. This sort of graph would suggest that the intervention has been successful for this patient.

When reporting the results of such studies we can supplement the description of the graphs with descriptive statistics for each phase of the study. We suggest providing minimum, maximum and mean (or median) values for each phase of the study.[3]

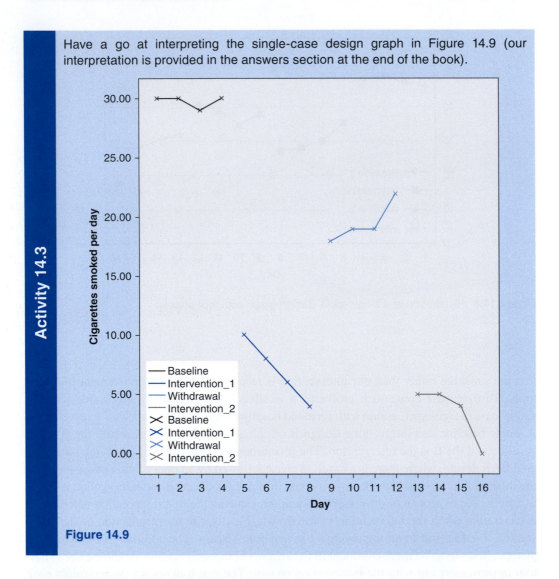

Have a go at interpreting the single-case design graph in Figure 14.9 (our interpretation is provided in the answers section at the end of the book).

Activity 14.3

Figure 14.9

Example from the Literature

A nice example of a single-case design is a study reported by Ownsworth et al. (2006). In this study they examined the errors that a severe traumatic brain injured patient made in two real life settings, at home cooking or when undertaking volunteering work. For the cooking task there were three phases to the study, baseline, intervention and maintenance, whereas for the volunteering task there was only a baseline and an intervention phase. The intervention in the study provided training for the participant to increase his error awareness and his self-correction behaviours. The authors presented their findings visually using a graph and we have reproduced their cooking task graph in Figure 14.10.

a, Cooking task

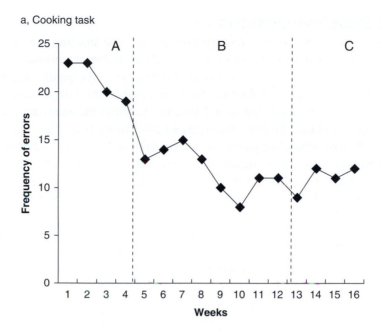

Figure 14.10   Frequency of errors of patient in the cooking task reported by Ownsworth et al. (2006). A = baseline, B = intervention and C = maintenance

You should notice from Figure 14.10 that the number of errors dropped quite substantially between the baseline and intervention phases and that this reduction was continued into the maintenance phases. The authors supplemented the graphical analyses with descriptive statistics for each phase.

We should note here that there are some problems with the ABAB design that we have just described. Perhaps the trickiest of these relates to the ethical concerns of withdrawing a treatment that may be effective in the second A phase of the study. This is a particularly important consideration for research in the health sciences where the intervention may have significant benefits to the long-term health of the patient. There are a number of ways of addressing this difficulty. One is to take advantage of situations where the patient him- or herself for some reason withdraws from the intervention temporarily. Although this does overcome some of the ethical concerns, it introduces potential bias to the study in that the reason for withdrawal may also influence the outcome measure during the withdrawal phase. An example might be a patient suffering from depression who may withdraw from a psoriasis intervention and may not look after themselves as they would usually do. The depression rather than the withdrawal of intervention might then be the cause of any changes in the outcome variable.

Multiple Baseline Designs

In multiple baseline designs there would typically be only one baseline phase and one intervention phase for each participant. However, the baselines and interventions are either introduced at different times across a number of single-case participants, or introduced in multiple settings, or assessed with multiple outcome variables for a single case. For the situation with multiple single cases we would take the baseline measures for varying times across participants and introduce the interventions at different times. So, for example, one participant might have a baseline phase starting on day 1 of the study and ending on day 7, and the intervention is introduced on day 8. The second participant might have the baseline phase starting on day 3 and ending on day 11, and the intervention is then introduced on day 12. A third participant might have the baseline starting on day 7 and finishing on day 14 (see Figure 14.11).

The variation in the start of the baseline and the intervention means that there are less likely to be variables outside the control of the researchers which have an impact upon the outcome variable consistently across all cases in the study. If we obtain improvements as a result of our intervention across all cases we can be more confident that our intervention has caused the improvements than if we included a single case. We also have the advantage in this design that we are not withdrawing a potentially beneficial intervention.

The other forms of multiple baseline design are multiple settings and multiple outcome measures. The example from the literature that we described previously is an example of a multiple setting design, as in this study the researchers looked at errors from their patient in a cooking task at home and in a volunteering setting too. An example of multiple outcome variables might be a study examining the effectiveness of a new drug for chest infections. In such a study you might look at the impact upon a subjective measure, such as ratings given by the patient of breathlessness and an objective measure such as peak expiratory flow rates.

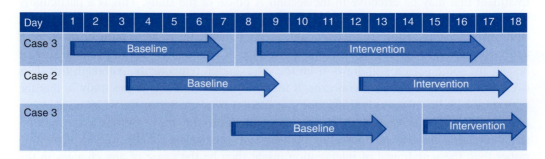

Figure 14.11   Illustration a multiple baseline single-case design study

GENERATING SINGLE-CASE DESIGN GRAPHS USING SPSS

Here we will show you how to generate a graph with the data presented in Figure 14.7. These data are 46, 47, 49, 48 for the baseline and 35, 30, 28, 27 for the intervention phases respectively. In SPSS you will need to set up three variables, one for the day of the trial, one for the baseline values and one for the intervention values. You then input the data as in Screenshot 14.14.

You can see that in the *Day* column we have numbered the days consecutively from 1 to 8. We then input the baseline values in the rows corresponding to days 1 to 4 and leave the other rows for this variable blank and input the intervention values in rows 5 to 8 and leave the other rows for this variable blank. To generate the graph you should select the *Graphs*, *Legacy Dialogs* and *Line* options and you will be presented with a dialogue box (Screenshot 14.15).

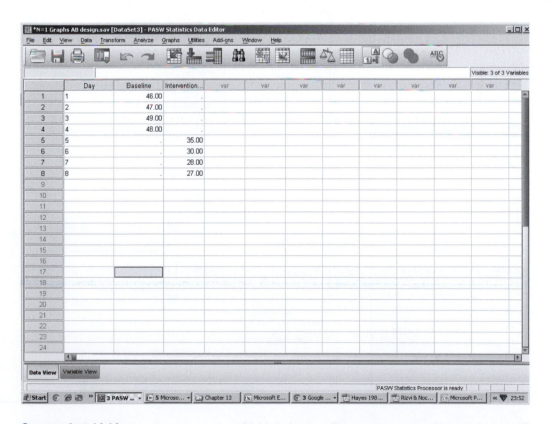

Screenshot 14.14

Select the *Multiple* and *Values of individual cases* options and then click on the *Define* button. You will be presented with another dialogue box (Screenshot 14.16).

In the *Category Labels* section you need to click on the *Variable* option and then move the *Day* variable to the relevant box. You should then move the *Baseline* and *Intervention* variables to the *Lines Represent* box and then click on the *OK* button. You will be presented with a graph that looks like Screenshot 14.17.

If you double click on the graph you can edit it to improve how it looks. For example you can adjust the *y*-axis scaling so that it starts at zero. To do this double click on the graph and this will open the graph editor. You should then double click on the *y*-axis itself and this will open up an options dialogue box for you (Screenshot 14.18).

You should change the value in the *Minimum* box to 0 and then click on *Apply* and *Close*.

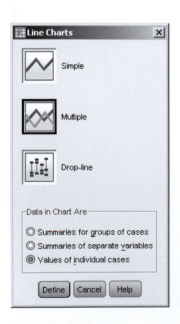

Screenshot 14.15

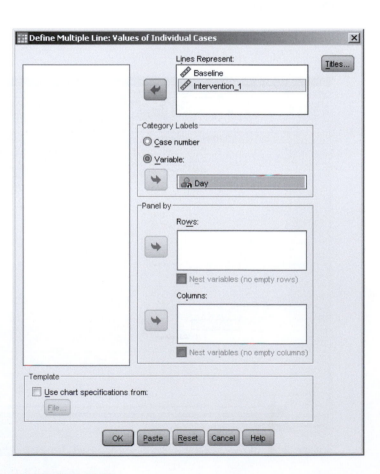

Screenshot 14.16

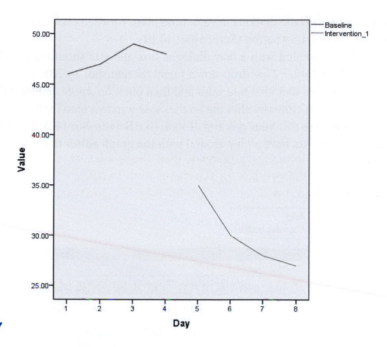

Screenshot 14.17

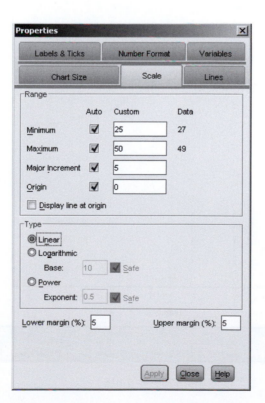

Screenshot 14.18

If you want to include markers at each time point for each phase you can do this by clicking on the *Add Markers* button (Screenshot 14.19).

You will be presented with a new dialogue box and you should click on the *Markers* tab and click on the *Marker Type* drop-down menu (Screenshot 14.20).

Select the marker style that you want and then click on *Apply* and then *Close*. You should then close the graph editor by clicking on the close window icon in the top right-hand corner. Once you have done this your graph will look like Screenshot 14.21.

If you wish you can have a play around with the graph editor to try to improve the look of the graph further.

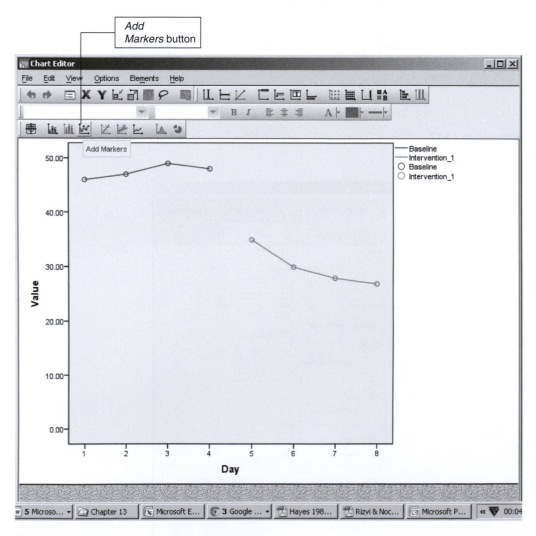

Screenshot 14.19

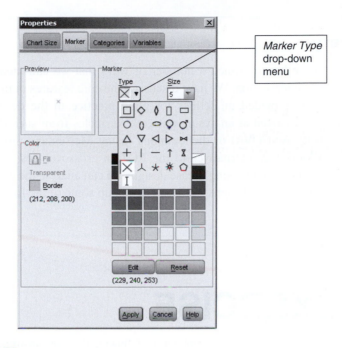

Screenshot 14.20

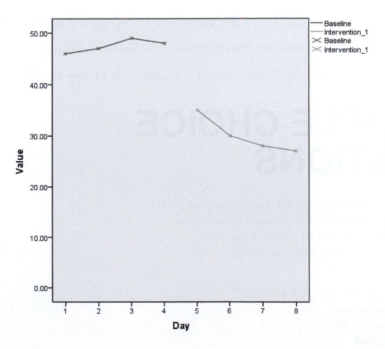

Screenshot 14.21

Summary

In this chapter we have outlined a number of ways that we can measure and analyse change due to an intervention. We have discussed the core features of randomised control trials (RCTs) and provided guidelines for good practice in the design and reporting of these. We have looked at analysing outcome variables from such designs which are continuous (using ANCOVA) or dichotomous (using McNemar's test or the sign test). We have also looked at alternatives to the RCT in crossover designs and single-case experimental designs, and for single-case designs we can analyse the data using graphical techniques. In all of these designs we have flagged up some of the limitations associated with them.

SPSS EXERCISE

Use SPSS to generate a single-case design graph for the following data (the answers are presented at the end of the book). The baseline data were collected on days 1 to 7. The data for the baseline phase were:

- day 1 = 17, day 2 = 15, day 3 = 19, day 4 = 21, day 5 = 19, day 6 = 18, day 7 = 18)

The intervention phase data were collected from days 8 to 14 and these data were:

- day 8 = 13, day 9 = 16, day 10 = 13, day 11 = 12, day 12 = 13, day 13 = 13, day 14 = 12)

MULTIPLE CHOICE QUESTIONS

1. Which of the following are *not* characteristics of RCTs?
   a) Random allocation of participants to conditions
   b) Blinding of all relevant people in the study
   c) Concealment of allocation sequence
   d) None of the above

2. McNemar's test is applicable to:
   a) Continuous data
   b) Dichotomous data
   c) Missing data
   d) All of the above

3. Which of the following applies to single-case designs?
    a) You cannot infer causation
    b) You need a baseline phase
    c) You cannot have multiple baselines
    d) You should never withdraw the intervention

4. Why do editors and research groups advise using the CONSORT guidelines?
    a) They improve the reporting of RCTs
    b) They improve the design of RCTs
    c) They improve the understanding of the outcomes of RCTs
    d) All of the above

5. A CONSORT flow chart is designed to:
    a) Make it clear which participants were included in each stage of the study and analysis of the data
    b) Make it clear who was running the study
    c) Make it clear where the money was spent when conducting a study
    d) Make it clear how the analyses were carried out

6. In an ABAB single-case design study:
    a) There is a staggered start to the intervention for different cases
    b) There is no baseline phase included
    c) There is a baseline phase, an intervention, a withdrawal of the intervention and then re-introduction of the intervention
    d) There is an intervention followed by withdrawal, followed by the intervention followed by withdrawal again

7. An intention to treat analysis should include:
    a) A power analysis of the number of participants you intended to include in the study
    b) All participants who were randomised
    c) All participants who completed the study
    d) All participants who adhered to the intervention instructions

8. According to Sutherland's ladder of evidence which rung do RCTs appear on?
    a) The top rung
    b) The second rung
    c) The third rung
    d) The bottom rung

9. Take a look at the following single-case design graph:

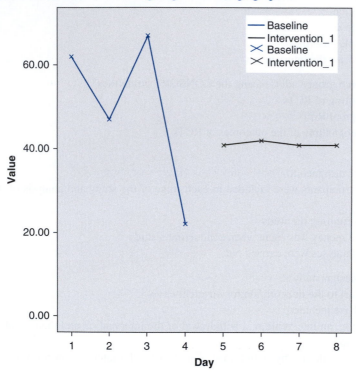

What would you say about the baseline phase?
a) The measures are not stable
b) The measures are stable
c) The measures are equivalent to the intervention phase
d) None of the above

10. Why is blinding used in RCTs?
    a) It helps minimise bias in participants' responses
    b) It helps minimise bias from researchers
    c) It helps minimise bias in the allocation of participants to conditions
    d) All of the above

11. How many items are there in the 2010 CONSORT checklist?
    a) 22
    b) 23
    c) 24
    d) 25

12. How would you analyse a pretest/posttest design with a continuous outcome measure?
    a) ANCOVA with the pretest scores included as a covariate
    b) Correlate the pretest with the posttest scores
    c) Run a McNemar test of change
    d) None of the above

13. How should you supplement visual graphical analysis for single-case designs?
    a) Include a detailed description of the method of generating your graphs
    b) Include descriptive statistics for each phase of the study
    c) Include alternative graphs in an appendix
    d) None of the above

14. Crossover designs are useful when:
    a) You cannot randomly allocate participants to conditions
    b) It is unethical to exclude participants from an intervention condition
    c) You have single cases
    d) All of the above

15. McNemar's test of change is used for pretest/posttest designs when:
    a) You have continuous outcome variables
    b) You have discrete outcome variables
    c) You have no outcome variables
    d) You have dichotomous outcome variables

Notes

1   It should be noted that many authors suggest that an ANOVA with one within-participants factor of time (pretest versus posttest) and one between-participants factor of group (intervention versus control) is the more appropriate way of analysing such RCTs. However, Rausch et al. (2003) have nicely demonstrated that this more complex ANOVA is mathematically equivalent to the simple ANOVA on change scores described here. In fact you would get exactly the same F- and p-values conducting the ANOVAs in these ways.

2   We could also conduct a slightly more complicated analysis called a factorial ANOVA where we have one within-participant variable called period and one between-participants factor called sequence. This sort of analysis is an extension of the ANOVAs that we covered in Chapter 8.

3   Increasingly researchers are being advised not to rely on the types of 'visual' analyses presented here. However, the statistical techniques that are suggested are beyond the scope of this text. For example see Brossart et al. (2006).

Survival Analysis: An Introduction

15

Overview

In this chapter we will introduce you to a slightly different perspective on data analysis, namely survival analysis. In the techniques we introduce here we are interested in the time to a particular event for participants. We will take you through the fundamental concepts underlying survival analysis, such as survival and hazard functions. We will also show you how to present such data in graphical forms through the use of survival and cumulative hazard curves, and we will show you how we can tell whether two survival curves are significantly different from one another. Finally, we will demonstrate how to run these survival analyses using SPSS.

In this chapter you will:

- Learn about survival and hazard functions
- Gain an understanding of the conceptual basis of survival curves and tables
- Learn about the difference between survival and hazard functions
- Gain a conceptual understanding of the Mantel–Cox (log rank) test which tests for differences between survival curves
- Acquire the skills for running survival analyses in SPSS

(Continued)

(Continued)

- Learn how to interpret and report these analyses in your own work as well as understand them in work produced by others

In order to understand the techniques we cover in this chapter it would be best that you ensure that you have a good understanding of probabilities and proportions, as well as chi-square analyses.

INTRODUCTION

One interesting analytical technique that is often used in the health sciences is survival analysis. In survival analysis we are interested in the times to a particular event happening. For example, we might be interested in when a person has a re-occurrence of a skin complaint after treatment, or when a particular cohort of interest first contact the medical services after an event, or when a person dies (hence survival analysis). Basically, the focus in survival analysis is the rate of occurrence of a particular event. In survival analysis we can compare these rates of occurrence across conditions if we so wished. So, for example, we might have two different treatments for eczema, and we might be interested in the differences between these in terms of the reappearance of the skin problems. Does treatment A lead to a longer time before re-occurrence than treatment B? Or perhaps we might be interested in whether treatment A leads to faster clearing of symptoms of eczema than treatment B. In the first example the event of interest is the reappearance of symptoms of eczema, whereas in the second example the event of interest is the absence of symptoms (clearing up of symptoms). We are often interested here in the time from the start of the study to a particular event occurring for participants in the study. Obviously, because people are different from one another, the time for an event to occur will vary across participants and potentially across treatment types. Thus we are interested in analysing the times to the event happening.

Generally when we are studying events we have a finite period of time within which to collect and analyse data. Thus we might only be able to track participants for a year after a particular intervention to see if the event of interest happens. In our eczema example we might track the participants in our study for one year in total to see how long it takes for symptoms to reappear. Or we might track them for three months to see how quickly symptoms disappear. It should be clear that it is not certain that the event will happen to all participants within the time-frame of the study. Not all participants will have a reoccurrence of symptoms within a year of treatment and not all participants will be symptom-free within three months of treatment. Where we have participants who do not experience the event of interest before the end of the study we call these *censored* cases. More specifically, we call these *right censored* cases. We can visualise this using a graph (Figure 15.1).

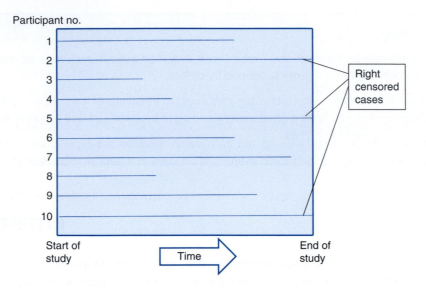

Figure 15.1   Illustration of the times to the event of interest for 10 participants in a study

In this study you can see that we have 10 participants. The lengths of the lines represent how long it took for each participant to experience the event of interest. We can see that participant no. 3 experienced the event the quickest and that three participants (nos 2, 5 and 10) did not experience the event at all. These three cases where they did not experience the event would be called right censored. Now let us have a look at Figure 15.2.

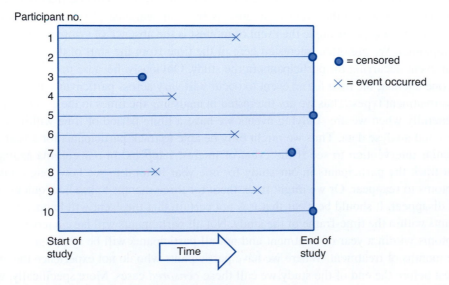

Figure 15.2   Distinguishing censored and non-censored data points

Here we have the same data as in Figure 15.1, but we have changed it slightly. You will now see that there are more participants who have censored data. When we have censored data it means that the participants did not experience the event of interest. We have the same three participants who are classed as right censored but we have an additional two participants (3 and 7) who are also censored. These two participants are marked down as not experiencing the event but their lines on the graph do not reach to the right-hand end ... Why is this so? These two participants dropped out of the study for some reason, thus the researchers were not able to follow them up and they are recorded as not experiencing the event of interest. These two participants are simply called censored data points. Now let us have a look at Figure 15.3.

Here we have a slightly different pattern for the participants. In this example not all of the participants started the study at the same point in time. You can see that the lines for participants 1, 6 and 8 begin some time into the time course of the study. When we present information in graphs similar to those above, we have to make it clear what the left-hand side of the graphs represent. Does it mean the start time for the study overall or does it mean the start time for each participant? If it means the start time for each participant we can change Figure 15.3 so that it now looks like Figure 15.4. In this figure we have simply shifted the lines for participants 1, 6 and 8 so that they too start at the left-hand side of the graph.

When presented in this way the left-hand side of the graph is often called the *time of randomisation*.

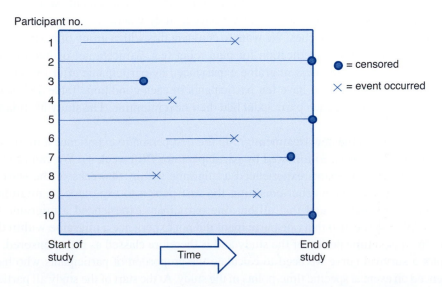

Figure 15.3 Illustration of participants who are included in the study after the start

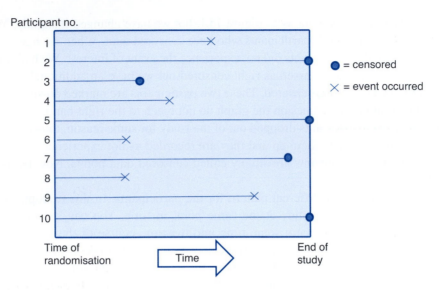

Figure 15.4   Information from Figure 15.3 presented as the time of randomisation

SURVIVAL CURVES

Often in survival analysis we want to compare the events of interest across two or more groups. A useful way of doing this is with survival curves. In a survival curve we plot the proportion of participants who have not experienced the event as a function of time. In the examples that we are going to give here it is assumed that all participants were available at the start of the study. Let us assume that we have a study where we are comparing a new treatment for migraine headaches. We want to compare this with a group of participants who only take over-the-counter medication for pain relief (e.g. paracetamol or ibuprofen). The event of interest here is the next migraine experienced by participants after the start of the study. Let us assume that we have ten participants in each condition. Table 15.1 shows us how long in weeks before each participant had their next migraine. The study itself lasted for six months.

We can see that in the new treatment group the first person to experience a migraine was participant no. 2 (in week 3) followed by participant no. 7 (in week 4). We can see that for this condition all participants experienced a migraine within 14 weeks of the start of the study. In the standard pain relief condition the first person to experience a migraine was participant 6 (in week 7) and that all but one participant experienced a migraine within 25 weeks. We can see also that one participant did not experience a migraine within the six-month (26 weeks) time period of the study and is therefore classed as right censored.

To plot a survival curve we need to calculate the proportion of participants who have not experienced an event at specific time-points in the study. At the start of the study all participants are migraine free, and so 100% of participants have not experienced the event of interest.

Table 15.1 Number of weeks for each participant in the new treatment and standard pain relief treatment conditions to experience the next migraine

New treatment		Standard pain relief	
Participant number	Weeks to event	Participant number	Weeks to event
1	12	1	14
2	3	2	17
3	14	3	19
4	9	4	21
5	7	5	12
6	5	6	7
7	4	7	18
8	7	8	Right censored
9	6	9	11
10	11	10	25

You should be able to see from Table 15.2 that the participants in the new treatment condition tend to experience their first migraine earlier than those in the standard pain relief condition. Presenting information in a table like this is fine, but presenting this information is much clearer in graphical form. This is where survival curves are useful. Figure 15.5 represents a survival curve for the information presented in Table 15.2.

Table 15.2 Details of which participants experienced a migraine in each week and also the weekly proportion of participants who had yet to experience a migraine

Week	New treatment		Regular pain killers	
	Participant experiencing first migraine in this week	Proportion not experienced migraine	Participant experiencing first migraine in this week	Proportion not experienced migraine
1		1		1
2		1		1
3	2	.90		1
4	7	.80		1

(Continued)

Table 15.2 Cont'd

Week	New treatment		Regular pain killers	
	Participant experiencing first migraine in this week	Proportion not experienced migraine	Participant experiencing first migraine in this week	Proportion not experienced migraine
5	6	.70		1
6	9	.60		1
7	5 and 8	.40	6	.90
8		.40		.90
9	4	.30		.90
10		.30		.90
11	10	.20	9	.80
12	1	.10	5	.70
13		.10		.70
14	3	0.0	1	.60
15		0.0		.60
16		0.0		.60
17		0.0	2	.50
18		0.0	7	.40
19		0.0	3	.30
20		0.0		.30
21		0.0	4	.20
22		0.0		.20
23		0.0		.20
24		0.0		.20
25		0.0	10	.10
26		0.0		.10

Traditionally, in a survival curve the curve drops vertically at a point where someone in the study experiences the event of interest, otherwise the graph stays horizontal. In Figure 15.5 you should be able to see that for the standard pain relief condition the line stays horizontal from the start of the study until week 7. This is the first point at which someone in this condition has a migraine. After this time the next person to experience a migraine is

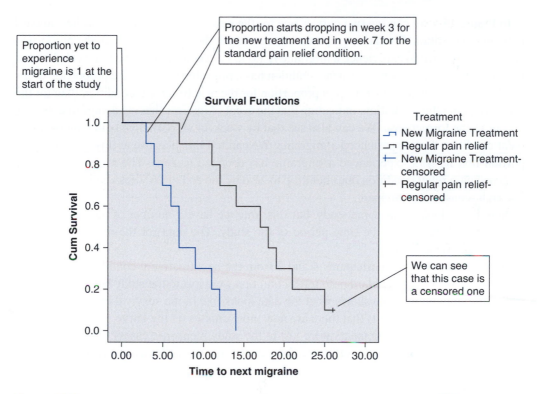

Figure 15.5 Survival curves for the new treatment and standard pain relief conditions

during week 11, and you can see that the graph stays horizontal again until this point in the study when it drops down. The survival curves are created in this way.

Activity 15.1

Plot the following data as a survival curve

Participant number	Weeks to event
1	4
2	3
3	10
4	9
5	7
6	5
7	4
8	7
9	6
10	8

In Figure 15.5 we can see two curves, one for the new treatment and one for the standard pain relief condition. From this graph we can see that at the start of the study the proportion of participants still to experience a migraine is 1.0 in both conditions. Then in week 3 one of the participants in the new treatment condition has a migraine and thus the proportion drops to 0.90. We can see a steeper drop in proportion for the new treatment condition than for the standard pain relief condition, indicating that the event of interest (having a migraine) occurs sooner in the former case. We can also see that by week 14 all participants in the new treatment condition have experienced a migraine. We can tell this because at this week the proportion that has not experienced a migraine has dropped to zero. The proportion for the standard pain relief condition does not drop to zero by the end of 26 weeks and thus we have one right-censored participant.

Now let us look at the same study, but this time we have a number of participants who have dropped out within the time period of the study. The data for these participants are presented in Table 15.3.

Here we can see that participants 4 and 7 from the new treatment condition and participants 1 and 3 from the standard pain relief condition were lost to the study before experiencing a migraine. Figure 15.6 shows what the data looks like in the survival curves.

The first thing to notice is that there are now more crosses on the curve. The little crosses indicate weeks where participants were lost to the study (censored cases). Also, the shapes of the curves are now slightly different. You can see this more clearly in Figure 15.7 where

Table 15.3 Number of weeks for each participant in the new treatment and standard pain relief treatment conditions to experience the next migraine (revised data)

New treatment		Standard pain relief	
Participant number	Weeks to event	Participant number	Weeks to event
1	12	1	Dropped out in week 14
2	3	2	17
3	14	3	Dropped out in week 19
4	Dropped out in week 9	4	21
5	7	5	12
6	5	6	7
7	Dropped out in week 4	7	18
8	7	8	Right censored
9	6	9	11
10	11	10	25

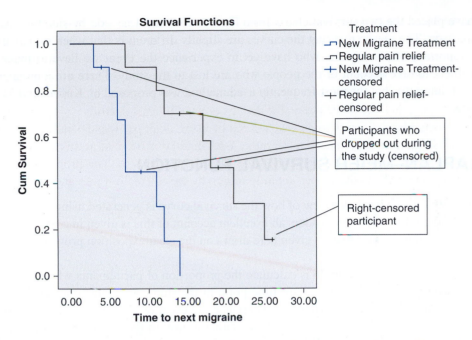

Figure 15.6 Survival curves for the new treatment and standard pain relief conditions showing participants who dropped out during the study

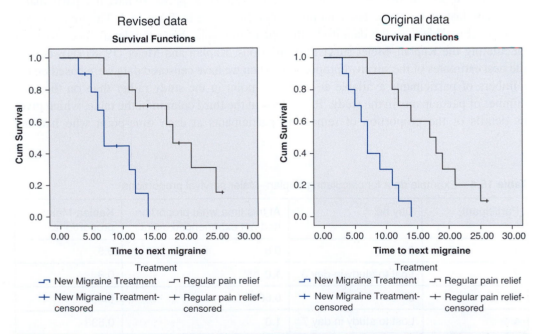

Figure 15.7 Survival curves for the new treatment and standard pain relief conditions (revised data) alongside those for the original data

we have placed the two survival charts from Figures 15.5 and 15.6 side-by-side for ease of comparison. The reason that that the curves are slightly different is that when we calculate the proportion of participants who have yet to experience the event we have to make an adjustment to take account of the people who are lost to the study. There are a number of ways of doing this but the most frequently used method was proposed by Kaplan and Meier in 1958.

THE KAPLAN–MEIER SURVIVAL FUNCTION

Here we will give a brief overview of how the survival curve is generated using the Kaplan–Meier method. For interested readers an excellent account of this is given in a paper by Peto et al. (1977) and the explanation given here draws on the clear exposition provided by those authors.

Basically, what we have to do is calculate the proportion of participants who could have experienced an event at each relevant time-point in the study. Relevant time-points in the study are classed as when a participant experiences an event or when someone is lost to the study. Thus on a survival curve you will see either a drop in the curve or a little cross to indicate a relevant time-point. What we have to do to work out the relevant proportions at each point is to think about how many participants are still in the study just prior to each relevant time-point in the study. Let us look at an example. Suppose we have five participants in a study lasting ten days. The data might look like those in Table 15.4. The first two columns of this table have the data itself, the rest of the table shows the details necessary for calculating the Kaplan–Meier survival proportions. Kaplan and Meier (1958) showed that the best estimates of the survival proportions when we have censored data were based on the numbers of participants available at each time-point in the study rather than on the total number of participants in the study. Take a look at the third column in the table, which gives us details of the proportion of remaining participants at each time-point who had not

Table 15.4   Example data for calculating Kaplan–Meier survival proportions

Participant	Day no.	At this time what proportion had not experienced event	Kaplan-Meier proportions
1	2	0.8	0.8
2	Lost to study in day 3	1.0	0.8
3	5	0.667	0.533
4	Lost to study in day 7	1.0	0.533
5	9	0.0	0.0

experienced the event of interest. For example, just before day 2 there were five people in the study and at day 2 itself, four out of five of the participants had not experienced the event of interest and so the proportion here is 4/5 or 0.8. Now let us move to the next relevant time-point, day 3. Just before day 3 there were four people in the study, however at day 3 none of these participants had experienced the event of interest and so the proportion not experiencing the event is 1.0. This is the case even though one participant was lost to the study. Now moving to the next relevant time-point, day 5, we see that just before this day there were three participants still in the study, and at day 5 two of these had not experienced the event, therefore the proportion here is 2/3 or 0.667. Moving on to day 7 we see that just before this day there were two people in the study and at day 7 none had experienced the event and so the proportion is 1.0. Finally, we move to day 9. Just before this day there was one person in the study and at day 9 this person experienced the event of interest and so none of the available people had not experienced event and thus this proportion is 0.0.

Now let us move to the Kaplan–Meier proportions column. This column contains the Kaplan–Meier proportions which are used to generate the survival curve. In order to understand these it is worthwhile thinking in terms of probabilities. The proportions presented in the table can be thought of as the probability that a person who has yet to experience the event at particular time-point will not actually experience the event at that time-point. Thus from the table we can see that on day number 2 a person has a 0.8 probability of not experiencing the event. Now we have to remember that when we combine probabilities they have to be multiplied together. For example, what is the probability that you will roll two sixes on two dice? The probability of rolling a six on each die independently is 1 in 6 or 0.167. But the probability of rolling a six on both dice is 0.167×0.167. Applying this idea of multiplying probabilities to the survival data, we can think in terms of the days in the study. What is the probability of survival (not experiencing the event) on day 1? In our case it is 1.0 as no participant experienced the event on this day. The probability of survival on day 2 is dependent upon surviving day 1 also, and so we have to multiply the probability of survival on day 1 by the probability of survival on day 2 to get our Kaplan–Meier probability (or proportion). The probability of survival on day 2 was 0.8 and if we multiply this by the probability of survival on day 1 (which is 1.0) we get 0.8, and this is the figure in the Kaplan–Meier column in the table. To calculate the Kaplan–Meier for day 3 we have to multiply the probability of surviving on day 3 (1.0) by the probability of surviving day 2 (0.8) and by the probability of surviving day 1 (1.0), leading to a figure of 0.8 again. Thus to calculate the Kaplan–Meier proportions we multiply all of the proportions in the third column down to the specific row that we are interested in. For example, if we look at row three (participant 3) in the table, to get the Kaplan–Meier proportion we multiply all the proportions in column three down to and including this row. Thus we multiply 0.8 by 1.0 by 0.667, and this gives us 0.533. Moving down to day 7 (fourth row in the table) we calculate the Kaplan–Meier proportion by multiplying 0.8 by 1.0 by 0.667 by 1.0, and this gives us 0.533.

When you conduct a survival analysis in SPSS you will get a survival curve based upon the Kaplan–Meier proportions. The survival curve for the data in Table 15.4 is presented in Figure 15.8.

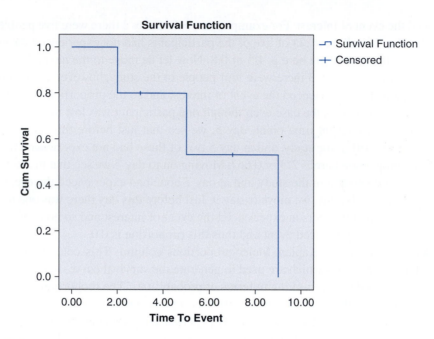

Figure 15.8   Survival curve for the data presented in Table 15.4

KAPLAN–MEIER SURVIVAL ANALYSES IN SPSS

In order to conduct a survival analysis in SPSS you need to set up your data file correctly. In this illustration we are going to set up an SPSS file using the data from Table 15.3. We need to set up three variables in the data file as we have done in the Screenshot 15.1. We have one variable with the condition that each participant is in (new treatment or standard pain relief), one variable which has the time the event happened to each participant (or the time they were lost to the study) and one variable which has information about the status of the participant. This last variable is incredibly important for ensuring that SPSS takes account of censored cases. This variable is where we record whether or not the participant experienced the event within the time-course of the study (i.e. whether or not they were censored). If they did have a migraine then they are recorded as 1, if they did not then they are recorded as 0.

To run the actual survival analysis you need to select the *Analyze, Survival, Kaplan-Meier* options (Screenshot 15.2).

You will then be presented with a dialogue box (Screenshot 15.3).

You should move the *Time* variable to the *Time:* box and the *Status* variable to the *Status:* box. You then should click on the *Define Event* button. This will open up a new dialogue box (Screenshot 15.4).

In this dialogue box you need to let SPSS know what values in the *Status* variable indicate that an event has occurred. Remember we typed a 1 in this variable for all those participants

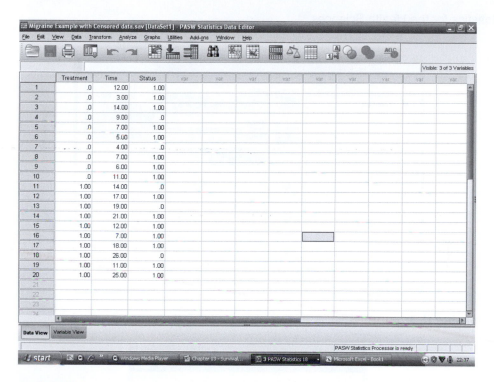

Screenshot 15.1

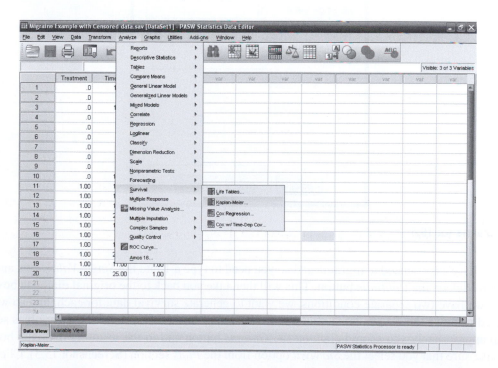

Screenshot 15.2

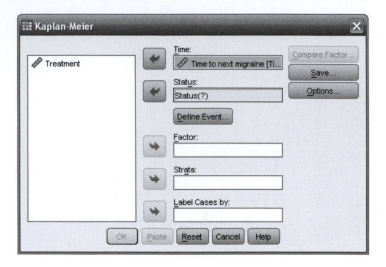

Screenshot 15.3

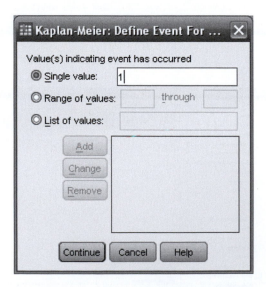

Screenshot 15.4

who have experienced a migraine and so you need to type a 1 into the *Single Value:* box and then click on the *Continue* button. This will then take you back to the original dialogue box. As we have two separate conditions, we want to generate survival data for each, and so we need to move the *Treatment* variable into the *Factor:* box. Once you have the variables set up appropriately you should click on the *Options* button and in the resulting dialogue box make sure that you select the *Survival* option from the *Plots* section (Screenshot 15.5). Click on *Continue* and then *OK* to run the analyses.

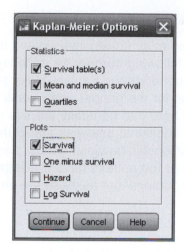

Screenshot 15.5

As part of the output you will get the a survival table (Screenshot 15.6). In this table the column of most interest is the *Estimate* column in the *Cumulative Proportion Surviving at the Time* section. This column contains the Kaplan–Meier survival proportions which are then presented in the survival plot.

Survival Table

Treatment		Time	Status	Cumulative Proportion Surviving at the Time		N of Cumulative Events	N of Remaining Cases
				Estimate	Std. Error		
New Migraine Treatment	1	3.000	1.00	.900	.095	1	9
	2	4.000	.00			1	8
	3	5.000	1.00	.788	.134	2	7
	4	6.000	1.00	.675	.155	3	6
	5	7.000	1.00	1.00		4	5
	6	7.000	1.00	.450	.166	5	4
	7	9.000	.00			5	3
	8	11.000	1.00	.300	.165	6	2
	9	12.000	1.00	.150	.134	7	1
	10	14.000	1.00	.000	.000	8	0
Regular pain relief	1	7.000	1.00	.900	.095	1	9
	2	11.000	1.00	.800	.126	2	8
	3	12.000	1.00	.700	.145	3	7
	4	14.000	.00			3	6
	5	17.000	1.00	.583	.161	4	5
	6	18.000	1.00	.467	.166	5	4
	7	19.000	.00			5	3
	8	21.000	1.00	.311	.168	6	2
	9	25.000	1.00	.156	.139	7	1
	10	26.000	.00			7	0

Screenshot 15.6

Example from the Literature

A study published by Burneo et al. (2008) investigated the role of gender and ethnicity on seizure outcome following surgery for epilepsy. The authors conducted survival analyses including generation of Kaplan–Meier survival curves. Their figure showing the survival curves for the gender analyses is presented in Figure 15.9. You should be able to see here that generally the two curves are similar to each other, and in fact in some additional analyses that Burneo et al. conducted they found that there was no relationship between gender and rate of seizures following surgery. You should note that the authors have presented percentages in the survival curves rather than proportions, but as these are equivalent this doesn't really matter.

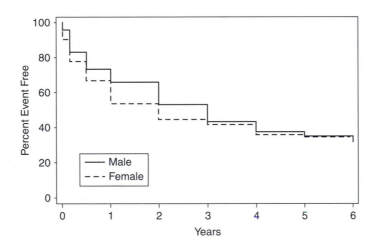

Figure 15.9   Survival curve from Burneo et al. (2008)

COMPARING TWO SURVIVAL CURVES – THE MANTEL–COX TEST

It is useful to compare two survival functions visually using survival curves, but what is often required is some formal test of whether two curves are statistically significantly different from each other. There are a number of ways of doing this but we are going to focus on one of the most frequently used techniques; the *Mantel–Cox* or *log rank* test. We will not be explaining the calculations in detail here but we want to give you a flavour of what lies behind this test. In order to understand this you need to think back to what you learned about chi-square tests in Chapter 9. Remember for chi-square you have to compare the observed frequencies with the expected frequencies. If there is little difference between the observed and expected frequencies we obtain a low value for chi-square, and we conclude that there are no differences between our conditions beyond that attributable to chance variations. A similar logic underlies the Mantel–Cox test, but this time instead of comparing observed and expected frequencies we are comparing observed and expected proportions at each time-point in the study. We then calculate a chi-square statistic from these observed and expected proportions and test this against a chi-square distribution with $k-1$ degrees of freedom where k is the number of survival curves that we are comparing. In our migraine example (with the censored data) the chi-square statistics come out at 9.64 with one degree of freedom. The probability associated with this chi-square value is .002 indicating that the two survival curves in this example are statistically significantly different from each other.

A worked example may help to conceptualise what the Mantel–Cox test is doing. Suppose that we have 20 participants and we are interested in how many experience mouth infection after they have wisdom teeth extracted. Half of the participants are asked to rinse their mouth regularly with salt water and the others are not asked to take any particular action to help prevent infection. We follow all participants for seven days after the extraction and record how many get an infection on each day. Some data for this are presented in Table 15.5.

Now, if there was no effect of rinsing the mouth with salt water on infection rates we would expect to have approximately equal numbers of participants getting infections on each day after tooth extraction. However, the calculation of this is somewhat complicated by the fact that at each time-point we don't necessarily have equal numbers of participants left in each condition who have yet to experience an infection. Thus because two participants got infections in the no action condition at time-point 2, there are now only eight participants who could get an infection at time-point 3, whereas for the salt water rinse condition there was only one person who had an infection at time-point 2, and thus nine participants could potentially get an infection at time-point 3. The Mantel–Cox test takes these factors into account and is calculated on the basis of how many participants could potentially get an

Table 15.5 Number of infections on each day for the salt water rinse group and the no action group after wisdom teeth extraction

Day no.	No action	Salt water rinse
1	0	0
2	2	1
3	1	0
4	3	1
5	2	1
6	0	0
7	0	0

Table 15.6   Observed and expected infections post wisdom teeth extraction

Day no.	No action			Salt water rinse		
	Observed	Expected	No. left in study	Observed	Expected	No. left in study
1	0	0	10	0	0	10
2	2	1.5	10	1	1.5	10
3	1	0.47	8	0	0.53	9
4	3	1.75	7	1	2.25	9
5	2	2	4	1	1	8
6	0	0	2	0	0	7
7	0	0	2	0	0	7
Totals	**8**	**5.72**		**3**	**5.28**	7

infection at each time-point. Thus, the test works by comparing the number of participants who haven't experienced infection at each time-point who then go on to actually experience an infection at that time-point (e.g. How many participants after day two who haven't yet got an infection go on to get an infection on day 3?). We have presented these numbers in Table 15.6 in the Observed column. We also have to work out how many participants we would expect for each condition on each day if there was no difference between the two conditions (i.e. if the salt water rinse was having no effect on infection rates). We have done this in Table 15.6 in the Expected column.

We then use the totals for the observed and expected numbers of infections across the time-points to calculate the chi-square statistic. This description is a simplification of what the Mantel–Cox test actually does, but it serves to illustrate what is going on here. In the case of the data in Table 15.6, the chi-square is calculated by SPSS as 4.77 and is statistically significant ($p < .05$).

MANTEL–COX USING SPSS

To conduct a Mantel–Cox analysis in SPSS we use the same dialogue box as we used to generate the survival curves earlier. So you need to click on the *Analyze, Survival, Kaplan-Meier* options and set up the dialogue box as we did earlier (see Screenshot 15.7).

You then need to click on the *Compare Factor* button and you will get another dialogue box (Screenshot 15.8).

Select the *Log rank* option and then *Continue* followed by *OK* to run the analysis. You will get the same survival curve and table output that we presented earlier in the chapter,

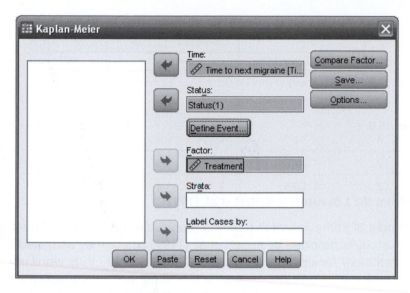

Screenshot 15.7

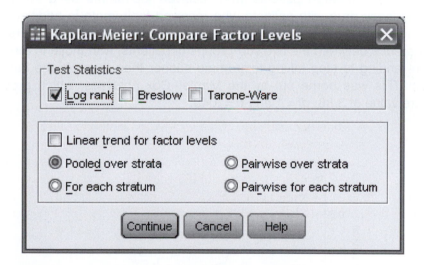

Screenshot 15.8

plus you will get a table which gives the relevant details of the Mantel–Cox analysis (Screenshot 15.9).

In this table you will see the chi-square statistic, the degrees of freedom (which is simply the number of curves that you are comparing minus one) and the *p*-value. Here we can see that for the migraine data that we presented earlier there is a significant difference between the new treatment and the standard pain relief conditions (*p* = .002).

Overall Comparisons

	Chi-Square	df	Sig.
Log Rank (Mantel-Cox)	9.694	1	.002

Test of equality of survival distributions for the different levels of Treatment.

Screenshot 15.9

Example from the Literature – Kellett et al. (1999)

As an example of some research that has reported the use of the Mantel–Cox (log rank) test a study is reported by Kellett et al. (1999) where they analysed the impact of a new treatment for epilepsy (topiramate). In the study they were interested in how long it took patients to stop using the new drug, and they present a number of survival curves for sub-groups of the patients that they included in the study. For example, they compared patients who received topiramate as a substitute for another epilepsy drug with patients who received topiramate in addition to other drugs. The survival curves are presented in Figure 15.10. There appears to be a clear difference between the two sub-groups of patients, with those in the 'add on' condition tending to stop taking topiramate sooner than those in the substitution condition. This was borne out by the Mantel–Cox analyses, which produced a chi-square value of 3.88, $df = 1$ and $p = .049$.

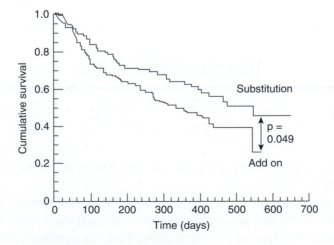

Figure 15.10   Survival curves presented for the analyses reported by Kellett et al. (1999)

HAZARD

A concept that is closely related to survival is *hazard*. When analysing survival data we can represent it in terms of the survival function as explained previously in this chapter, or in terms of the *hazard function*. The hazard function is defined as the instantaneous death (event) rate. That is, it is the rate of the event at a particular moment in time after the start of the study (time of randomisation). Thus whilst the survival function focusses on the proportion who survive (or don't experience the event of interest) at a particular time-point, the hazard function is the rate of death (event) at a particular time-point. A definition of the hazard function provided by Everitt and Pickles (1999) suggests that it is the probability of a person experiencing the event of interest at a particular time, given that they have survived (not experienced the event) up to that particular time.

HAZARD CURVES

We can generate a curve similar to the survival curve to represent the hazard function; the easiest form of this curve is something called the *cumulative hazard function* and this is the one that is generated in SPSS. The cumulative hazard curves for the migraine data presented earlier in the chapter are presented in Figure 15.11.

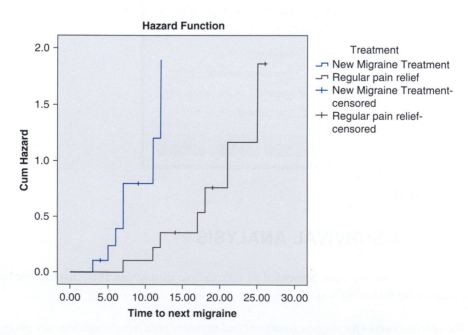

Figure 15.11   Cumulative hazard curves for the migraine treatment example

You should be able to see that the curves represented in Figure 15.11 suggest that the rate of the event happening seems to increase over time, that is the curve is flatter in the earlier months and steeper in the later months. The clear thing from this though is that the curves for the two conditions are fairly well separated over time, and suggest that the rates of events increase at an earlier time for the new treatment condition compared to the standard pain relief condition.

HAZARD FUNCTIONS IN SPSS

In order to generate the hazard curve in SPSS you follow the procedure above for generating survival curves. Click on the *Options* button and make sure that you select the *Hazard* option from the *Plots* section of the dialogue box. Click on *Continue* followed by *OK* to generate the graph (Screenshot 15.10).

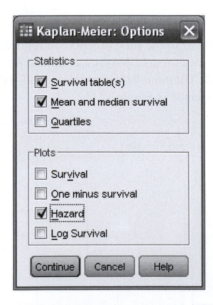

Screenshot 15.10

WRITING UP A SURVIVAL ANALYSIS

For the analyses that we have presented as an example throughout this chapter you might write it up in the following way:

The survival curves for the new treatment and standard pain relief conditions are presented in Figure 1. These suggest that contrary to expectation the participants in the new

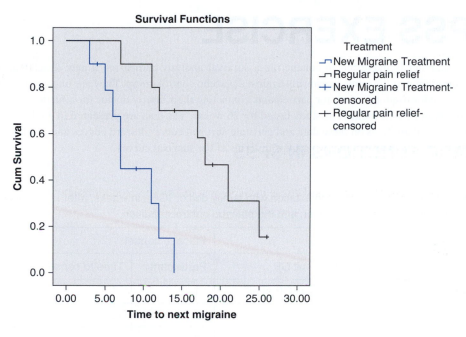

Figure 1   Survival curves for the new treatment and standard pain relief conditions

treatment condition tended to experience migraines sooner after the time of randomisation than those participants in the standard pain relief condition. Mantel–Cox analysis of the survival functions confirmed that the two survival curves were significantly different from each other $\chi^2 = 9.69$, df = 1, p = .002.

Summary

In this chapter we have given you a grounding in basic survival analysis. You will find the concepts and techniques presented here reported in many research papers where survival analysis has been used. We have shown how we can represent survival data in terms of proportions of participants surviving to specified time-points in the study in the form of survival tables and survival curves. We have shown you how you can use the Mantel–Cox test to discover whether two survival curves are significantly different from one another. This is important, as it allows us to find out if the rate of survival (or not experiencing an event) is different across two conditions in a study or across two sub-groups of participants (e.g. males and females). Finally, we have briefly described another way of looking at survival data by generating hazard functions and curves.

SPSS EXERCISE

A researcher is interested in conducting a survival analysis comparing a new drug treatment for inflammation of the joints in arthritis against a placebo control group. They are interested in the time from randomisation to time for participants contacting their family doctor for a further consultation about pain in their joints. The study lasted for 26 weeks. The data are presented in Table 15.7. Please run survival analyses on these data and generate survival curves, hazard curves and test for a significant difference between the two groups in terms of the survival curves.

Table 15.7 Times to first consultation with family doctor (GP), in weeks, after randomisation for the new drug treatment condition and the placebo control condition

New drug		Placebo control	
Participant	Time to consult GP	Participant	Time to consult GP
1	Did not consult GP at all	1	1
2	3	2	10
3	Lost to study in week 22	3	4
4	22	4	1
5	Did not consult GP at all	5	15
6	Did not consult GP at all	6	26
7	26	7	9
8	19	8	Lost to study in week 7
9	12	9	12
10	Lost to study in week 12	10	Did not consult GP at all

MULTIPLE CHOICE QUESTIONS

1. In a survival curve the y-axis represents:
   a) The time taken for participants to experience the event
   b) The proportion of participants yet to experience the event
   c) The probability of experiencing the event
   d) None of the above

2. The definition of the hazard function is:
   a) The rate of survival at each time-point
   b) The rate of the event of interest at a specified time-point
   c) The dangers associated with the conditions in the study
   d) All of the above

3. Another name for the Mantel–Cox test is:
   a) The cumulative hazard function
   b) The survival function
   c) The log rank test
   d) The log fire test

4. The calculations for the Mantel–Cox test are:
   a) Based upon comparing the observed number of events with the expected number of events at each time-point
   b) Based only on the numbers of participants who are lost to the study or who do not experience the event
   c) Based upon the mean number of events for each condition
   d) None of the above

5. When a person does not experience the event within the time-frame for the study they are called:
   a) Surplus to requirements
   b) An invalid case
   c) An outlier
   d) Right censored

6. Which of the following represents the best definition of censored cases?
   a) People who do not want to join the study
   b) Participants who drop out of the study and/or have not experienced the event of interest
   c) Participants who don't read the instructions carefully enough
   d) Both b) and c) above

7. The beginning of the time-period for a survival analysis is often called:
   a) The start of the study
   b) The time of randomisation
   c) Time zero
   d) Let's get started

8. Take a look at the following survival curves. What can you say about the person indicated in the graph by the circle around the cross?
   a) The person had a migraine in week 14
   b) The person did not have a migraine in week 14 but had it at a later time
   c) The person did not have a migraine at all within the time-frame of the study
   d) The person was lost to the study in week 14

Survival Functions

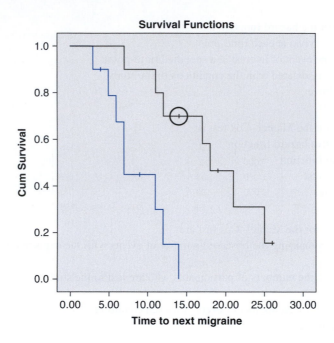

9. Referring back to the graph in question 8, what term is given to the person highlighted?
   a) They are unimportant
   b) They are censored
   c) They are right censored
   d) They are a hazard

10. How might we calculate the probability of a participant surviving until the fifth day in the study?
   a) It is the probability of not experiencing the event divided by the probability of experiencing the event
   b) It is the probability of surviving until the fourth day multiplied by the probability of surviving the fifth day
   c) It is the probability of surviving the first day, times the probability of surviving the second day, times the probability of surviving the third day, times the probability of surviving the fourth day, times the probability of surviving the fifth day
   d) Both b) and c) above

11. From the following SPSS survival table work out how many participants in each condition are censored:
   a) 7 and 5
   b) 0 and 1
   c) 4 and 4
   d) 3 and 5

Survival Table

Treatment		Time	Status	Cumulative Proportion Surviving at the Time		N of Cumulative Events	N of Remaining Cases
				Estimate	Std. Error		
New Migraine Treatment	1	3.000	1.00	.900	.095	1	9
	2	4.000	.00			1	8
	3	5.000	1.00	.788	.134	2	7
	4	6.000	1.00	.675	.155	3	6
	5	7.000	1.00			4	5
	6	7.000	1.00	.450	.166	5	4
	7	9.000	.00			5	3
	8	11.000	1.00	.300	.165	6	2
	9	12.000	.00			6	1
	10	14.000	1.00	.000	.000	7	0
Regular pain relief	1	7.000	1.00	.900	.095	1	9
	2	11.000	.00			1	8
	3	12.000	.00			1	7
	4	14.000	.00			1	6
	5	17.000	1.00	.750	.158	2	5
	6	18.000	1.00	.600	.184	3	4
	7	19.000	.00			3	3
	8	21.000	1.00	.400	.204	4	2
	9	25.000	1.00	.200	.174	5	1
	10	26.000	.00			5	0

12. What does the following output from SPSS say about the two survival curves?

Overall Comparisons

	Chi-Square	df	Sig.
Log Rank (Mantel-Cox)	10.436	1	.001

Test of equality of survival distributions for the different levels of Treatment.

a) They are different but not significantly so
b) They are identical
c) They are significantly different
d) None of the above

13. Given the following survival curves what would be a good interpretation?
   a) That the two survival curves are different from each other but there are too many censored cases to make them valid
   b) The two survival curves are the same but not enough participants had a migraine within the time-frame of the study
   c) The two survival curves are the same but new treatment participants had migraines about two weeks earlier than the standard pain relief participants
   d) All of the above

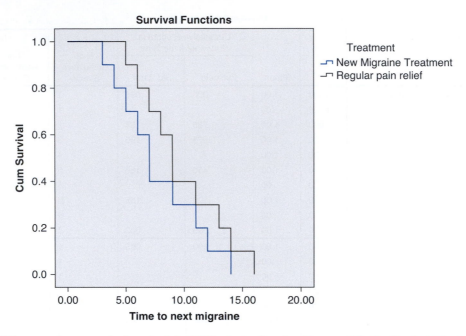

Survival Functions

14. When running a survival analysis in SPSS what value should you put in the *Single Value* box in the dialogue box below if you have coded those who have not experienced the event of interest as 1 and those who have as 2?

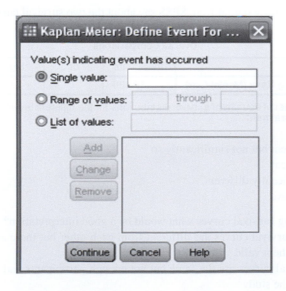

a) 1
b) 2
c) 1 or 2
d) Neither 1 or 2

15. In a survival analysis if you have ten participants at the start of the study and at 3 weeks you have a proportion surviving of 0.8, how many participants have experienced the event in that week?
    a) 2
    b) 8
    c) 10
    d) We can't tell from the above information

Answers to Activities and Exercises

CHAPTER 1

Activity 1.1

The conceptualisation of research in Figure 1.1 suggests that research ideas come from reading the relevant literature in a field. However, research ideas can often precede a survey of the literature. You might have an idea out of the blue about ways of helping nurses deal with obese patients. You would then read the literature relevant to this to see how best to implement and test your idea.

Activity 1.2

- Types of jobs undertaken by staff in an intensive care ward – *Nominal*
- Ratings for job satisfaction of A & E staff – *Ordinal (or could be interval)*
- Number of visits to a family doctor after a hospital stay for heart transplant patients – *Ratio*
- Length of time to regain consciousness after a general anaesthetic – *Ratio*

- Number of fillings given to primary school children – *Ratio*
- Temperatures of children after being given 5 ml of ibuprofen – *Interval*
- Ethnicity of patients – *Nominal*

Activity 1.3

1. Examining the difference between paracetamol and aspirin in the pain relief experienced by migraine sufferers – Independent variable is type of pain relief and dependent variable is measured experience of pain relief.
2. Examining the effects of consultants providing full information about a surgical procedure to patients (rather than minimal information) prior to surgery on time to be discharged post surgery – Independent variable is amount of information given prior to surgery and dependent variable is length to time to discharge post surgery.
3. Examining the difference between wards with matrons and those without on in-patient satisfaction – Independent variable is whether or not wards have matrons and dependent variable is in-patient satisfaction.
4. Examining the uptake of chlamydia screening from family doctor surgeries with and without chlamydia health promotion leaflets – Independent variable is whether or not GP surgeries have chlamydia health promotion leaflets and dependent variable is how many people are screened for chlamydia.

Activity 1.4

Remember, for an experimental design you need to randomly allocate participants to the conditions of the independent variable. Therefore, you might have two conditions of your independent variable (e.g. an exercise regime versus no exercise) and you would randomly allocate children to one of these conditions to see what effect this has on ADHD symptoms. For a quasi-experimental design you will probably be comparing already pre-defined groups, and so you might recruit children who already undertake regular exercise and compare them for ADHD symptoms to children who do not undertake regular exercise. Finally, for a correlational study you might record how much exercise each participant undertakes per week and see if this is related to the severity of symptoms of ADHD.

MCQs

1b, 2d, 3c, 4d, 5b, 6d, 7a, 8d, 9c, 10b, 11a, 12d, 13a, 14a, 15c

CHAPTER 2

SPSS Exercise 1

You should set up two variables in SPSS. One for the *occupation* variable and one for the stress scores. Remember, when you set up the *occupation* variable to use the *Values* characteristic to give meaningful labels to the occupations (e.g. 1 = nurses, 2 = junior doctors and 3 = consultants). The data file should look like this:

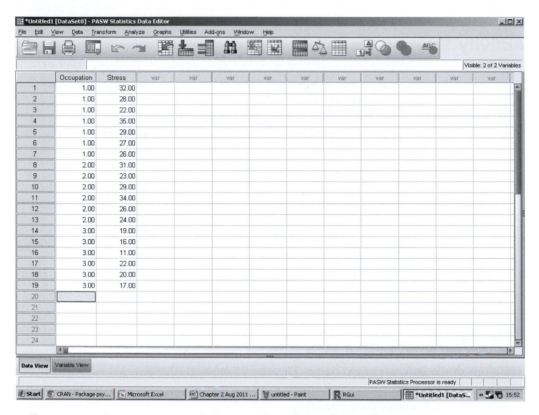

To generate the summary statistics you should use the *Analyse*, *Descriptive Statistics*, *Explore* menu options and set up the dialogue box like this:

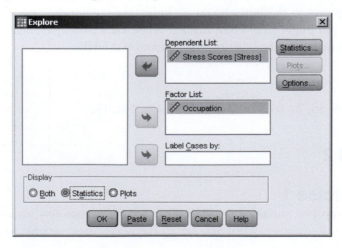

Then click on *OK* and you will be presented with the following table:

Descriptives

Occupation				Statistic	Std. Error
Stress Scores	Nurse	Mean		28.4286	1.58651
		95% Confidence Interval for Mean	Lower Bound	24.5465	
			Upper Bound	32.3106	
		5% Trimmed Mean		28.4206	
		Median		28.0000	
		Variance		17.619	
		Std. Deviation		4.19750	
		Minimum		22.00	
		Maximum		35.00	
		Range		13.00	
		Interquartile Range		6.00	
		Skewness		.147	.794
		Kurtosis		.274	1.587
	Junior Doctor	Mean		27.8333	1.74005
		95% Confidence Interval for Mean	Lower Bound	23.3604	
			Upper Bound	32.3063	
		5% Trimmed Mean		27.7593	
		Median		27.5000	
		Variance		18.167	
		Std. Deviation		4.26224	
		Minimum		23.00	
		Maximum		34.00	
		Range		11.00	
		Interquartile Range		8.00	
		Skewness		.358	.845
		Kurtosis		−1.326	1.741
	Consultant	Mean		17.5000	1.56525
		95% Confidence Interval for Mean	Lower Bound	13.4764	
			Upper Bound	21.5236	
		5% Trimmed Mean		17.6111	
		Median		18.0000	
		Variance		14.700	
		Std. Deviation		3.83406	
		Minimum		11.00	
		Maximum		22.00	
		Range		11.00	
		Interquartile Range		5.75	
		Skewness		−.894	.845
		Kurtosis		1.020	1.741

SPSS Exercise 2

First of all you need to set up two variables in SPSS. One will contain the patient satisfaction ratings and the other the length of time they stayed in hospital. The file should look like this:

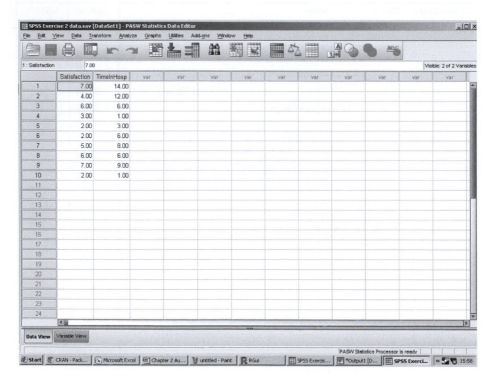

To generate the summary statistics you can use the *Analyze*, *Descriptive Statistics*, *Explore* commands and set up the dialogue box as we have below:

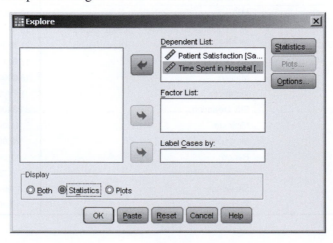

Make sure you select the *Statistics* option in the *Display* section and then click on *OK* to obtain the following table:

Descriptives

Occupation			Statistic	Std. Error
Patient Satisfaction	Mean		4.4000	.65320
	95% Confidence Interval for Mean	Lower Bound	2.9224	
		Upper Bound	5.8776	
	5% Trimmed Mean		4.3889	
	Median		4.5000	
	Variance		4.267	
	Std. Deviation		2.06559	
	Minimum		2.00	
	Maximum		7.00	
	Range		5.00	
	Interquartile Range		4.25	
	Skewness		−.011	.687
	Kurtosis		−1.845	1.334
Time Spent Hospital	Mean		6.6000	1.36789
	95% Confidence Interval for Mean	Lower Bound	3.5056	
		Upper Bound	9.6944	
	5% Trimmed Mean		6.5000	
	Median		6.0000	
	Variance		18.711	
	Std. Deviation		4.32563	
	Minimum		1.00	
	Maximum		14.00	
	Range		13.00	
	Interquartile Range		7.25	
	Skewness		.310	.687
	Kurtosis		−.586	1.334

To generate the scattergram you should select the *Graphs*, *Legacy Dialogs*, *Scatter/Dot* commands and select the *Simple* option and click on the *Define* button. You should then set up the dialogue box as we have below:

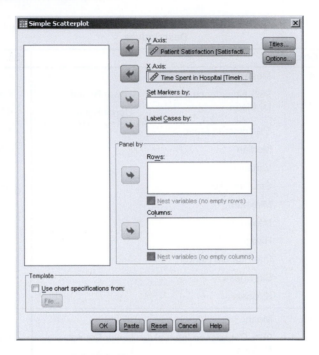

Then click on *OK* to generate the scattergram:

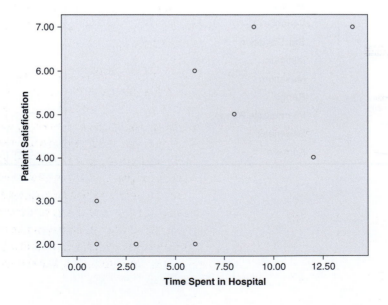

R Exercise 1

To set up the data in R you should code the occupation variable, e.g. nurses = 1, junior doctors = 2 and consultants = 3. You should then type in the following:

```
>Occupation <- c(1, 1, 1, 1, 1, 1, 1,2, 2, 2, 2, 2, 2, 3,
                 3, 3, 3, 3, 3)
```

and then:

```
>Stress <- c(32, 28, 22, 35, 29, 27, 26, 31, 23, 29, 34,
             26, 24, 19, 16, 11, 22, 10, 17)
```

Then to let R know that the occupation variable is a grouping or categorical variable you need to type the following:

```
> Occupation <- factors(Occupation)
```

Now to generate the summary statistics you need to refer to the package called psych but you don't need to re-install this as it should be already installed. So you simply type in the following:

```
> library(psych)
> describe.by(Stress, Occupation)
```

You will then be presented with the following summary statistics:

```
group: 1
   var n   mean   sd median trimmed   mad min max range skew kurtosis   se
1   1 7 28.43 4.2      28    28.43 2.97  22  35    13 0.09    -1.26 1.59
------------------------------------------------------------
group: 2
   var n   mean    sd median trimmed   mad min max range skew kurtosis   se
1   1 6 27.83 4.26    27.5   27.83 5.19  23  34    11  0.2    -1.83 1.74
------------------------------------------------------------
group: 3
   var n   mean    sd median trimmed   mad min max range  skew kurtosis   se
1   1 6 15.83 4.62    16.5   15.83 5.93  10  22    12 -0.07    -1.81 1.89
> |
```

R Exercise 2

To enter the data for R Exercise 2 you could try creating an Excel file first and then saving it as a .CSV file. We have set up the data in Excel as follows and then used *File*, *Save As*, and chosen the CSV file type to save the data. We have called it Patients.csv:

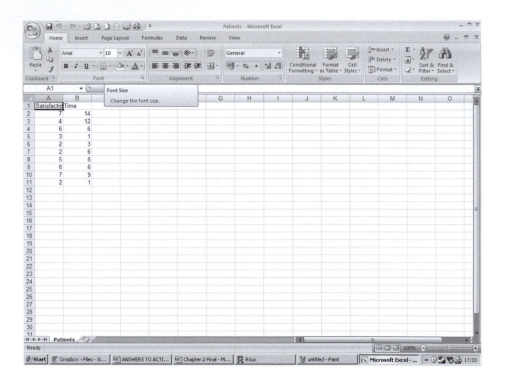

You now need to read the data into R. You do this by typing the following command:

```
> Patients <- read.csv(file="Patients.csv",head=TRUE,sep=",")
```

Don't forget to make sure that your working directory is the same as the one that you have saved your file in by clicking on the *File, Change dir* options:

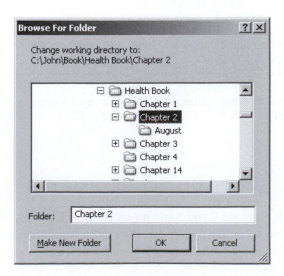

To generate the summary statistics for each variable you can use the following summary command but remember you will need to reference the data frame (in our example 'Patients') followed by the variable name separated by a $ sign:

```
> summary (Patients$Satisfaction)
>summary (Patients$Time)
```

You will be presented with the following:

```
> summary (Patients$Satisfaction)
   Min. 1st Qu.  Median    Mean 3rd Qu.    Max.
   2.00    2.25    4.50    4.40    6.00    7.00
> summary (Patients$Time)
   Min. 1st Qu.  Median    Mean 3rd Qu.    Max.
   1.00    3.75    6.00    6.60    8.75   14.00
>
```

To generate the scattergram, type in the following command:

```
> plot(Patients$Satisfaction, Patients$Time, main="Scatterplot
                Satisfaction by Time")
```

You will be presented with the following:

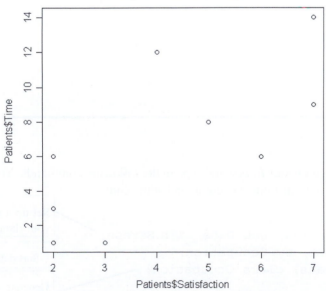

Scatterplot Satisfaction by Time

SAS Exercise 1

The first thing you need to do is open up a new data file. Go to your library and click on *File* and *New* and then double click on the *Table* icon. You will need to set up two variables, one for the stress levels and one for the occupation. Your file should look like the one below (don't forget to save it to your library):

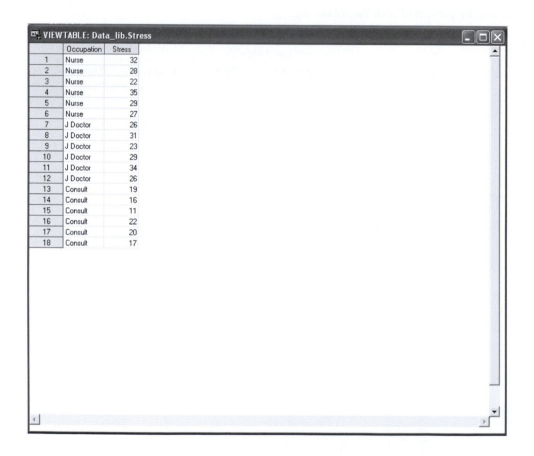

You should then go to your *Editor* and type in the following commands. You can type them all in one go and have just one *run* command at the end:

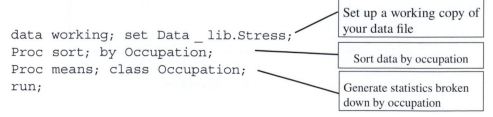

```
data working; set Data _ lib.Stress;
Proc sort; by Occupation;
Proc means; class Occupation;
run;
```

Set up a working copy of your data file

Sort data by occupation

Generate statistics broken down by occupation

You will be presented with the following table.

The SAS System   17:09 Friday, August 12, 2011   1

The MEANS Procedure

Analysis Variable : Stress

Occupation	Obs	N	Mean	Std Dev	Minimum	Maximum
Consult	6	6	17.5000000	3.8340579	11.0000000	22.0000000
J Doctor	6	6	28.1666667	3.9707262	23.0000000	34.0000000
Nurse	6	6	28.8333333	4.4459720	22.0000000	35.0000000

SAS Exercise 2

The first thing you need to do is open up a new data file. Go to your library and click on *File* and *New* and the double click on the *Table* icon. You will need to set up two variables, one for the satisfaction scores and one for the length of time spent in hospital. Your file should look like the one below (don't forget to save it to your library):

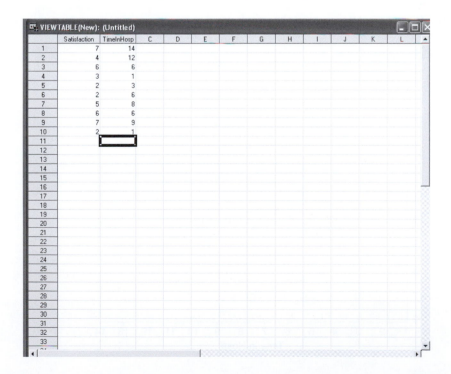

In order to generate the summary statistics and scattergram you can type in all the commands in one mini-program (this is one of the advantages of SAS over R). Type in the following:

```
data working; set Data _ lib.Patients;
Proc means;
Proc gplot;
plot Satisfaction*TimeInHosp;
run;
```

The statistics will be presented in a table like the one below:

The SAS System   17:09 Friday, August 12, 2011   2

The MEANS Procedure

Variable	N	Mean	Std Dev	Minimum	Maximum
Satisfaction	10	4.4000000	2.0655911	2.0000000	7.0000000
TimeInHosp	10	6.6000000	4.3256342	1.0000000	14.0000000

You will also get a scattergram in the graph window:

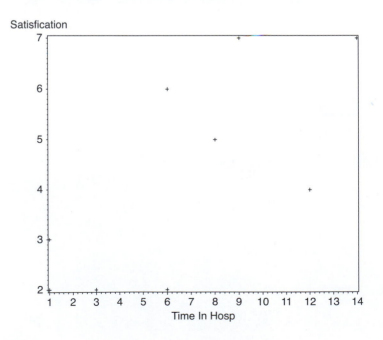

CHAPTER 3

SPSS Exercise

You should set up your data file like this:

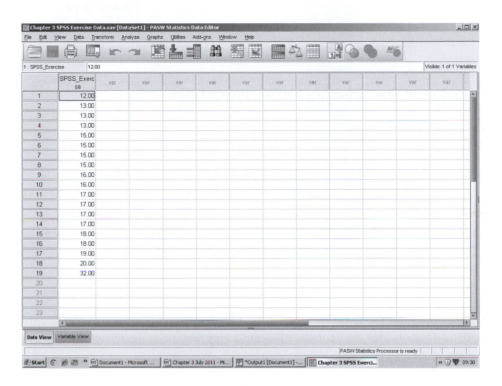

You can generate the histogram and the box-plot using the *Analyze*, *Descriptive Statistics*, *Explore* options. You would need to set up the dialogue box like this:

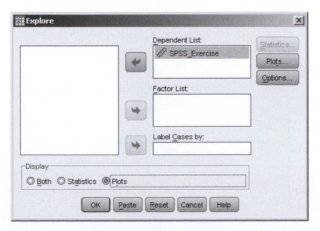

Then click on the *Plots* button and select the *Histogram* option and deselect the *Stem and leaf* option. Click on *Continue* followed by *OK*. The histogram should look like this:

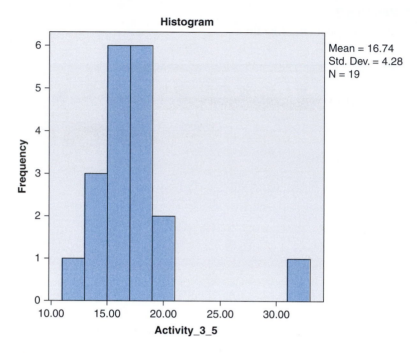

You can see from this that there are more scores between 16 and 19 than towards the extremes of the data. There is also one score that is quite a long way from the rest of the scores.

The box-plot looks like this:

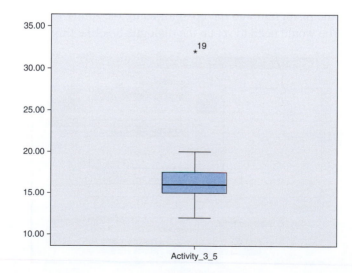

It looks from this that 50% of the scores fall between 15 and 17.5. Also, there is one extreme score which falls a long way above the top whisker. This is the score from row 19 in the data file.

To generate the numerical statistics you could use the *Explore* menu again and select the *Statistics* option. However, this would not give you the quartiles and so you can use the *Analyze*, *Descriptive statistics*, *Frequencies* option and set up the dialogue box like this:

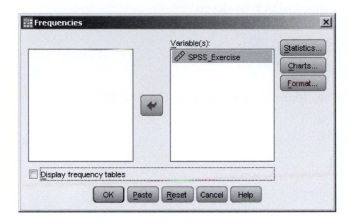

Then click on the *Statistics* button and select all of the statistics that you need. When you have finished click on *Continue* followed by *OK*. You will be presented with a table like that below:

Statistics

SPSS_Exercise

N	Valid	19
	Missing	0
Mean		16.7368
Median		16.0000
Mode		15.00[a]
Std. Deviation		4.27970
Variance		18.316
Range		20.00
Percentiles	25	15.0000
	50	16.0000
	75	18.0000

a. Multiple modes exist. The smallest value is shown.

Activity 3.3
The median for the stroke patient scores is 23, and for the heart attack scores it is 27.

Activity 3.4
The mean, median and mode for the first dataset are 19.2, 20.5 and 21 respectively, and for the second dataset they are 15.7, 16 and 20.

MCQs
1d, 2b, 3c, 4c, 5d, 6b, 7b, 8c, 9b, 10c, 11c, 12a, 13c, 14d, 15b

CHAPTER 4

Activity 4.3
- Rolling a number greater than two on a die: $4 \div 6 = 0.67$ or 67%
- Selecting an ace from a pack of cards: $4 \div 52 = 0.077$ or 7.7%
- Getting tails when tossing a coin: $1 \div 2 = 0.5$ or 50%
- The probability of selecting a red ball from a bag which contains four red balls, five blue balls, seven green balls and four white balls: $4 \div 20 = 0.20$ or 20%
- The probability of obtaining a difference of three or greater from the data in Table 4.4: $3 \div 50 = 0.06$ or 6%

Activity 4.4
The bottom five scores in Table 4.1 are presented below along with the calculation of the z-scores:
- 10 – z-score calculated as: $(10-14.95)/5.46 = -0.91$
- 13 – z-score calculated as: $(13-14.95)/5.46 = -0.36$
- 12 – z-score calculated as: $(12-14.95)/5.46 = -0.54$
- 19 – z-score calculated as: $(19-14.95)/5.46 = 0.74$
- 15 – z-score calculated as: $(15-14.95)/5.46 = 0.01$

SPSS Exercise

You should set up your data file as we have done in the image below:

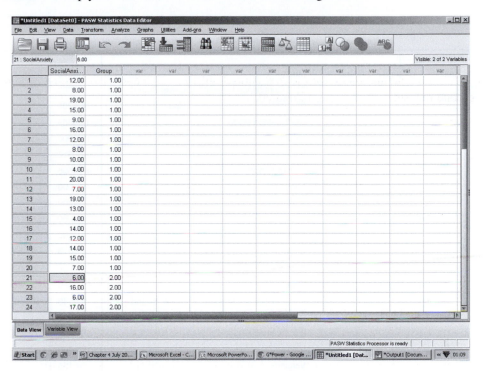

To generate the actual numerical values of the confidence intervals you should use the *Analyze*, *Descriptive statistics*, *Explore* options and set up the dialogue box as we have done below:

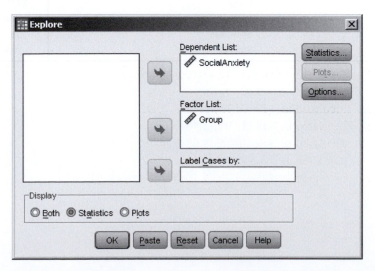

When you run the analysis you will be presented with the following output:

Descriptives

Group				Statistic	Std. Error
Social Anxiety	Hearing Aid Group	Mean		11.9000	1.06103
		95% Confidence Interval for Mean	Lower Bound	9.6792	
			Upper Bound	14.1208	
		5% Trimmed Mean		11.8889	
		Median		12.0000	
		Variance		22.516	
		Std. Deviation		4.74508	
		Minimum		4.00	
		Maximum		20.00	
		Range		16.00	
		Interquartile Range		7.00	
		Skewness		.013	.512
		Kurtosis		−.777	.992
	Waiting List Control Group	Mean		15.9000	1.30681
		95% Confidence Interval for Mean	Lower Bound	13.2148	
			Upper Bound	18.6852	
		5% Trimmed Mean		15.8333	
		Median		16.0000	
		Variance		34.155	
		Std. Deviation		5.84425	
		Minimum		6.00	
		Maximum		28.00	
		Range		22.00	
		Interquartile Range		7.50	
		Skewness		.253	.512
		Kurtosis		.045	.992

To generate the bar chart select the *Graphs*, *Legacy Dialogs*, *Bar* options and then click on *Define* in the first dialogue box. Then set up the dialogue box as we have below:

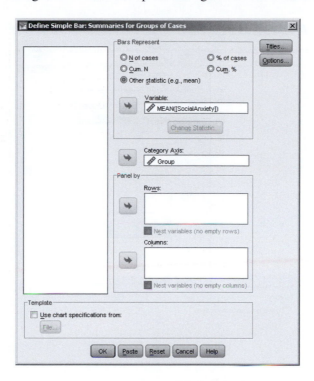

Don't forget to click on the *Options* button and select the *Display Error Bars* option. When you have done this you can run the analysis and you will be presented with the following bar chart:

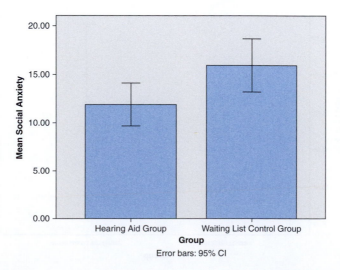

To generate the error bar chart select the *Graphs*, *Legacy Dialogs* and *Error Bar* options and click on *Define*. Then set up the dialogue box as we have done below:

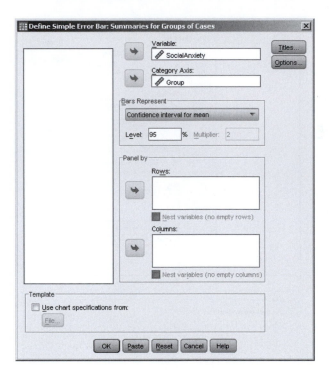

You will be presented with the error bar chart given below:

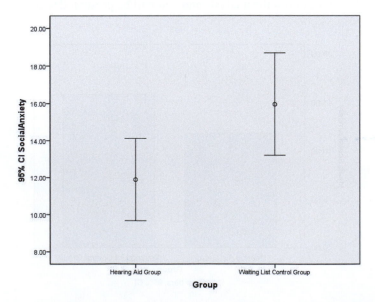

If you compare this one to the error bar chart we presented in the confidence interval section you should be able to see that there is slightly less overlap in the confidence intervals in this example.

MCQs

1d, 2c, 3c, 4a, 5b, 6c, 7b, 8d, 9b, 10d, 11c, 12d, 13d, 14b, 15c

CHAPTER 5

Activity 5.1

You should have found that exposure to inconsistent parenting is associated with increased risk of conduct disorder:

- Risk in consistent discipline group: $420/9000 = .047$
- Risk in inconsistent discipline group: $80/1000 = .08$
- Risk ratio: $.08/.047 = 1.70$

Activity 5.2

a) Total cases divided by total sample, multiplied by 100: $(231/2000) \times 100 = 11.6\%$
b) Regular high heel wearers: 20.3%. Irregular high heel wearers: 2.4%
c) Risk ratio $= .203/.024 = 8.5$ (there may be some rounding error here)
d) Odds in regular high heel wearers: $.203/(1-.203) = .255$
   Odds in irregular high heel wearers $= .024/(1-.024) = .025$
   Odds-ratio $= .255/.025 = 10.2$

MCQs

1b, 2b, 3a, 4a, 5a, 6b, 7c, 8a, 9c, 10d, 11d, 12b, 13a, 14c, 15d

CHAPTER 6

Activity 6.1

The two most important issues to be considered when data screening and cleaning are:
a) accuracy of data entry
b) missing data

Activity 6.2

a) case 10
b) case 15

Activity 6.3

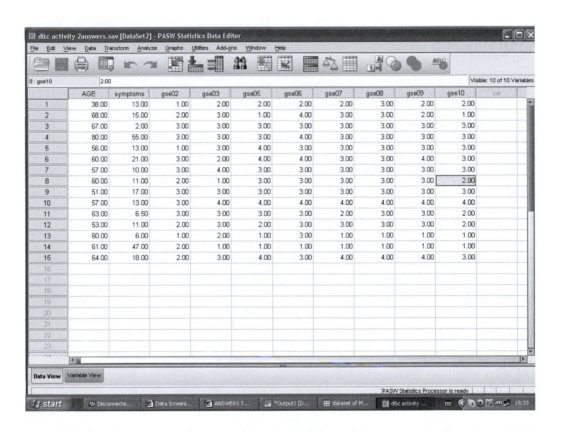

Check your answers with ours – note that you might have made different decisions to us.

MCQs

1d, 2b, 3c, 4c, 5d, 6a, 7b, 8a, 9a, 10a, 11c, 12b, 13d, 14c, 15c

CHAPTER 7

Activity 7.1

At baseline, the control group scored significantly higher on the recognition test (mean 11.34 versus 10.73 respectively, $p < .05$) and the six-letter cancellation test (mean 17.31 versus 14.11 respectively, $p < .01$).

Activity 7.2

The patient group showed improvements on some cognitive measures from baseline to the three-month follow-up test. They improved on immediate recall, recognition, six-letter cancellation test, delayed recall test (all $p < .001$) and on word list memory ($p < .05$). Other slight improvements were not statistically significant.

Activity 7.3

Blake and Batson:

Descriptive Statistics

	N	Mean	Std. Deviation	Minimum	Maximum
GHQ-12 at follow up, patients	20	1.75	2.314	0	8
Group	20	.50	.513	0	1

Ranks

	Group	N	Mean Rank	Sum of Ranks
GHQ-12 at follow up, patients	control	10	13.30	133.00
	Exercise	10	7.70	77.00
	Total	20		

Test Statistics[b]

	GHQ-12 at follow up, patients
Mann-Whitney U	22.000
Wilcoxon W	77.000
Z	−2.227
Asymp. Sig. (2-tailed)	.026
Exact Sig. [2*(1-tailed Sig.)]	.035[a]

a. Not corrected for ties.

b. Grouping variable: group

Activity 7.4

There is not enough evidence, based on this study, that the noise reduction programme reduced sound levels and disturbance due to sound, as a Wilcoxon test found that the difference between the pre and post scores was not statistically significant ($p = .67$).

MCQs

1b, 2a, 3c, 4c, 5a, 6b, 7b, 8b, 9c, 10a, 11c, 12b, 13a, 14a, 15c

CHAPTER 8

Activity 8.1

Scarpellini et al. (2008):	**independent design**
Button (2008):	**independent design**
Paterson et al. (2009):	**repeated measures design**
Gariballa and Forster (2009):	**independent design**

Activity 8.2

Group 3 has the most variability; group 1 has no variability at all.

Activity 8.3

Factor A (type of illness) has four levels (CFS, IBS, IBD and RA). The cortisol level is the dependent variable.

Activity 8. 4

Cohen's *d* for IBS and controls:

$$\frac{97.48 - 107.87}{11.26 + 11.67/2}$$

$$= \frac{-10.39}{22.93/2}$$

$$= 10.39/11.47$$

$$= .91$$

.91 is a strong effect.

Cohen's *d* for IBD and controls:

$$\frac{93.21 - 107.87}{13.42 + 11.67/2}$$

$$= \frac{-14.66}{25.09/2}$$

$$= 14.66/12.55$$

$$= 1.17$$

1.17 is an even stronger effect.

We could report this in a results section as follows:

> *A one-way (between-participants ANOVA showed that there were significant difference between the illness groups in terms of IQ ($F_{2,85} = 11.40$, $p < .001$) A post-hoc test (Bonferroni correction) showed that controls had significantly higher IQ than both the IBS and IBD groups (Cohens d = .91, $p = .004$ and Cohen's d = 1.17, $p < .001$ respectively). The differences between IBS and IBD groups were not statistically significant ($p = .551$).*

Activity 8.5

Conditions 1 and 2; 1 and 3; 2 and 3.

Activity 8.6

You should have carried out a Wilcoxon test in order to look at whether there was a statistically significant difference between scores at baseline and scores 12 months later. The output looks like this:

Ranks

		N	Mean Rank	Sum of Ranks
Fatigue at twelve months follow up - Fatigue before intervention	Negative Ranks	6[a]	3.50	21.00
	Positive Ranks	0[b]	.00	.00
	Ties	0[c]		
	Total	6		

a. Fatigue at twelve months follow up < Fatigue before intervention

b. Fatigue at twelve months follow up > Fatigue before intervention

c. Fatigue at twelve months follow up = Fatigue before intervention

Test Statistics[b]

	Fatigue at twelve months follow up - Fatigue before intervention
Z	−2.201[a]
Asymp. Sig. (2-tailed)	.028
Exact Sig. (2-tailed)	.031
Exact Sig. (1-tailed)	.016
Point Probability	.016

a. Based on positive ranks.

b. Wilcoxon Signed Ranks Test

This means that there is a significant difference between the two conditions (z= -2.201; p=.031). Note that we have used a two-tailed value, but if you have chosed he asymp. Sig or the exact 1-tailed sig you would be correct.

MCQs

1d, 2a, 3a, 4c, 5a, 6a, 7a, 8a, 9b, 10 yes, 11a, 12c, 13b, 14c, 15a

CHAPTER 9

Activity 9.2

The screenshot shows value labels

	gender	crashtype	freq	
1	women	no crash	51.00	
2	women	no blame c...	5.00	
3	women	blame-wort...	3.00	
4	men	no crash	29.00	
5	men	no blame c...	15.00	
6	men	blame-wort...	16.00	
7				
8				

*gendercrash3x2.sav [DataSet6] - PASW Statistics Data Edit

File   Edit   View   Data   Transform   Analyze   Direct Marketing

MCQs

1d, 2c, 3d, 4a, 5c, 6b, 7a, 8d, 9c, 10a, 11a, 12b, 13a, 14c, 15d

CHAPTER 10

Activity 10.1

a) The strongest relationship is between appearance schemas inventory and self-esteem (−.64). This means that as scores increase on the appearance schemas inventory, scores tend to increase on the self-esteem scale. This relationship is strong and statistically significant at $p < .01$

b) The weakest relationship is between the body satisfaction scale and the GAS (.30). Although this is a weak correlation, it is statistically significant ($p < .01$). As scores on the body satisfaction scale increase, scores on the GAS increase. This means they were *less* satisfied with their genital appearance

c) There is a negative relationship between scores on the self-esteem scale and the GAS (−0.41). This is statistically significant at $p < .01$. The correlation is moderate. As scores on the self-esteem scale increase, scores on the GAS decrease. Remember that high scores on the GAS mean lower satisfaction, so the more self-esteem increases, the higher the genital appearance satisfaction!

Activity 10.2

a) The correlation coefficient for the mean diastolic BP with paternal sensitivity in girls is −0.11

b) This correlation coefficient is very weak – in fact, near to zero. It is not statistically significant, and the −0.11 is highly likely to be due to chance (sampling error)

Activity 10.3

The correct answer is: c)

MCQs

1a, 2c, 3d, 4a, 5b, 6b, 7b, 8a, 9a, 10c, 11c, 12a, 13d, 14a, 15b

CHAPTER 11

Activity 11.1

Give the following information :

a) The value of a – zero

b) The value of r^2 – .71

c) For every increase in 10,000 of total blood culture sets, the number of MRSA bacteriaemias increases by approximately 50.

Activity 11.2

.735 × 8 = 5.88
5.88 + 2.330 = 8.21

Thus someone who scored 8 on worry about 'transmission of infection' is predicted to score 8.21 on the perception of the importance of handwashing.

Activity 11.3

Case	Predicted CFQ	Score you would enter instead of missing score
24	36.29	36
38	26.25	26
42	37.41	37

MCQs

1a, 2a, 3d, 4b, 5a, 6b, 7c, 8c, 9d, 10a, 11c, 12a, 13b, 14b, 15c

CHAPTER 12

Activity 12.1

In respect of the perceived 'risk to others', the unstandardised *b* weights show that for every one-unit increase in perceived 'risk to others', the frequency of handwashing increases by .453. The standardised weight, beta, means that for every one SD increase in perceived 'risk to others', frequency of handwashing increases by .24 SD in the sample. This was statistically greater than would be expected by sampling error alone ($t = 2.15$, $p = .035$). We are 95% confident that the true regression line lies somewhere between .03 and .87.

Activity 12.2

The explanatory variables together accounted for 29% of the variance in General Adjustment (TAPES subscale). This was statistically significant at $p < .05$. The Hope Scale was statistically significant at $p < .01$, showing that as hope increased by 1 SD, general adjustment increased by 0.29 SD. A stronger predictor was the social support Scale, which showed that for every 1 SD increase in social support, general adjustment rose by .36 SD. This was statistically significant at $p < .001$. The other explanatory variables had little predictive value, as the slopes of the lines were almost flat.

MCQs

1b, 2b, 3d, 4a, 5a, 6c, 7c, 8a, 9d, 10a, 11d, 12a, 13b, 14d, 15a

CHAPTER 13

Activity 13.2

Logit (heart attack´) = $-3.37 + (.09 \times 42) = .41$

(We don't expect you to calculate it, but this can be converted into a .60 probability of heart attack.)

MCQs

1a, 2d, 3d, 4c, 5a, 6b, 7d, 8c, 9b, 10c, 11a, 12b, 13c, 14d, 15c

CHAPTER 14

Activity 14.1

To discount a placebo interpretation of a positive effect of our new treatment for halitosis you should include the design feature that we described early in the chapter. You should have a control group and an intervention group. You need to ensure that the participants cannot tell whether they are getting the intervention or are in the control condition. Often researchers try to make the control condition as similar to the intervention condition as possible. And so if we had a mouthwash as the new intervention we would give participants in the control condition a similar mouthwash, but which didn't have the active ingredient that is in the intervention mouthwash. You should also ensure that participants either all think that they are in the control condition or all think that they are in the intervention condition, or you could have half your participants (half of those in the intervention and half in the control) think they are in the control condition, and the other half think that they are in the intervention condition. In this way we would have a better chance of being able to discount the placebo effect.

Activity 14.3

Our interpretation would that at baseline the participant was smoking about 30 cigarettes per day. During the first intervention phase there was a sudden drop to ten cigarettes per day and then a steady decline over the next three days. When the intervention was withdrawn there was a big increase in number of cigarettes smoked per day but this was not up to the baseline levels. Finally, during the next intervention phase, numbers of cigarettes smoked per day reduced dramatically until on the final day no cigarettes were smoked.

SPSS exercise

You should enter you data into SPSS as we have in the screenshot below:

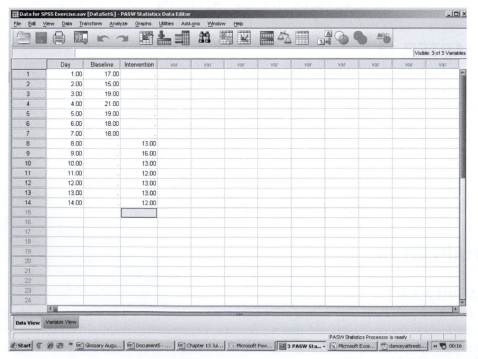

You should then select the *Graphs*, *Legacy Dialogs*, *Line* options and set out the dialogue box as we have below:

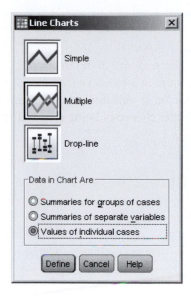

Then click on *Define* and set out the dialogue box as we have here:

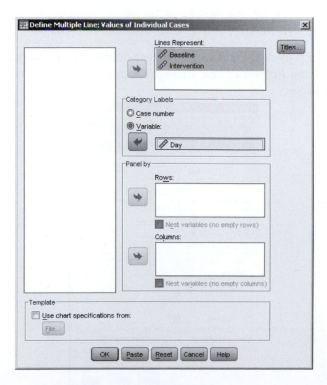

Then click on *OK* to get the graph.

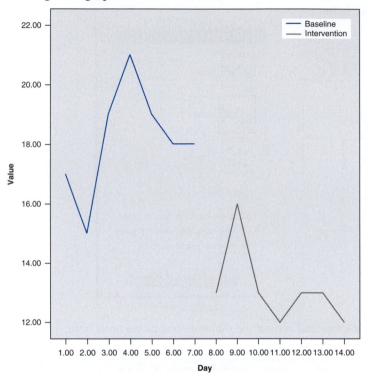

You can edit the graph by double clicking on it, then double click on the *y*-axis and then click on the *Scale* tab in the *Properties* box. Change the minimum value to 0 and then click on *Apply* and close this box:

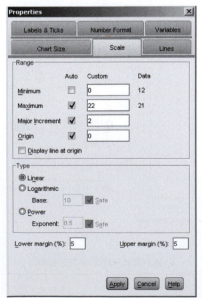

Then you can click on the *Add Markers* button and then select the markers that you want.

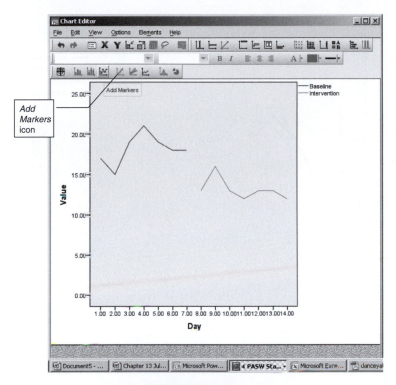

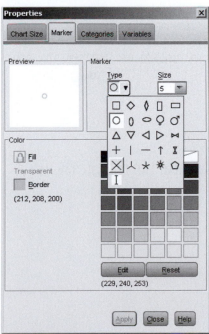

Finally, close down the chart editor and you should have a graph that looks like this:

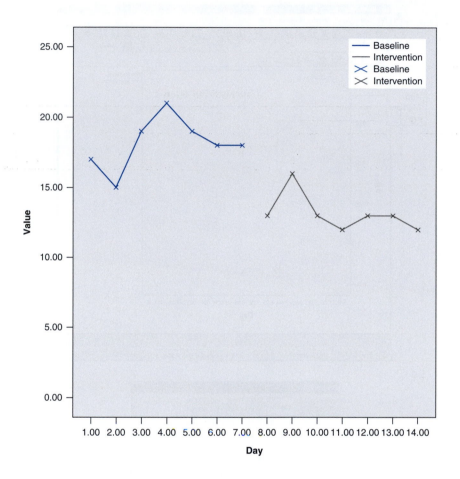

MCQs
1d, 2b, 3b, 4d, 5a, 6c, 7b, 8b, 9a, 10d, 11d, 12a, 13b, 14b, 15d

CHAPTER 15

Activity 15.1

Here is the survival curve for the data presented in the data table:

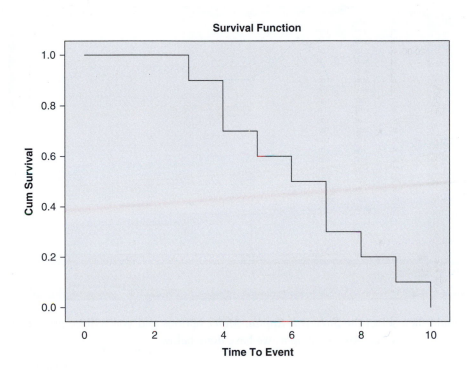

You should be able to see from this table that all participants experienced the event of interest by week 10, that is the proportion not experiencing the event has moved down to zero at this point. Also, you can see two steeper steps down during weeks 4 and 7, in each of these weeks two participants experienced the event of interest and so obviously, the proportion not experiencing the event has decreased more than in the other weeks.

SPSS Exercise

You should set up your SPSS file as we have done in the screenshot below:

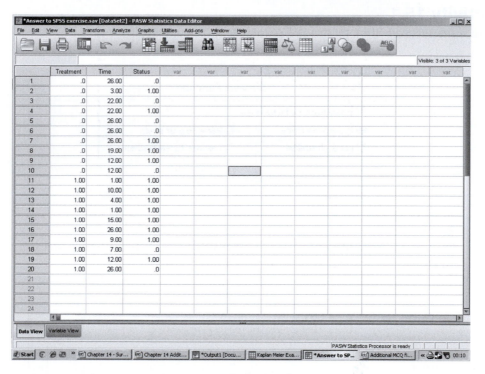

You should then select the *Survival*, *Kaplan-Meier* options and you will be presented with the following dialogue box. Set it up as we have done below:

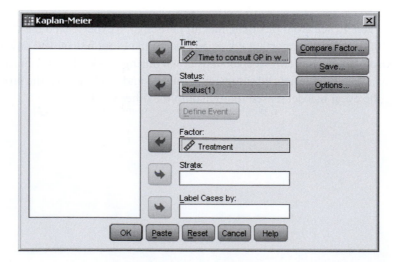

Click on the *Compare Factor* button and select the *Log rank* option:

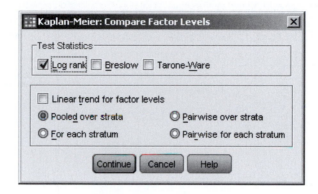

Click on *Continue* and then click on the *Options* button and make sure that you select the *Survival* and *Hazard* options:

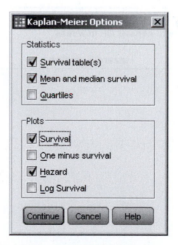

Click on *Continue* and *OK* and you will be presented with the following curves and Mantel–Cox test output:

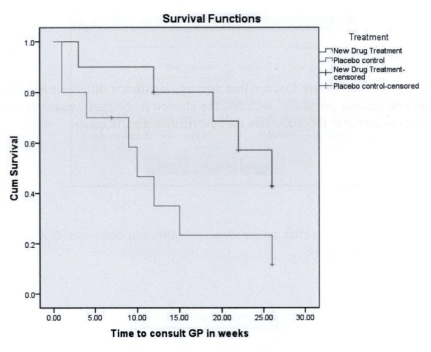

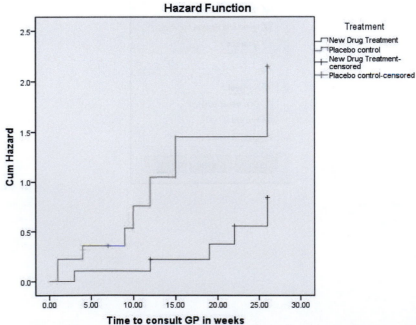

Overall Comparisons

	Chi-Square	df	Sig.
Log Rank (Mantel-Cox)	3.889	1	.049

Test of equality of survival distributions for the different levels of Treatment.

You can see from the Mantel–Cox test that there is a significant difference between the new treatment and placebo conditions, such that the placebo participants tended to consult their family doctors earlier in the study than the new treatment participants.

MCQs

1b, 2b, 3c, 4a, 5d, 6b, 7b, 8d, 9b, 10c, 11d, 12c, 13c, 14b, 15d

Glossary

–2 log likelihood – A measure of goodness of fit in logistic regression. Lower scores indicate a better fit between the model and observed data.

Analysis of Covariance (ANCOVA) – A statistical technique where differences between the conditions are analysed after controlling for of partialling out a specified variable (the covariate).

Analysis of Variance (ANOVA) – A statistical technique which shows whether there are significant differences between the conditions or groups.

Assumption of sphericity – In a repeated measures design, analysed by ANOVA, we assume that the variances of the pairwise differences are similar.

A symmetrical/Asymptotic methods for calculation of p values – Statistical significance is based on the assumption that we have a large, normally distributed dataset.

Bar chart – Graph representing means by the length of vertical or horizontal bars.

Baseline model – In logistic regression a model containing no predictors, only a constant term. Models including predictors are compared to this baseline.

Between-groups / between-participants / independent groups designs – Research designs where different participants are allocated to each of the conditions in the study.

Between-groups variance – A measure of the variation in scores between two or more groups.

Bimodal distribution – A distribution of scores with two modes.

Bins – Range of scores represented by one bar in a frequency histogram.

Bivariate correlational analysis – A measure of the relationship between two sets of scores.

Blinding – Any procedure which prevents people involved in a trial from knowing the condition to which participants has been allocated.

Bonferroni correction/adjustment – When multiple comparisons are made, or multiple tests are carried out, the Bonferroni correction (.05/number of comparisons) decreases the likelihood of making a Type I error.

Bootstrapping – Method of taking thousands of repeated samples from a study sample to generate 95% confidence intervals around a statistic.

Box-plots – Graphs representing the interquartile range, median and any outlying or extreme scores.

Case-control study – A study which recruits a group of cases of disease and a group of control participants. These are then compared to identify risk factors for the disease.

Categorical variables – Variables that are made up of categories and involve frequency counts.

Chi-square statistic – An inferential statistic. In this book it has most prominently featured in the assessment of the association of two categorical variables in a contingency table analysis. The chi-square statistic was also involved in significance testing within logistic regression.

Cluster sampling – Sampling where the population is divided into smaller identifiable clusters and one or more of these clusters are then randomly selected. Participants are then randomly selected from these smaller clusters to take part in a study.

Clustered bar chart – Graph displaying the means of several variables grouped together for each group.

Concepts – Ideas about phenomena of interest.

Conditional probability – The probability of some event occurring under certain specified conditions.

Confidence intervals – Interval within which we can be confident that the population parameter will be found.

Cohen's *d* – A measure of effect: $\dfrac{Mean\ 1 - Mean\ 2}{Mean\ of\ SDs}$.

Cohen's Kappa – A measure of inter-rater reliability.

Cohort Study – A longitudinal study that follows a sample of participants over time.

Confounding variable – A variable in a study that is not controlled by the researcher and is related to both the independent and the dependent variable.

CONSORT – Consolidated Standard of Reporting Trials: standard guidelines for designing and reporting RCTs.

Contingency table – A table to represent the association of two categorical variables. The cells show the number of participants falling into each combination of categories.

Continuous variables – Variables that can take on any value on a scale and are not limited to whole numbers.

Correlational designs – Designs which measure variables to see how they are related.

Counterbalancing – A technique to reduce bias in within-group designs where half the participants are presented with one order of conditions and the other half are presented with the reverse order of conditions.

Co-variate – A variable which is related to another variable.

Cox and Snell R-square – A measure of model fit in logistic regression.

Cramer's *V* – A measure of effect size in contingency table analysis.

Criterion variable – Dependent variable.

Cronbach's alpha – A measure of the reliability or internal consistency of a questionnaire.

Criterion for significance – The probability below which researchers decide they have enough evidence to reject the null hypothesis.

Crossover design – A design where all participants receive an intervention but one group of participant receive the control condition followed by the intervention and another group receive the intervention followed by the control.

Data Screening & Cleaning – A set of techniques used to ensure the accuracy and suitability of the dataset for carrying out statistical analyses.

Dependent variable – A variable measured by a researcher in a study that is hypothesised to be influenced by the independent variable.

Descriptive statistics – Statistical techniques which help us describe our data.

Discrete variables – Variables that are measured using a whole number scale.

Epidemiology – The study of the causes and distribution of disease in society.

Exact method of calculating p values – The statistical significance is based on the distribution of the sample which we have, i.e. the exact distribution.

Evidence-based practice – Treatments and procedures which are based upon research evidence.

Experiment – A type of design where the researcher manipulates an independent variable to see what effect this has on a dependent variable.

Experimental hypothesis – A hypothesis which states that there is an effect in the population.

Explanatory variable – Predictor or independent variable.

F ratio – In ANOVA, a measure of the between groups variability divided by a measure of the within groups variability.

Fisher's Exact Test – An alternative to the chi-square test of association of categorical variables when assumptions are violated.

Frequency counts – The number of participants in a category or who have a particular value on a variable.

Frequency histogram – Graph of the frequency of occurrence of scores or a range of scores in a sample.

Friedman's ANOVA – A non-parametric ANOVA used for a repeated measures design where there are three or more conditions.

Gain scores – Difference between a pre-test value on a variable and a post-test value on the same variable.

Graphical descriptive – Techniques for describing data using graphs and charts.

Hierarchical multiple regression – Model in which the researcher determines the order in which variables are entered into the equation.

Incidence – The rate of onset of new cases of disease in a particular population over a defined timeframe.

Independent variable – A variable manipulated by a researcher in an experimental or quasi-experimental design.

Inferential statistics – Statistical techniques devised to allow us to generalise from our data to populations.

Intention to treat analysis – A statistical analysis which includes all participants who were originally randomised to conditions and where in the analysis every participant is included in the group to which they were originally allocated.

Interquartile range – The range within a dataset which contains 50% of the scores.

Interval level data – Scales that are ordered and there are equal intervals between adjacent scores on the scale.

Kruskal-Wallis test – A non-parametric ANOVA used for an independent groups design where there are three or more groups.

Levene's test of equal variances – Used in the independent t-test, Levene's test shows whether the groups have equal variances.

LOCF – Last Observation Carried Forward: a missing data technique used in longitudinal repeated measures research, whereby missing data is replaced with the last recorded value.

Levels of measurement – Classification system for the types of variables that we encounter in research.

Line graph – Graph to illustrate the means of different conditions in which the means are linked by lines.

Linear relationship – A relationship between two variables which can be best described by a straight line.

Linear regression – A correlational technique in which a straight line is drawn through a set of datapoints on a scatterplot, in order to obtain a measure of the strength of association between two variables which are related linearly.

Listwise deletion – A method of excluding participants by deleting them from the dataset if they have a missing value on any of the variables.

Mauchley's test of Sphericity – A test which shows whether the variances of related variables are similar or dissimilar.

Logistic regression – Regression model suitable for dichotomous outcome variables.

McNemar's test – Statistical technique for analysing dichotomous outcome variables in a repeated measures design.

Mann–Whitney U test – A non-parametric test for two independent conditions which uses the ranking of scores in a formula which calculates the test statistic 'U'.

Maximum likelihood estimation – An approach to estimating the parameters in a statistical model.

MAR (Missing at random) – Data which is missing at random, i.e. when missingness is related to another variable in the dataset, but not related to the variable which is missing.

MCAR (Missing completely at random) – Data which is missing completely at random, i.e. the missing data has nothing to do with any of the measured or observed variables.

Mean – A measure of central tendency where the scores in a sample are added together and then this sum is divided by the number of scores in the sample.

Measures of central tendency – Descriptive statistics which give an indication of the typical or average score in a sample.

Median – A measure of central tendency which is the middle score after all of the scores in a sample are ranked.

The median test – A little used test which shows whether the medians of two or more conditions or groups are different from each other.

Mode – A measure of central tendency which is the most frequently occurring score in a sample.

Multiple baseline designs – Are single case designs where either multiple single cases have different baseline durations and different times for the intervention to start; or for a single case that has multiple outcome measures or outcome measured in different circumstances.

Multiple regression – An advanced correlational technique which assesses the relationship between a set of explanatory or predictor variables and a criterion variable.

Multi-stage clustering – Where clusters within clusters are identified and selected at random to form the pool of participants which are then randomly selected for inclusion in a study.

Nagelkerke R-square – A measure of model fit in logistic regression.

NMAR (Not missing at random) – Data which is not missing at random.

Nominal level data – Lowest level of measurement and constitutes unordered categories.

Non-parametric tests – Inferential statistical tests that make no assumptions about the distributions in populations.

Normal distribution – A distribution of scores which is symmetrical, peaked in the middle, is bell-shaped and tails off equally on both sides of the peak.

Null hypothesis – The hypothesis that there is zero effect in the population.

Null Hypothesis Significance Testing (NHST) – The process of calculating the probability of obtaining a particular pattern of data by chance if there was no effect in the population.

Numerical descriptives – Statistical techniques that describe data using numbers.

Odds-ratio – The ratio of the odds of disease in two groups.

One-tailed hypotheis – A research hypothesis where we have specified the direction of the predicted difference or relationship.

Operationalisation – The process of deciding how to measure a concept.

Opportunity sampling – Sampling from those people who are available at a particular time and place.

Ordinal level data – Scales that consist of ordered categories.

Outlier – Extreme score in your dataset, a score that is markedly larger or smaller than the majority of other scores in the dataset.

Overfitting (in Multiple Regression) – Fits the sample much better than it would a new sample. This often happens when there are many variables and not enough participants. The predictive value of the exploratory variables may be good in the sample, but may not be generalisable.

Pairwise deletion – A method of excluding participants by deleting them from the dataset if they have a missing value for the variable being analysed.

Parameters – Statistical descriptions of populations.

Parametric tests – Inferential statistical tests that make assumptions about the distributions in populations.

Partial correlation – The relationship between two variables which remains after a third (or more) variables have been co-varied (accounted, for, partialled out).

Pearson's *r* – A parametric test to assess the relationship between two or more variables.

Placebo – Is a treatment that has no active ingredient which is often used in clinical trials.

Planned comparisons – Pairwise comparisons which the researchers decide they will carry out in advance of the analyses.

Population – All items, objects or people with a particular characteristic.

Post-hoc tests – Pairwise comparisons which the researchers decide they will carry out after the main analyses have been run. There are many post-hoc tests.

Power – The sensitivity of a study to detect effects that are existent in the population.

Prevalence – The existing level of disease in a specified population.

Probability distribution – A mathematical distribution where we know the probability of randomly selecting scores from any part of the distribution.

p-value – Probability of obtaining a pattern of data if the null hypothesis were true.

Quartiles – Values which divide a dataset into exactly four equal parts.

Random allocation – Allocation of participants to conditions by use of a random procedure.

Random allocation sequence – A list of how participants are going to be allocated to conditions produce prior to the randomised control trial beginning.

Randomised Control Trial – Study where participants are randomly assigned to an intervention and control condition and that includes blinding of all people likely to introduce bias into the study.

Range – Maximum score in a sample minus the minimum score.

Ratio level data – Scales with equal intervals and a fixed zero.

Regression line/slope – In a regression analysis, the regression line (b) shows the strength of the relationship between two variables.

Reliability – A reliable measure is one which is consistent.

Replacement randomisation – The repeated generation of random allocation sequences until a sequence is generated that falls within the pre-specified condition disparity limits.

Research Hypothesis – Precise, testable statement concerning the relationship between variables or differences between conditions.

Risk factors – Factors that increase the likelihood of disease.

Risk ratio – The ratio of the risk of disease in one group compared to another.

Sample – A selection of items, objects or people from a particular population.

Sampling – Selecting individuals from a population.

Sampling error – Biases in the estimation of population parameters that arise from using samples.

Scatterplot/scattergram – A graphical method of showing the relationship between two variables.

Simple random selection – A sampling technique where each member of a particular population has an equal chance of being randomly selected for inclusion in a study.

Single case design – An experimental study involving only one participant.

Skewness – A deviation from a normal distribution such that the peak is shifted to one side and the tail is extended to the opposite side.

Snowball sampling – A sampling technique where individuals who have taken part in a study provide details of people they know who might also be willing to participate.

Spearman's rho – A non-parametric correlational technique.

Standardised slope of the regression line – β (beta). Shows the results of the unstandardised b weights after conversion to z-scores.

Stacked bar chart – Bar chart where several variables are indicated within one bar for each group.

Standard deviation – A standardised measure of the deviation of scores in a sample from the mean.

Standard Multiple regression – Model in which all explanatory variables are entered into the equation together.

Statistical power – The ability of a proposed study to detect an effect that exists in the population.

Statistical significance – Where the p-value calculated for a statistical test is small enough to allow a researcher to reject the null hypothesis.

Statistics – Descriptions applied to samples.

The Standard Normal Distribution – The distribution of z-scores which has a mean of zero and a standard deviation of 1.

Stepwise Multiple Regression – Model in which the order of entry is determined on mathematical grounds.

t-test – A parametric test which is used to determine whether there are significant differences between two independent groups or two repeated measures conditions.

Transformed scores – In situation in which a mathematical calculation is carried out on a set of scores e.g. the simplest transformation is to add a constant to all participants' scores on a variable (e.g. adding 50 to everyones score).

Two-tailed hypotheis – A research hypothesis where we have not specified the direction of the predcited difference or relationship.

Type I error – Where a researcher rejects the null hypothesis when it is true.

Type II error – Where a researcher fails to reject the null hypothesis when it is false.

Unstandardised slope of the regression line – b, the slope of the line in the original units.

Validity – Usually used to refer to scales or questionnaires which measure what they are supposed to measure, and which agree with other similar instruments which measure the same constructs.

Variables – Measured concepts.

Variability – The extent to which scores vary from the mean of the group.

Variance – The average of the squared deviations from the mean.

Volunteer sampling – Sampling which relies on participants coming forward to volunteer to take part in a study usually in response to an advert.

Wald statistic – The test statistic used to test the significance of individual predictors in logistic regression.

Wilcoxon signed rank test – A non-parametric test for a two-condition repeated measures design which uses the ranking of scores in a formula which calculates the test statistic 'W' and/or z.

Within-groups/within-participants/repeated measures designs – Research designs where one group of participants takes part in all conditions of the study.

Within-groups variance – A measure of the extent to which scores given by participants in the same condition vary.

Zero-order correlation – Full correlation between variables.

z-test – A test which shows whether groups differ from each other, given in standardised scores.

References

Al-Faris, E.A. (2000). Students' evaluation of a traditional and an innovative family medicine course in Saudi Arabia. *Education for Health*, 13(2), 231–235.

Andrews, T. & Waterman, H. (2008). What factors influence arterial blood gas sampling patterns? *Nursing in Critical Care*, 13(3), 132–137.

Anzalone, P. (2008). Equivalence of earlobe site blood glucose testing with finger stick. *Clinical Nursing Research*, 17, 251–261.

Armitage, C.J. (2006). Evidence that implementation intentions promote transitions between the stages of change. *Journal of Consulting and Clinical Psychology*, 74(1), 141–151.

Arnold, S., Herrick, L.M., Pankratz, V.S. & Mueller, P.S. (2007). Spiritual well-being, emotional distress, and perception of health after a myocardial infarction. *Internet Journal of Advanced Nursing Practice*, 9(1).

Attree, E.A., Dancey, C.P., Keeling, D. & Wilson, C. (2003). Cognitive function in people with chronic illness: Inflammatory Bowel Disease and Irritable Bowel Syndrome. *Applied Neuropsychology*, 10(2), 96–104.

Baumhover, N. & Hughes, L. (2009). Spirituality and support for family presence during invasive procedures and resuscitations in adults. *American Journal of Critical Care*, 18(4), 357–367.

Begg, C., Cho, M., Eastwood, S., Horton, R., Moher, D., Olkin, I. et al. (1996). Improving the quality of reporting of randomized controlled trials: the CONSORT statement. *Journal of the American Medical Association*, 276, 637–639.

Bell, B.G. & Belsky, J. (2008). Parenting and children's cardiovascular functioning. *Child Care Health & Development*, 34(2), 194–203.

Bize, R. & Plotnikoff, R.C. (2009). The relationship between a short measure of health status and physical activity in a workplace population. *Psychology, Health & Medicine*, 14(1), 53–61.

Blake, H. & Batson, M. (2008). Exercise intervention in brain injury: a pilot randomized study of Tai Chi Qigong. *Clinical Rehabilitation*, 23, 589–598.

Booij, L., Merens, W., Markus, C.R. & Van der Does, A.J.W. (2006). Diet rich in α-lactalbumin improves memory in unmedicated recovered depressed patients and matched controls. *Journal of Psychopharmacology*, 20, 526–535.

Brace, N., Kemp, R. & Snelgar, R. (2009). *SPSS for Psychologists*, 4th edn, Basingstoke: Palgrave.

Bramwell, R. & Morland, C. (2009). Genital appearance satisfaction in women: the development of a questionnaire and exploration of correlates. *Journal of Reproductive and Infant Psychology*, 27(1), 15–27.

Brossart, D.F., Parker, R.I., Olson, E.A. & Mahadeven, L. (2006). The relationship between visual analysis and five statistical analyses in a simple AB single-case research design. *Behavior Modification*, 30(5), 531–563.

Bruscia, K., Shultis, C., Dennery, K. & Cherly, D. (2008). The sense of coherence in hospitalized cardiac and cancer patients. *Journal of Holistic Nursing*, 26, 286–294.

Buhi, E.R., Goodson, P. & Neilands, T.B. (2008). Out of sight, not out of mind: strategies for handling missing data. *American Journal of Health Behavior*, 32(1), 83–92.

Burneo, J.G., Villanueva, V., Knowlton, R.C., Faught, R.E. & Kuzniecky, R.I. (2008). Kaplan–Meier analysis on seizure outcome after epilepsy surgery: do gender and race influence it? *Seizure*, 17, 314–319.

Button, L.A. (2008). Effect of social support and coping strategies on the relationship between health care-related occupational stress and health. *Journal of Research in Nursing*, 13(6), 498–524.

Byford, S. & Fiander, M. (2007). Recording professional activities to aid economic evaluations of health and social care services. *Unit Costs of Health and Social Care*, 19–24 (accessed at: http://www.pssru.ac.uk/pdf/uc/uc2007/uc2007_recordingactivities.pdf).

Carvajal, A., Ortega, S., Del Olmo, L., Vidal, X., Aguirre, C., Ruiz, B. et al. (2011). Selective serotonin reuptake inhibitors and gastrointestinal bleeding: a case-control study. *Plos One*, 6(5), 6.

Castle, N.G. (2005). Nursing home closures and quality of care. *Medical Care Research Review*, 62, 111–132.

Chiou, S.S. & Kuo, C.D. (2008). Effect of chewing a single betel-quid on autonomic nervous modulation in healthy young adults. *Journal of Psychopharmacology*, 22(8), 910–917.

Cohen, J. (1988). *Statistical Power Analysis for the Behavioral Sciences,* 2nd Edn. Hillsdale, NJ: Erlbaum.

Cohen, J. (1990). Things I have learned (so far). *American Psychologist*, 45, 1304–1312.

Cohen, J. (1992). A power primer. *Psychological Bulletin*, 112(1), 155–159.

Cohen, J.H., Kristal, A.R. & Stanford, J.L. (2000). Fruit and vegetable intakes and prostate cancer risk. *Journal of the National Cancer Institute*, 92(1), 61–68.

Costello, E.J., Angold, A., Burns, B.J., Stangl, D.K., Tweed, D.L., Erkanli, A. & Worthman, C.M. (1996). The Great Smoky Mountains Study of youth – Goals, design, methods, and the prevalence of DSM-III-R disorders. *Archives of General Psychiatry*, 53(12), 1129–1136.

Costello, E.J., Compton, S.N., Keeler, G. & Angold, A. (2003). Relationships between poverty and psychopathology – A natural experiment. *Journal of the American Medical Association*, 290(15), 2023–2029.

Dancey, C.P. & Reidy, J.G. (2011). *Statistics without Maths for Psychology*, 5th edn. Harlow: Pearson.

Dancey, C.P., Hutton-Young, S., Moye, S. & Devins, G. (2002). The relationship among stigma, illness intrusiveness and quality of life in men and women with IBS. *Psychology, Health & Medicine*, 7(4), 381–395.

Dancey, C.P., Attree, E.A. & Brown, K.F. (2006). Nucleotide supplementation: a randomised double-blind placebo controlled trial of IntestAidIB in people with Irritable Bowel Syndrome [ISRCTN67764449] *Nutrition Journal*.

Dariusz, A. & Jochen, R. (2009). Increased prevalance of colorectal adenoma in patients with sporadic duodenal adenoma. *European Journal of Gastroenterology & Hepatology*, 21(7), (816–818), 1473–5687.

Department of Health. (2003). The second year of the Department of Health's mandatory MRSA bacteraemia surveillance scheme in acute NHS Trusts in England: April 2002–March 2003. *CDR Weekly*, 13(25), 1–9.

Dimitrov, D.M. & Rumrill Jr, P.D. (2003). Pretest-posttest designs and measurement of change. *Work*, 20, 159–165.

Dingle, G.A. & King, P. (2009). Prevalence and impact of co-occurring psychiatric disorders on outcomes from a private hospital drug and alcohol treatment program. *Mental Health and Substance Use*, 2(1), 13–23.

Doest, L. ter., Dijkstra, A., Gebhardt, W.A. & Vitale, S. (2007). Cognitions about smoking and not smoking in adolescence. *Health Education and Behaviour*, 36, 660–672.

Ebbutt, A.F. (1984). Three-period crossover designs for two treatments. *Biometrics*, 40, 219–224.

Emerson, E., Graham, H. & Hatton, C. (2006). Household income and health status in children and adolescents in Britain. *European Journal of Public Health*, 16(4), 354–360.

Everitt, B.S. & Pickles, A. (1999). *Statistical Aspects of the Design and Analysis of Clinical Trials*. London: Imperial College Press.

Farren, A.T. (2010). Power, uncertainty, self-transcendence and Quality of Life in Breast Cancer Survivors. *Nursing Science Quarterly*, 23(1), 63–71.

Field, A. (2009). *Discovering Statistics Using SPSS*, 3rd edn. London: Sage.

Gabriel, S.E. (2001). The epidemiology of rheumatoid arthritis. *Rheumatic Disease Clinics of North America*, 27(2), 269–281.

Gariballa, S. & Forster, S. (2009). Effects of smoking on nutrition status and response to dietary supplements during acute illness. *Nutrition in Clinical Practice*, 24, 84–90.

Gheissari, A., Sirous, M., Hajzargarbashi, T., Kelishadi, R., Merrikhi, A. & Azhir, A. (2010). Carotid intima-media thickness in children with end-stage renal disease on dialysis. *Indian Journal of Nephrology*, 20(1), 1–33.

Giovannelli, M., Borriello, G., Castri, P., Prosperini, L. & Pozzilli, C. (2007). Early physiotherapy after injection of botulinum toxin increases the beneficial effects on spasticity in patients with multiple sclerosis. *Clinical Rehabilitation*, 21(4), 331–337.

Goldacre, B. (2008). *Bad Science*. London: Fourth Estate.

Green, H., McGinnity, A., Meltzer, H., Ford, T. & Goodman, R. (2005). *Mental Health of Children and Young People in Great Britain, 2004*. London: The Stationary Office.

Gunstad, J., Paul, R.H., Brickman, A.M., Cohen, R.A., Arns, M., Roe, D., Lawrence, J. & Gordon, E., (2006). Patterns of cognitive performance in middle-aged and older adults; a cluster examination. *Journal of Geriatric Psychiatry & Neurology*, 19, 59–64.

Halpern, S.D., Karlawish, J.H.T. & Berlin, J.E. (2002). The continuing unethical conduct of unethical clinical trials. *Journal of the American Medical Association*, 288(3), 358–361.

Hanna, D., Davies, M. & Dempster, M. (2009). Psychological processes underlying nurses' handwashing behaviour. *Journal of Infection Prevention*, 20(3), 90–94.

Harris, A.H.S., Reeder, R. & Kyun, J.K. (2009). Common statistical and research design problems in manuscripts submitted to high-impact psychiatry journals: what editors and reviewers want authors to know. *Journal of Psychiatric Research*, 43, 1231–1234.

Hibbeln, J. R., Davis, J. M., Steer, C., Emmett, P., Rogers, I., Williams, C., et al. (2007). Maternal seafood consumption in pregnancy and neurodevelopmental outcomes in childhood (ALSPAC study): an observational cohort study. *Lancet*, 369(9561), 578–585.

Howell, D.C. (2009). *Statistical Methods for Psychology*. New York: Wadsworth.

Howitt, D. & Cramer, D. (2008). *Introduction to Statistics in Psychology*, 4th edn. Harlow: Pearson Prentice Hall.

Hrobjartsson, A. & Gotzsche, P.C. (2001). Is the placebo powerless: an analysis of clinical trials comparing placebo with no treatment. *The New England Journal of Medicine*, 344(21), 1594–1603.

Hrobjartsson, A. & Gotzsche, P.C. (2004). Is the placebo powerless: update of a systematic review with 52 randomized trials comparing placebo with no treatment. *Journal of Internal Medicine*, 256, 91–100.

Jaiswal, A., Bhavsar, V. & Jaykaran, Kantharia, N.D. (2010). Effect of antihypertensive therapy on cognitive function of patients with hypertension. *Annals of Indian Academy of Neurology*, 13(3), 180–183.

Janszky, I., Ahnve, S., Lundberg, I. & Hemmingsson, T. (2010). Early-onset depression, anxiety, and risk of subsequent coronary heart disease: 37-year follow-up of 49,321 young Swedish men. *Journal of the American College of Cardiology*, 56(1), 31–37.

Kaplan, E.L. & Meier, P. (1958). Nonparametric estimation from incomplete observations. *Journal of the American Statistical Association*, 53, 457–481.

Kazdin, A.E. (1978). Methodological and interpretive problems of single-case experimental designs. *Journal of Consulting and Clinical Psychology*, 46(4), 629–642.

Kellett, M.W., Smith, D.F., Stockton, P.A. & Chadwick, D.W. (1999). Topiramate in clinical practice: first year's postlicensing experience in a specialist epilepsy clinic. *Journal of Neurology, Neurosurgery & Psychiatry*, 66, 759–763.

Kelly, M., Steele, J. Nuttall, N., Bradnock, G., Morris, J., Nunn, J. Pine, C., Pitts, N. & Treasure, E. (2000). *Adult Dental Health Survey: Oral Health in the United Kingdom 1998.* London: Office of National Statistics.

Knutson, J.F. & Lansing, C.R. (1990). The relationship between communication problems and psychological difficulties in persons with profound acquired hearing loss. *Journal of Speech and Hearing Disorders*, 55, 656–664.

Lester, H., Schmittdiel, J., Selby, J., Fireman, B., Campbell, S., Lee, J., Whippy, A. & Madvig, P. (2010). The impact of removing financial incentives from clinical quality indicators: longitudinal analysis of four Kaiser Permanente indicators. *British Medical Journal*, 340, c1898.

Lipton, R.B., Manack, A., Ricci, J.A., Chee, E., Turkel, C.C. & Winner, P. (2011). Prevalence and burden of chronic migraine in adolescents: results of the chronic daily headache in adolescents study (C-dAS). *Headache*, 51(5), 693–706.

Logan, P.A., Coupland, C.A.C., Gladman, J.R.F., Sahota, O., Stoner-Hobbs, V., Robertson, K. et al. (2010). Community falls prevention for people who call on an emergency ambulance after a fall: randomised controlled trial. *British Medical Journal*, 340, c2102.

Meltzer, H., Gatward, R., Goodman, R. & Ford, T. (2000). *Mental Health of Children and Adolescents in Great Britain.* London: The Stationary Office.

Merline, A.C., O'Malley, P.M., Schulenberg, J.E., Bachman, J.G. & Johnston, L.D. (2004). Substance use among adults 35 years of age: prevalence, adulthood predictors, and impact of adolescent substance use. *American Journal of Public Health*, 94(1), 96–102.

Meyer, T.A. & Gast, J. (2008). The effects of peer influences on disordered eating behavior. *The Journal of School Nursing*, 24(1), 36–42.

Mlodinow, L. (2008). *The Drunkard's Walk: How Randomness Rules Our Lives.* London: Allen Lane.

Moher, D., Hopewell, S., Schulz, K.F., Montori, V., Gotzsche, P.C., Devereaux, P.J. et al. (2010). CONSORT 2010 explanation and elaboration: updated guidelines for reporting parallel group randomised trials. *British Medical Journal*, 340: c869.

Mok, L.C. & Lee I.F.-K. (2008). Anxiety, depression and pain intensity in patients with low back pain who are admitted to acute care hospitals. *Journal of Clinical Nursing*, 17, 1471–1480.

Morbidity and Mortality Weekly Report. (2009). May 1st, 58, 16, 421–426. Department of Health & Human Services, Centers for Disease Control and Prevention.

Newgard, C.D., Haukoos, J.S. & Lewis, R.J. (2006). Missing data: what are you missing? Society for Academic Emergency Medicine Annual Meeting. San Francisco, CA.

Oman, D., Shapiro, S.L., Thoresen, C.E., Plante, T.G. & Flinders, T. (2008). Meditation lowers stress and supports forgiveness among college students: a randomized controlled trial. *Journal of American College Health*, 56(5), 569–578.

Ownsworth, T., Flemming, J., Desbois, J., Strong, J. & Kuipers, P. (2006). A metacognitive contextual intervention to enhance error awareness and functional outcome following traumatic brain injury: a single case experimental design. *Journal of the International Neuropsychological Society*, 12, 54–63.

Paloutzian, R. & Ellison, C. (1982). Loneliness, spiritual well-being and the quality of life. In Peplau, L. & Perlman, D. (eds.). *Loneliness: A Sourcebook of Current Theory, Research and Therapy.* (pp. 224–237). NY: John Wiley and Sons.

Patel, A.B. (2009). Impact of weight, height and age on blood pressure in children. *The Internet Journal of Family Practice*, 7(2).

Paterson, L.M., Nutt, D.J., Ivarsson, M., Hutson, P.H. & Wilson, S.J. (2009). Effects on sleep stages and microarchitecture of caffeine and its combination with zolpidem or trazodone in healthy volunteers. *Journal of Psychopharmacology*, 23, 487–494.

Peto, R., Pike, M.C., Armitage, P., Breslow, N.E, Cox, D.R., Howard, S.V. et al. (1977). Design and analysis of randomized clinical trials requiring prolonged observation of each patient II: analysis and examples. *British Journal of Cancer*, 35, 1–39.

Pine, C.M., Pitts, N.B., Steele, J.G., Nunn, J.N. & Treasure, E. (2001). Dental restorations in adults in the UK in 1998 and implications for the future. *British Dental Journal*, 190(1), 4–8.

Porter, S.R. & Scully, C. (2006). Oral malodour (halitosis). *British Medical Journal*, 333, 632–635.

Price, D.D., Finniss, D.G. & Benedetti, F. (2008). A comprehensive review of the placebo effect: recent advances and current thought. *Annual Review of Psychology*, 59, 565–590.

Quirynen, M., Mongardini, C. & van Steenberghe, D. (1998). The effect of a 1-stage full-mouth disinfection on oral malodour and microbial colonization of the tongue in periodontitis: a pilot study. *Journal of Periodontology*, 69, 374–382.

Rausch, J.R., Maxwell, S.O. & Kelly, K. (2003). Analytic methods for questions pertaining to a randomised pretest, posttest, follow-up design. *Journal of Clinical Child and Adolescent Psychology*, 32(3), 467–486.

Rowe, R., Maughan, B. & Goodman, R. (2004). Childhood psychiatric disorder and unintentional injury: findings from a national cohort study. *Journal of Pediatric Psychology*, 29, 93–104.

Ryder-Lewis, M.C. & Nelson, K.M. (2008). Reliability of the Sedation-Agitation Scale between nurses and doctors. *Intensive & Critical Care Nursing*, 24, 211–217.

Scarpellini, M., Lurati, A., Marrazza, M., Re, K.A., Bellistri, A., Galli, L. & Riccardi, E. (2008). Clinical value of antibodies to cyclic citrullinated peptide in osteoarthritis, rheumatoid arthritis and psoriatic arthritis. *International Journal of Health Science*, 1(2), 49–51.

Schulz, K.F. & Grimes, D.A. (2002). Generation of allocation sequences in randomised trials: chance, not choice. *The Lancet*, 359, 515–519.

Shearer, A., Boehmer, M., Closs, M., Rosa, R.D., Hamilton, J., Horton, K. et al. (2009). Comparison of glucose point-of-care values with laboratory values in critically ill patients. *American Journal of Critical Care*, 18(3), 224–229.

Silveira, P., Vaz-da-Silva, M., Dolgner, A. & Almeida, L. (2002). Psychomotor effects of mexazolam vs placebo in healthy volunteers. *Clinical Drug Investigation*, 22(10), 677–684.

Simon, J.A. & Hudes, E.S. (1998). Serum ascorbic acid and other correlates of gallbladder disease among US adults. *American Journal of Public Health*, 88, 1208–1212.

Skumlien, S., Skogedal, E.A., Bjørtuft, O. & Ryg, M.S. (2007). Four weeks' intensive rehabilitation generates significant health effects in COPD patients. *Chronic Respiratory Diseases*, 4, 5–13.

Sutherland, S.E. (2001). Evidence-based dentistry: Part IV. Research design and levels of evidence. *Journal of the Canadian Dental Association*, 67(7), 375–378.

Tabachnick, B.G. & Fidell, L.S. (2007). *Using Multivariate Analysis*. Harlow: Pearson.

Taylor-Ford, R., Catlin, A., LaPlante, M. & Weinke, C. (2008). Effect of a noise reduction program on a medical surgical unit. *Clinical Nursing Research*, 17, 74–88.

Todman, J. & Dugard, P. (2007). *Approaching Multivariate Analysis*. East Sussex: Psychology Press.

Tukey, J.W. (1977). *Exploratory Data Analysis*. Boston: Addison-Wesley.

Unwin, J., Kacperek, L. & Clarke, C. (2009). A prospective study of positive adjustment to lower limb amputation. *Clinical Rehabilitation*, 23, 1044–1050.

van der Colff, J.J. & Rothmann, S. (2009). Occupational stress, sense of coherence, coping, burnout and work engagement of registered nurses in South Africa. *SA Journal of Industrial Psychology*, 35(1), 1–10.

Vermeer, S.E., Prins, N.D., den Heijer, T., Hofman, A., Koudstaal, P.J. & Breteler, M.M.B. (2003). Silent brain infarcts and the risk of dementia and cognitive decline. *The New England Journal of Medicine*, 348, 1215–1222.

Watson, D. & Friend, R. (1969). Measurement of social evaluative anxiety. *Journal of Consulting and Clinical Psychology*, 33(4), 448–457.

Williamson, D.A., Rejeski, J., Lang, W., Van Dorsten, B. Fabricatori, A.N. & Toledo, K. (2009). The impact of a weight-management program on health related quality of life in overweight adults with type 2 diabetes. *Archives of Internal Medicine*, 169(2), 163–171.

Yaghmaie, F., Khalafi, A., Majd, H.A. & Khost, N. (2008). Correlation between self-concept and health status aspects in haemodialysis patients at selected hospitals affiliated to Shaheed Benesht, University of Medical Sciences. *Journal of Research in Nursing*, 13(3), 198–205.

Yu, M., Song, L, Seetoo, A., Cai, C., Smith, G. & Oakley, D. (2007). Culturally competent training program: a key to training lay health advisors for promoting breast cancer screening. *Health Education & Behavior*, 34, 928.

Yusuf, S., Hawken, S., Ounpuu, S., Dans, T., Avezum, A., Lanas, F. et al. (2004). Effect of potentially modifiable risk factors associated with myocardial infarction in 52 countries (the INTERHEART study): case-control study. *Lancet*, 364(9438), 937–952.

Index